EXCITOTOXINS

The Taste that Kills

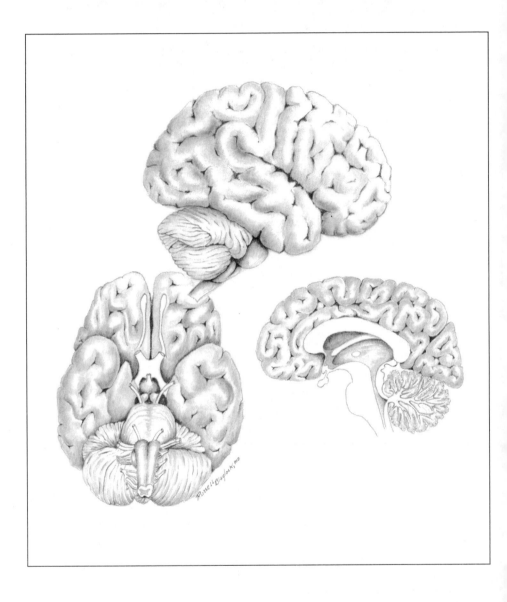

The Brain

EXCITOTOXINS

The Taste that Kills

∎

HOW MONOSODIUM GLUTAMATE, ASPARTAME (NUTRA-
SWEET®) AND SIMILAR SUBSTANCES CAN CAUSE HARM
TO THE BRAIN AND NERVOUS SYSTEM AND THEIR RELA-
TIONSHIP TO NEURODEGENERATIVE DISEASES SUCH
AS ALZHEIMER'S, LOU GEHRIG'S DISEASE (ALS)
AND OTHERS.

∎

Russell L. Blaylock, M.D.
Foreword by George R. Schwartz, M.D.

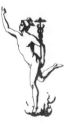

Health Press
Santa Fe, New Mexico

Copyright 1997 by Russell L. Blaylock, MD

Published by Health Press
P.O. Drawer 1388
Santa Fe, NM 87504

Library of Congress Cataloging in Publication Data

Blaylock, Russell L., 1945-
Excitotoxins: the taste that kills / by Russell L. Blaylock
p. cm.
Includes bibliographical references and index.
ISBN 0-929173-14-7
1. Neurotoxic agents. 2. Excitatory amino acids. 3. Nervous
system—Degeneration.   I. Title
RC347.5.B53 1994
616.8'047—dc20   93-34412 CIP
ISBN 0-929173-25-2

Illustrations by Russell L. Blaylock, MD
Design by Jim Mafchir

I dedicate this book to my dad, C.D. Blaylock, who has always been an inspiration to me, an exemplar, and without whose guidance and encouragement I would never have gone as far as I have. And to my mother who likewise always pushed me to excel and guided me through the rough seas of life.

Disclaimer

The information presented in this book has been obtained from authentic and reliable sources. Although great care has been taken to ensure the accuracy of the information presented, the author and the publisher cannot assume responsibility for the validity of all the materials or the consequences for their use. Before starting any regimen of vitamins or supplements you should consult with your physician.

Contents

Acknowledgements

I would like to thank several people who made this work possible. First, I would like to thank my wife, Diane, who has been a continuous source of encouragement in this project. I also thank my two sons, Ron and Damien who so frequently saw me disappear for hours behind the door of my study. To my sister, Linda Pender, I owe an unpayable debt of gratitude for reading my manuscript with a critical eye and making many helpful suggestions. For all of his help in checking the accuracy of my biochemical terms and cell physiology I want to thank Bob Smith, who is working on his PhD degree in biochemistry and cell biology at Rice University.

I would also like to thank the librarians at the Mississippi Baptist Medical Center and Mrs. Nyla Stevens, head librarian at the Luther Manship Library, St. Dominic Hospital, for their invaluable help in doing literature searches and in retrieving scientific papers.

It was the research of Dr. John Olney which led me on my way to understanding excitotoxicity of these taste-enhancing compounds. And it was because of his strong sense of duty and courage in pointing out the dangers of putting excitotoxins in baby foods that many children have been spared the ravages of excitotoxin brain damage.

A special note of thanks to Dr. Adrienne Samuels and her husband Jack for their courage in carrying on the battle to alert all of us about the adverse effects of excitotoxins added to our food. They have given me encouragement and support during the writing of this book, as well as extremely useful information.

Finally, I would like to thank Dr. George Schwartz and his wonderful wife, Kathleen, for believing in this project and making it happen.

Foreword

There are some discoveries which come when the time is ripe; when science, understanding and research come together to allow a new synthesis. For example, understanding aerodynamics would have had limited use, indeed, in the early 19th century since other components necessary for flight were undeveloped. In this context, Dr. Blaylock's book is a remarkable achievement and the timing is right. The research, scientific understanding, observation of disease, coupled with the increased use of neurological excitotoxins in our food supply have allowed Dr. Blaylock to create this cutting-edge synthesis. Also gratifying is that Dr. Blaylock is a highly qualified professional. He is a practicing board-certified neurosurgeon with a deep understanding of the structure and function of the brain and nervous system. He brings his credibility to this critical topic.

When Dr. Blaylock writes of neurodegenerative diseases such as Alzheimer's, Lou Gehrig's (ALS), and others, his voice comes from one who has studied and treated these conditions and offers many years of experience. Thus, his is a voice which cannot be dismissed by those who seek financial gain from the use of excitotoxins and who show little or no concern for long-term damage to consumers.

When Dr. Blaylock shows how excitotoxins such as monosodium glutamate, aspartic acid, aspartame (Nutrasweet®) and others can affect the developing brain, we can see how our children are at risk. Is there a relationship between these deleterious substances in our foods and the diminution in educational test scores? Perhaps all the educational approaches to such societal problems are, very simply, ''off-base''.

Scientific research has demonstrated many receptors in the nervous system which can be affected by excitotoxins. In some cases, the excitation can lead to death of the nerve cells. The research correlation between these effects and the neurodegenerative disease are truly alarming. This is not the first time that toxic substances have been allowed entry into the human system, despite forewarnings. As a physician practicing for well over twenty years and with a special interest in toxicology, I have seen the effects of long-term lead and mercury exposure in children resulting in neurological damage. We have witnessed the pollution of Great Lake's fish. I am frequently reminded of the "DDT" trucks on beaches with innocent children following after the sprays, having been assured of the harmlessness. This was a wide-spread practice in the 1940's and 1950's to try to rid the beaches of insects. I have witnessed defective medical products such as medical devices and silicone breast implants creating serious medical problems having been assured by those with financial ties to the industry that they were safe. I believe we are witnessing a very similar event in the case of the excitotoxins. Our "watchdogs" have become industry "pussy cats" and the "research" supposedly demonstrating safety is deeply flawed. What is even more disconcerting is that many researchers have demonstrated just how these studies are flawed.

Some educated people have advised caution in that they have said, "We don't want to scare people, so tone it down." I ask them to read Dr. Blaylock's remarkable and detailed book to see if they can still urge this caution. To them I ask, "Is it prudent to keep your voice low and scare nobody when poisoning is occurring on a day to day basis? Certainly, if you know that the airplane you are riding in is defective, it is the least prudent thing you can do not to bring it to attention. The future of many of our citizens can be affected in subtle yet deep ways and there are some who can be affected seriously on a day to day basis. Many of these substances added to foods can rightfully be called "poisons". What concerned parent would knowingly sprinkle poison on food destined for the metabolism of their children. Yet this is just what is now occurring.

I believe the words of this expert, Dr. Blaylock, are correct. Our society is spending billions of dollars more than is needed on long-term medical care for those with neurological diseases. What is the good of detailed "health care reform" if toxic substances are not taken into account?

Dr. Russell Blaylock has given us a unique and compelling work which literally can affect the health and well being of millions of people as well as future generations. His is a voice not easily dismissed. *Excitotoxins: The Taste that Kills* is a book which must be read and reread by the educated public, by researchers, by teachers and dieticians, members of PTA groups, industry representatives, and others concerned with the foods we are giving to our society.

I take my hat off to Dr. Blaylock. He has gone from where I left off in my book, *In Bad Taste: the MSG Syndrome* (Health Press, 1988). He has provided the needed research underpinning as well as his unique perspective. In future years, his work *Excitotoxins: The Taste that Kills* will be seen as a landmark work akin to the remarkable books by Rachel Carson published in the 1950's. Will the lessons be heeded? We cannot know that yet. Certainly, the lessons of cigarette smoking have had limited effect on people's behavior. Yet this book will be seen, regardless, as a milestone, a marker of our time. From this moment on, **the word is out**. All concerned people must spread the message far and wide.

George R. Schwartz, M.D., FACEP, FAAEM
Author, *In Bad Taste: The MSG Syndrome*
Editor, *Principles and Practice of Emergency Medicine*
Visiting Associate Professor of Emergency Medicine
Medical College of Pennsylvania
Private Consultative Practice, Santa Fe, NM

Introduction

What if someone were to tell you that a chemical added to food could cause brain damage in your children, and that this chemical could effect how your children's nervous systems formed during development so that in later years they may have learning or emotional difficulties? What if there was scientific evidence that these chemicals could damage a critical part of the brain known to control hormones so that later in life your child might have endocrine problems? How would you feel?

Suppose evidence was presented to you strongly suggesting that the artificial sweetener in your diet soft drink may cause brain tumors to develop, and that the number of brain tumors reported since the widespread introduction of this artificial sweetener has risen dramatically? Would that affect your decision to drink these products and especially to allow your children to drink them? What if you could be shown overwhelming evidence that one of the main ingredients in this sweetener (aspartate) could cause the same brain lesions as MSG? Would that affect your buying decisions?

And finally, what if it could be demonstrated that all of these types of chemicals (called excitotoxins) could possibly aggravate or even precipitate many of the neurodegenerative brain diseases, such as Parkinson's disease, Huntington's disease, ALS, and Alzheimer's disease? Would you be concerned if you knew that these excitotoxin food additives are a particular risk if you have ever had a stroke, brain injury, brain tumor, seizure, or have suffered from hypertension, diabetes, meningitis or viral encephalitis?

I would think that all of us would be more than just concerned to learn that well known powerful brain toxins were being added to our food and drink to boost sales. We would be especially upset to learn that these additives have no other purpose than to enhance the taste of food and the sweetness of various diet products.

You would also be upset to learn that many of these brain lesions in your children are irreversible and can follow a single exposure of a sufficient concentration. And I would bet that you would be incredulous to learn that the food industry disguises many of these "excitotoxin additives" so that they will not be recognized. In fact, many foods that are labeled "No MSG" not only contain MSG, but also contain other excitotoxins of equal potency. Now let us look at the history of this group of food additives.

For thousands of years Japanese cooks have added a special ingredient to their recipes to magnify the desired taste of foods. This ingredient was made from a sea weed known as "sea tangle" or kombu. Yet, it was only in this century that the active chemical of this "taste enhancing" ingredient was isolated. Most of you will immediately recognize the chemical which has this almost magical property—it's called monosodium glutamate, or MSG.

Shortly after its isolation, the chemists who discovered MSG turned it into a worldwide multi-million dollar industry. At the center of this empire is the Ajinomoto Company which today produces most of the world's supply of MSG and a related taste-enhancing substance called hydrolyzed vegetable protein, which also contains MSG.

After World War II, American food manufacturers also discovered the virtues of this taste-enhancing substance. Soon all of the giants of the food industry, such as Pillsbury, Oscar Mayer, Libby's and Campbell's, were adding millions of pounds of MSG each year to processed foods. At the time of its discovery, it was thought to be perfectly safe, since it was a natural substance (an amino acid).

The amounts of MSG and similar additives being added to foods increased throughout the post-war period. In fact, the amount of MSG alone added to foods has doubled in every decade since the 1940's. By 1972 262,000 metric tons of MSG were produced. Many cookbooks recommended adding MSG to their recipes, especially for soups and sauce recipes.

Throughout this period, few suspected that these taste enhancing additives could be doing serious harm to individuals eating these foods. But, by the end of the 1960's, research data began to appear demonstrating the dangers of MSG as a food additive. This scientific data should have alerted those responsible for public safety to the danger.

Until this time, neuroscientists assumed that glutamate supplied the brain with energy. Based on this idea scientists in one clinical study, fed large doses of MSG to retarded children to see if it would improve their IQ. The experiment failed. Then, in 1957, two ophthalmologists, Lucas and Newhouse, decided to test MSG on infant mice in an effort to study an eye disease known as hereditary retinal dystrophy. But, when they examined the eye tissues of the sacrificed animals, they made a startling discovery. The

MSG had destroyed all of the nerve cells in the inner layers of the animal's retina which are the visual receptor cells of the eye.

Despite this frightening discovery, MSG continued to be added to food in enormous amounts and cookbooks continued to recommend it as a taste enhancing additive for recipes. But the worst was yet to be disclosed about this compound. Some ten years later John W. Olney, MD, a neuroscientist working at the Department of Psychiatry at Washington University in St. Louis, repeated Lucas and Newhouse's experiment in infant mice.

His findings indicated that MSG was not only toxic to the retina, but also to the brain. When he examined the animals' brains he discovered that specialized cells in a critical area of the animals' brain, the hypothalamus, were destroyed, after a single dose of MSG.

The implications of Dr. Olney's findings should have been earth-shaking to say the least. Why? Because millions of babies all over the world were eating baby foods containing large amounts of MSG and hydrolyzed vegetable protein (a compound which contains three excitotoxins). In fact, the concentrations of MSG found in baby foods was equal to that used to create brain lesions in experimental animals. And in all of these experiments, immature animals were found to be much more vulnerable to the toxic effects of MSG than were older animals. This was true in all animal species tested.

Yet, food manufacturers continued to add tons of this excitotoxic additive to foods of all kinds, including baby foods. Even the government's public health watch-dog agency, the Food and Drug Administration, refused to take action. Dr. Olney, one of the leading researchers in this area, felt compelled to do something to protect unsuspecting mothers and their infants from this danger. First he informed the FDA of the real danger to human infants and encouraged them to take action. But they refused. His only recourse was to go public with what he knew to be true—that MSG was a dangerous compound that should not be added to infant foods. It was only after his testimony before a Congressional committee that the food manufacturers agreed to remove MSG from baby foods. But did they really?

Instead of adding pure MSG they added a substance known as hydrolyzed vegetable protein that contains three known excitotoxins and has added MSG. As we shall see later this substance is even more dangerous than MSG. They continued this practice for seven more years, and there is evidence that excitotoxins are still added to baby foods today. Usually these are in the form of caseinate, beef or chicken broth, or flavoring.

Another type of food sold by these manufacturers is directed at toddlers. At least some of these foods contain hydrolyzed vegetable protein. Experimentally we know that the brain is extremely vulnerable to excitotoxins even at this stage of development.

In this book I shall present research findings and discuss experiments that will demonstrate that glutamate and other excitotoxins can alter the way the brain is formed during development. It is hypothesized by some neuroscientists that exposure to these powerful compounds early in life could cause developmental brain defects that would produce learning difficulties and behavioral problems as the child grows older. There is also some evidence that it may contribute to violent behavior as well.

In experimental animals "MSG babies" are found to be short in stature, obese, and to have difficulty reproducing. This effect only becomes evident long after the initial MSG exposure. More detailed studies have found that "MSG babies" have severe disorders involving several hormones normally produced by the hypothalamus.

Unfortunately, MSG is not the only taste enhancing food additive known to cause damage to the nervous system. In fact, there is a whole class of chemicals that can produce very similar damage—they all share one important property. When neurons are exposed to these substances, they become very excited and fire their impulses very rapidly until they reach a state of extreme exhaustion. Several hours later these neurons suddenly die, as if the cells were excited to death. As a result, neuroscientists have dubbed this class of chemicals "excitotoxins".

Several of these "excitotoxins" are man made and are used as research tools. Others are found in nature, such as glutamate, aspartate and cysteine— all of which are amino acids. MSG is a modified form of glutamic acid in which sodium is added to the molecule. But the toxic portion is the glutamic acid, not the sodium. Often food manufacturers will mix MSG with other substances to disguise it, or use substances known to contain high concentrations of glutamate and/or aspartate. For example, the label designation "natural flavoring" may contain anywhere from 20 to 60 percent MSG.

Earlier I mentioned a substance called hydrolyzed vegetable protein, also referred to as vegetable protein or plant protein. This powerful excitotoxin mixture is often portrayed as a perfectly safe and "natural" substance. "After all," manufacturers say, "it's made from plants."

Actually, this mixture is made from "junk" vegetables that are unfit for sale. They are especially selected so as to have naturally high contents of glutamate. The extraction process of hydrolysis involves boiling these vegetables in a vat of acid. This is followed by a process of neutralization with caustic soda. The resulting product is a brown sludge that collects on the top. This is scraped off and allowed to dry. The end product is a brown powder that is high in three known excitotoxins—glutamate, aspartate, and cystoic acid (which converts in the body to cysteine). It is then added by the food industry to everything from canned tuna to baby food.

So what is it that these "excitotoxins" actually do that is so important to the food manufacturers? All of these chemicals stimulate the taste cells in the tongue, thereby greatly enhancing the taste of whatever food to which it is added. It is what gives soups the scrumptious taste that we all love so much. Today they are used extensively in sauces, soups, gravy mixes, and especially frozen diet foods. Low fat foods are often tasteless. To help sell them to the public, food manufacturers add "excitotoxin" taste enhancers to these foods to improve the taste.

Another excitotoxin additive that is familiar to all of us is the artificial sweetener NutraSweet®. Actually, 40 percent of the compound is composed of the excitotoxin aspartate. Like glutamate, aspartate is a powerful brain toxin which can produce similar neuron damage. NutraSweet® is used in many diet foods and beverages. It is well recognized that liquid forms of excitotoxins are much more toxic to the brain than dry forms as they are absorbed faster and produce higher blood levels than when mixed with solid foods.

But the negative effects of excitotoxins are not limited to small children. There is growing evidence that excitotoxins play a major role in a whole group of degenerative brain diseases in adults—especially the elderly. These diseases include Parkinson's disease, Alzheimer's disease, Huntington's disease, Amyotrophic Lateral Sclerosis (ALS), as well as several more rare disorders of the nervous system.

What all of these diseases have in common is a slow destruction of brain cells that are specifically sensitive to excitotoxin damage. Neurons that use glutamate for a transmitter are destroyed by these high concentrations of glutamate, while other neurons that use other transmitters are spared.

While there is little evidence that food borne excitotoxins are the cause of these disorders, there is growing evidence that they can aggravate these conditions and that they may even precipitate them in sensitive individuals. Certainly the scientific evidence is far too strong to ignore the possibility that excitotoxic food additives may cause such conditions to appear sooner and to a more serious degree.

More and more diseases of the nervous system are being linked to excitotoxin build-up in the brain. For example disorders such as strokes, brain injury, hypoglycemic brain damage, seizures, migraine headaches, hypoxic brain damage, and even AIDS dementia have been linked to excitotoxin damage. There is also evidence that some individuals born with metabolic defects in certain brain cells may be particularly susceptible to excitotoxin damage.

In this book I have tried to compile some of the vital research linking excitotoxins to injury and diseases of the nervous system. This area of research is growing by leaps and bounds. I feel that this new information linking excitotoxins with disease must reach the general public so that each of you can make up your own mind on this issue. Unfortunately, most of this critical information is buried in technical and scientific journals, far from the public's eye.

Despite what the defenders of MSG and NutraSweet® will scream, this book is not unduly alarmist. There are far too many false environmental alarms being sounded today. It was only after a year of careful examination and debate that I decided to write this book. I felt that the information concerning the dangers to small children and older persons was too important to withhold. Each person must decide for themself if they choose to believe that the danger is real.

The book is written mainly for the lay public, but also for those trained in medical science and biology. I have provided references for those who seek either to check the accuracy of my statements or to delve deeper into the subject themselves. Of course, the book does not claim to be an exhaustive study of each area of controversy, but leading experts are quoted in each case. The field is far too vast for such a review.

This first chapter of the book is optional. It is primarily for those unfamiliar with the central nervous system and the terms used to describe the various diseases and conditions associated with excitotoxin damage. You may choose to refer back to it when reading the other chapters. A glossary of terms is also provided for quick reference.

I was warned when I submitted the manuscript for this book to my publisher that I should prepare for the backlash from the food industry, and especially from the representatives of the glutamate manufacturers. These two industries have joined together to fight anyone who would dare criticize the use of flavor enhancers. In fact, they have formed a special lobby group to counter any negative claims about their product. This group, called The Glutamate Association, is made up of representatives of major US food manufacturers and the Ajinomoto Company, which, based in Japan, is the chief manufacturer of MSG and hydrolyzed protein.

Many have been scared off by these powerful businesses and organizations. But I feel that the message is too important to be left alone. The FDA has failed in its stated purpose of protecting the public from harmful substances being added to the food supply. Millions of lives are at stake— including those of future generations. People must be warned.

A NOTE JUST BEFORE PUBLICATION: IT HAS RECENTLY BEEN DISCLOSED THAT EXCITOTOXINS ARE BEING ADDED TO SMOKING TOBACCO. THESE COULD CONCEIVABLY PASS THROUGH THE ABSORPTIVE SURFACES OF LUNG TISSUE AND ENTER THE BLOOD STREAM.

EXCITOTOXINS

The Taste that Kills

· 1 ·

A Crash Course in How the Brain Works

The human brain is one of the most complex entities in the known universe. Within this three pound mass of jelly-like tissue there exist over ten billion nerve cells, billions more nerve pathways, and a million trillion connections. Often the brain is compared to a computer. But the organization of this remarkable organ is infinitely more complex than any computer system known. At best, it can be compared to a living computer.

Such a living computer would have to be able to change its circuits according to the problems to be solved, and, in addition, respond to thousands or even millions of outside influences. Plus, it must be able to protect itself from overloads, wear and tear, and even repair itself should injury result. It would have to learn to adapt in a span of milliseconds. But even more remarkable it must develop circuits that would make it capable of feeling. Not just rudimentary sensations, but be able to feel the deeper emotions of love, hate, wonder, compassion, jealousy, and all the other emotions that make us human. And it would have to have a curiosity about its own inner workings. This computer must be able to control the entire spectrum of the endocrine system, the immune system, and the circulatory system, and all the other systems of the body. Its feedback control systems must be exact, all the while computing a quadrillion other functions.

To fully understand all that we presently know about this remarkable organ would fill thousands of volumes. And what we still do not know about the brain would fill all the books in the Library of Congress. The purpose of this introductory chapter on the brain is to supply the reader with enough basic knowledge so that you will have a clearer understanding of the devastating effect of excitotoxins on this complicated organ.

THE CEREBRAL HEMISPHERES
The bulk of the brain consists of two large masses called hemispheres which

are covered by deep folds of grey matter. These worm-like wrinkles are termed convolutions and the grooves in between are termed sulci. The purpose of these sinuous folds is to provide the brain with a large surface area within a small volume. If these convolutions were flattened out, the surface area of the human brain would cover such an enormous area that it would not fit within the skull.

THE FRONTAL LOBES

If you examine these hemispheres you will see that they can be roughly divided into anatomical pairs of lobes, each with its own name. (FIG 1-1) Those in the front, called the frontal lobes, are of considerable importance in humans in that they allow us to learn and to restrain our "negative" emotions. You can remember the functions of the frontal lobes by memorizing the three "T's"—tension, tact and tenacity of endeavor.

Most important are the last two "T's". Tact allows us to engage in socially acceptable behavior. Recently scientists have found that the major malfunction in children suffering from hyperactivity is that their frontal lobes seem to be tuned down. As a result, they have difficulty controlling their behavior; they act out inappropriately. They also have difficulty with the last "T", tenacity of endeavor, as they find it difficult to focus their minds on one single tasks for any length of time. It is our ability to focus our attention on one task at a time that allows us to learn.

So we see that the frontal lobes are very complicated and play a major

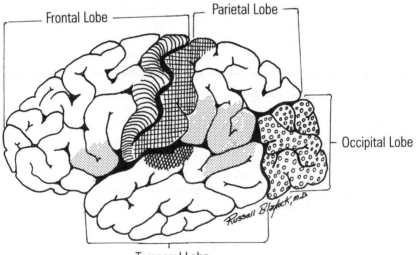

1-1 *Lobes of the Brain*

role in our ability to function in a complex world. The back edge of the frontal lobes contain two strips of cortex that are also very important. They contain nerve cells that control movement on the opposite side of the body. The left hemisphere controls movement of the right side of the body and vice versa. Actually it is much more complicated than that, but for the sake of simplicity let us leave it there. Many of these "motor" neurons are quite large. They are called the giant cells of Betz.

THE PARIETAL LOBES: THE ASSOCIATION CORTEX

These lobes are actually continuous with the other lobes of the brain, and for a very good reason. They sit tucked between the temporal lobes below, the frontal lobes in front, and the occipital lobes behind. The reason this is a perfect location is that the parietal lobes must have intimate communication with all other areas of the brain so that it can integrate this information into a clear picture. This is why it is called the association cortex. It must also connect to the primary memory lobe of the brain, the temporal lobe, so as to check for previous memories of what is being seen, heard or felt. It thumbs through the files and if it finds a previous record of what is being presently analyzed, it says, "ah ha!".

It is the parietal lobes that keep us oriented not only to our surroundings, but also to our own body parts. Right after birth we begin to learn the layout of our body. This is why a baby stares at and explores its hands and feet. The infant is discovering its new body and registering that memory for later use. When it is time, for example, to write with a pencil, the association cortex draws the memory of the hand from the temporal lobes and then formulates an internal visual and tactile picture on how to carry out the activity using the hand. It then contacts the appropriate sections of the brain and gives commands as how best to carry this out.

When we travel by car to the store for our weekly trip to get groceries, it is our association cortex that tells us how to get there and back. It records a map in our brain and stores it there for later use. This internal map requires the use of the visual lobes of the brain (the occipital lobes), which record visual cues. When the parietal lobe of the brain is damaged, the person gets lost in otherwise familiar surroundings. This is the part of the brain destroyed in Alzheimer's disease that causes the elderly to wander away from home and become lost.

OCCIPITAL LOBE

This is the visual lobe of the brain. It receives impulses from our eyes in a rather complex manner, that at first seems not to make sense. The fiber from the retina travels through the optic nerves of each eye and then enters an x-shaped structure just underneath the brain called the chiasm. Here something strange happens. The fibers receiving light from the inner half of the visual field travel straight back to the occipital lobes on the same side, but the fibers receiving light from the outer visual field cross in the chiasm and travel to the opposite occipital lobe. That is, the image is split and registered on opposite sides of the brain.

Why was the brain designed in such a complicated manner? Well, it may be that it gives us maximum protection for our vision should the brain pathways be damaged, for example by a stroke. That is, it allows us to retain at least some vision in both visual fields should an injury result.

The physiology of vision is very complex and is beyond our discussion. Suffice it to say that nerve cells of the visual cortex connect to many areas of the brain, including the association cortex and the temporal lobes.

TEMPORAL LOBES: THE MEMORY LOBES

With the advent of neurosurgery it was found that surgeons could remove almost one entire temporal lobe with little adverse effect. This was done when treating tumors and epilepsy. However, in 1937 two scientists, Kluver and Bucy, found that when both temporal lobes of monkeys were removed the animals exhibited quite unusual behavior, including a loss of visual memory. It was then found that in human cases of bilateral temporal lobe destruction (as seen with herpes encephalitis) the person exhibited a complete loss of recent memory—they were unable to remember anything that had occurred in the recent past.

Later a neurosurgeon by the name of Wilder Penfield operated on a seizure patient while the patient was awake. During this surgery Dr. Penfield began stimulating the exposed temporal lobe with tiny jolts of electricity. As he moved the probe along the surface of the temporal lobe the patient suddenly reported a clear visual memory. It was as if a movie of the memory was being shown before the patient's very eyes. When the probe was removed the memory suddenly disappeared.

Dr. Penfield repeated this experiment many times and discovered that all sorts of memories could be called up, including musical memories. One patient heard a tune that he recalled hearing as a child each time the probe was activated on his temporal lobe. These memories were not just vague recollections—it was more as if the events were being relived at the very moment. It appears that memories are stored in the temporal lobes of the brain, even those long forgotten consciously.

When we combine these two observations we discover that short term memories, like what you had a for breakfast this morning, and long term memories are both generated within the temporal lobes of the brain. Later it was discovered that recent memory processes were further localized to a special area in the temporal lobes called the hippocampus. These are curled cortical areas tucked beneath the temporal lobes. Herpes encephalitis, a type of brain inflammation caused by the herpes simplex virus, tends to attack this area of the brain, often leaving its victims unable to make new memories.

The memory process remains a mystery, but seems to involve wide areas of the entire brain as well. This has been referred to as the hologram theory of memory. Destruction of critical nerve cells in the temporal lobes also plays an important role in Alzheimer's disease. Because of its role in elaborating memories and combining them into emotional patterns, Dr. Penfield referred to this enigmatic lobe of the brain as the "interpretive cortex".

THE INTERIOR OF THE BRAIN

THE VENTRICLES: CAVERNS IN THE BRAIN

The brain, as we have seen, is divided into two hemispheres that are connected deep in the middle by a broad band of nerve fibers called the corpus callosum. The fibers going to and coming from the hemispheres travel by way of the brain stem. If you were to hold a fresh brain you would instantly notice its jelly-like consistency and its weight. Although it would feel solid, it is not a solid mass. Deep within its core there exists a series of caverns called the ventricles. Like most caverns, the ventricles connect to each other by way of several narrow passages, each having its own special name. Anatomists love to give every hole and bump a name; usually their own.

The ventricles are filled with a fluid that is as clear as spring water, called cerebrospinal fluid, or CSF for short. This fluid is produced by specialized structures, called the choroid plexus, located primarily within the main caverns (the lateral ventricles). This fluid circulates through the narrow openings, passing into each successive cavern, until it escapes to the outside, where it then circulates over the surface of the brain and is absorbed back into the blood.

The ancient Greeks thought the brain was a cooling system because of the fluid filled cavities in the brain. But we now know that the CSF is far more than just a cooling system for the brain. Recent studies indicate that it can act as a transport mechanism for important chemicals, hormones and electrolytes. These chemicals can travel through the walls of the ventricles of the brain itself.

RELAY STATIONS BELOW THE SURFACE

Generally we are told that grey matter is on the surface of the brain and white matter is below. But this is not entirely true. In fact, there is a considerable amount of grey matter below the surface of the brain. The grey matter is grey because it consists mainly of nerve cells called neurons and specialized non-nerve cells called glia. The white matter consists of the billions of nerve fibers (axons) coming from and going to the grey matter.

The grey matter below the surface of the brain is arranged into compact spheroids called nuclei. (FIG 1-2) Usually these nuclei blend together at various points even though we speak about them as if they were isolated. Many of the strange sounding names given to these nuclei are based on their early anatomical descriptions and are not always related to functional arrangements. For example, the striatum refers to the putamen, globus pallidus, and the caudate nucleus. (FIG 1-3) As scientists have learned more about these strange nuclei they begin to appreciate that they do not function as independent units. Most beginners of brain study want to know what a certain nucleus does. Well, often, by itself, it does very little. It is just part of a whole.

Thalamus

This is the largest of the paired nuclei found deep in the brain. It is located just above the brain stem into which it appears to blend. "Thalamus" is Greek for *inner chamber*. When I took neuroanatomy in medical school I was taught that it was merely a relay nucleus concerned with the sensation of touch and other sensory functions. In other words, it was like an electrical substation that redirected impulses to other parts of the brain. Now we know that it is much more than that. It is what we call an integration unit, more like a miniature brain, performing quite complex functions, including the independent appreciation of some sensations.

Birds, for example, can function without a cortex, purely on a thalamic level. In humans, pain and crude touch sensations can be felt solely from the thalamus. It also plays a part in language function and possibly in memory. It still has not revealed all of its secrets.

The Striatum

This actually consists of three large nuclei, called the putamen, globus pallidus, and the caudate nucleus. The caudate sits right next to the outer wall of the front part of the lateral ventricle. The putamen is a wedge-like nucleus that rests behind and lateral to the caudate. In fact, it is attached to another nucleus called the globus pallidus. Below this is a whole array

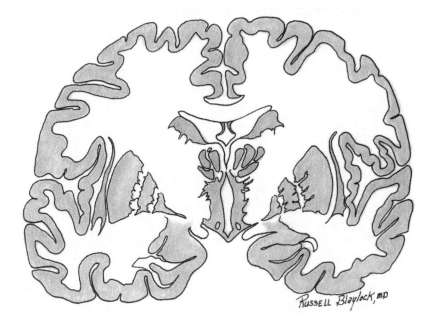

1-2 Cross Section of the Brain Demonstrating the Grey Matter and the White Matter—the nuclei lie below the cortex, deep in the brain.

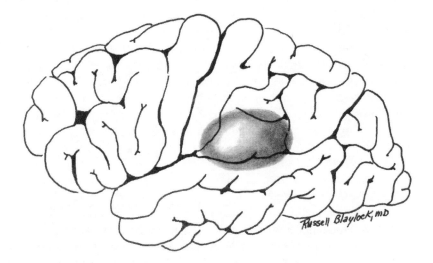

1-3 Location of Basil Ganglion Deep in the Brain

of smaller nuclei that interconnect to all the others. All of these connections are extremely complex.

The striatum plays a major role in what we call automatic movements, such as swinging our arms when we walk. When you walk you automatically swing your arms to counterbalance the shifting of your center of gravity. This is all done unconsciously. In fact, many of our more complex movements are already pre-programmed within the striatal system, even the conscious ones. When we consciously will to carry out a movement our brain merely activates one of these complex circuits. It is really an incredibly clever system.

When one of these circuits is injured some very bizarre events can occur. For example, when a small stroke destroys a tiny nucleus, called the subthalamic nucleus, the person will have uncontrollable flinging movements of one arm. It will just fly out, giving the appearance that they are purposely trying to strike out at someone. What has happened is that the stroke has damaged the control mechanism that holds this automatic movement in check.

This system of interconnecting nuclei consists of a multitude of such circuits that are carefully balanced by both negative and positive feedback control systems. The negative feedback dampens, or shuts off the circuit, and the positive feedback system either releases the circuit or stimulates it to activity. This carefully regulated and balanced system of circuits gives our movements a smooth action. If you have ever seen a person with cerebral palsy you can get a good idea of what can happen when this system is out of control. These writhing, jerky movements are the result of motor circuits that have lost their negative feedback control systems.

Huntington's chorea is an inherited disease that also produces similar movements of the arms, legs, and body. Ironically these patients start out their life as normal people. But around age 30 they began to show uncontrollable writhing movements, and within a decade they are confined to a nursing home. Something causes the control system in their brain to go berserk. This will be discussed in greater detail later in the book.

No Lobe is an Island

While we talk about certain areas of the brain carrying out specific functions, in reality no part acts alone. Every part of the brain depends on many other parts for its function. Often these sections of the brain are relatively far apart. These various parts must talk to each other by way of nerve fibers, which are like very sophisticated electrical cables. They can alter the signals under various circumstances, making the signal smoother and more understandable.

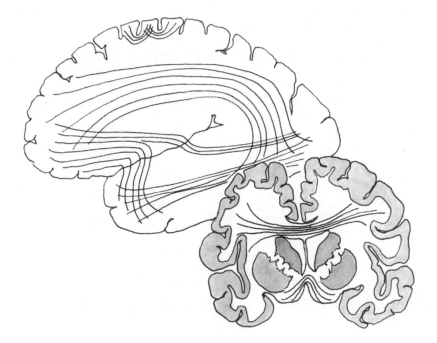

1-4 *Fibers Connecting Various Brain Regions*

These fiber tracts travel in all directions. (FIG 1-4) Some travel long distances, even to the opposite hemisphere of the brain. The same lobe of one hemisphere of the brain connects to its mirror image on the opposite hemisphere. These billions of fiber pathways make up the white matter of the brain. Hidden to the naked eye is the fact that billions of microcircuits also exist throughout the brain; small ones, large ones, simple ones, and extremely complex ones.

CONNECTIONS

Thanks to many new techniques in neurochemistry and neuroanatomy, we now know a lot more about how brain cells and their connections are arranged. For example, we know that in the cortex, neurons are arranged in functional columns, each interacting with its neighbor.

We should also appreciate that not all neurons fire so as to produce some type of action. Some brain cells are inhibitory—they stop other neurons from firing. Still others merely modulate and modify the action of the primary neurons. Everything in the brain is very carefully regulated and finely tuned, right down to the subcellular level. Some single brain cells may connect to thousands of others.

THE BRAIN STEM: THE GATEWAY TO THE BRAIN

The brain stem is actually arranged in three levels, based on increasing degrees of sophistication. The higher up the more sophisticated the circuits become. Some smaller animals are able to function entirely with no more than a brain stem. Attached primarily to the back portion of the brain stem, is two cauliflower looking hemispheres of brain called the cerebellum. Each of the three levels of the brain stem connect to the cerebellum by fiber bundles.

The cerebellum is a very complex, yet, at the same time, simply constructed structure. Its circuitry's repertoire of actions is enormously complex, but its basic mode of action is relatively simple. The input from the primary cerebellar neurons, strangely enough, is completely inhibitory. But it is how these inhibitory impulses are "played" that makes the music that controls the other parts of the brain. Until recently it was thought that the cerebellum produced no impulses itself, but rather reacted to input from other parts of the brain. It was considered to be the coordination center, making all of our movements smooth and well coordinated. But recent studies indicate that it can do much more than that. In fact, impulses do originate from the cerebellum.

Within the brain stem we see a multitude of nuclei scattered about. Some control breathing, heart rate, and balance. Others operate the various sensory and motor nerves of the face and neck called cranial nerves. Scattered throughout the brain stem is a cloud of nerve cells that make up what is called the reticular formation, or reticular activating system. This loosely organized system not only integrates impulses from all the various areas of the brain stem, but it is also responsible for our alertness. That is, it keeps us awake. Sometimes we see injuries to this reticular activating system such as in cases of head injury or strokes. This can result in prolonged comas.

The remainder of the brain stem is made of fibers passing to the upper brain and those coming down into the spinal cord and cerebellum from the cortex. One pair of nuclei located in the upper segment of the brain stem that is particularly important, is called the substantia nigra. It is unusual in that these nuclei contains a very dark pigment. Under the microscope we see that the black color comes from a substance located within the nerve cells of the nucleus. This nucleus is important in the causation of Parkinson's disease, and plays a vital role in the functioning of the striatal system.

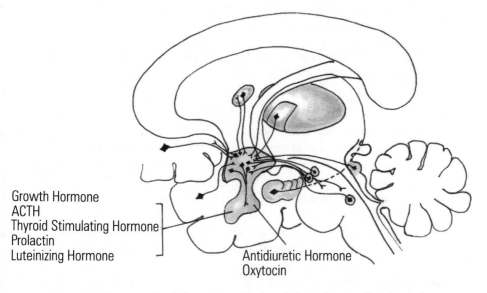

Growth Hormone
ACTH
Thyroid Stimulating Hormone
Prolactin
Luteinizing Hormone

Antidiuretic Hormone
Oxytocin

1-5 *Drawing demonstrating the importance of the hypothalamus in controlling the pituitary gland. The hypothalamus receives many fiber inputs from various brain regions. The neuron system within the hypothalamus appears to use glutamate as a neurotransmitter.*

THE MASTER GLAND AND ITS CONTROL

The pituitary gland has been called the master gland, because it is the central control center for most of the endocrine glands located throughout the body. (FIG 1-5) This tiny gland, no bigger than the tip of your little finger, sits at the bottom of the brain, encased in a bony pocket above the nose. Basically, the pituitary gland controls the other endocrine glands, such as the adrenal glands, the thyroid, and the reproductive organs, by releasing small amounts of its controlling hormones into the blood, which then circulates to the various endocrine organs and causes them to secrete their hormones. By using this control, the brain can regulate growth, metabolism, and the onset of puberty. This is why this tiny gland is often called the "master gland".

But what controls the pituitary gland? If we examine the brain, with the pituitary gland still attached, we see that the pituitary is connected to a wedge shaped piece of brain called the hypothalamus. This tiny piece of brain, despite its size, is immensely important. It controls hormone releasing factors that travel only a few centimeters to the pituitary gland, where they stimulate the pituitary to release its hormones. By a clever system of feedback controls, the hypothalamus regulates the hormone balance in the body. It's sort of a hormone thermostat.

But the hypothalamus is much more. It also controls hunger and satiety, sleep and waking cycles, the autonomic system, emotions, and even our biological clocks. Even minor injuries to the hypothalamus can be fatal. It is extremely delicate both physically and biochemically.

THE ELECTROCHEMICAL BRAIN

Normally we think of the nervous system as a vast array of electronic circuits; living circuits, but circuits none the less. But in reality the nervous system is much more than that. It is a system which can generate impulses and convey those impulses over long distances by way of special self-propagating biochemical events. And it is an endocrine gland.

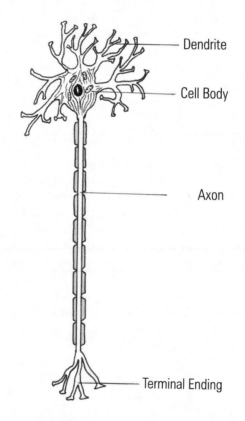

1-6 *A Neuron: the dendrite, the cell body, and the axon with its terminal ending. Glutamate receptors appear to be located primarily on the dendrite and less so on the cell body.*

The typical nerve cell is made of three parts: a dendrite, which receives the information, a cell body, which acts as the central command headquarters, and the axon, a single fiber which carries the information to the next nerve cell in line. (FIG 1-6) This transmission along nerve fibers begins in the dendrite, which looks like a spiny tree in the winter. These spiny receiving fibers can connect to hundreds, even thousands of other neurons. The cell body contains all of the necessary equipment for the second by second operation of the nerve cell. It supplies the genetic code, the energy, and even special internal messenger substances for the rest of the neuron. Like all cells of the body, it contains a system to supply energy for maintenance of the cell, support for repair mechanisms, and energy necessary for the generation and propagation of impulses. The brain consumes 20% of the body's oxygen and 25% of the body's glucose, yet makes up only 2% of the body's weight. The majority of this energy is spent supporting impulse generation and transmission. The brain never rests, even during deep sleep. In fact, during deep anesthesia the brain is still consuming enormous amounts of energy.

We know that the nerve impulses begin at one spot on the dendrite or axon and spreads from there like falling dominos. The axon acts as a semipermeable membrane, keeping sodium ions on the outside and chloride and potassium ions on the inside. This produces a net positive charge on the outside of the axon and a net negative charge on the inside. When the site on the axon is stimulated, the membrane suddenly changes its properties so that sodium rushes into the interior of the nerve fiber and depolarizes the axon. This is called the axon potential. This process of sodium rushing into the interior of the nerve fiber, continues down the axon until it reaches the end of the fiber. Some axons conduct these impulses at speeds up to 200 miles per hour. While there is an electric current generated, the impulse is actually a chemical message. In order for this chemical message to reach the next neuron down the line, a gap must be bridged. This gap is called the synapse.

SYNAPTIC TRANSFER OF INFORMATION

While occasionally the gap is crossed by true electrical conductance, in most cases it occurs by a chemical transfer of information. This is referred to as neurotransmission and the chemical messenger is called a neurotransmitter. Trillions of chemical messages are being transmitted throughout the brain every second.

Basically, this process requires that the impulse stimulates the release of chemical transmitters from microscopic packets located in the bulbous

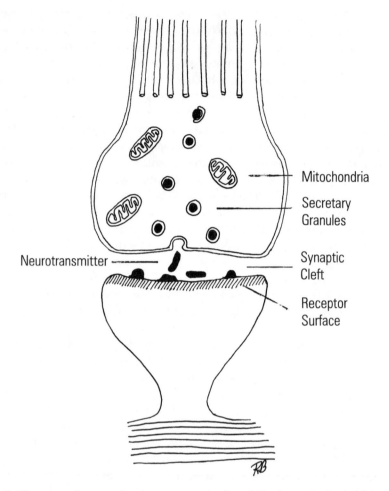

1-7 *The synapse, demonstrating the secretory mechanism within the terminal end of the axon which packages the transmitter and excretes it into the synaptic cleft. Here it attaches to the receptor surface on the next neuron, causing the cell to fire.*

end of the axon. This neurotransmitter is released into the space between the synapse and the next neuron receptor called the synaptic cleft. This, in turn, causes the next neuron in line to fire and send its message on down the line. Release of the neurotransmitter is triggered by the sudden flow of calcium ions into the bulbous end of the axon. (FIG 1-7)

So why doesn't the neuron just keep firing as long as the neurotransmitter remains in the synaptic cleft? Well, it will unless something is done to remove this transmitter chemical. The brain has several clever mechanisms to carry this out. One method is to reabsorb the chemical back into the neuron bulb that released it in the first place. Another method is for the neuron to use special enzymes to change the transmitter into a harmless by-product. That is, it is inactivated. In some instances it just diffuses away.

Many anti-depressants work by inactivating the neurotransmitter inactivator enzyme. For example, some brain cells have a neutralizing enzyme called monoamine oxidase, or MAO for short, which neutralizes several of the amine neurotransmitters. One of the treatments of depression is aimed at increasing the amount of the neurotransmitter that elevates mood. This mood elevating neurotransmitter is called norepinephrine. MAO normally inactivates norepinephrine. Some anti-depressants also prevent re-uptake of the transmitter, thereby allowing mood elevating neurons to be stimulated longer.

In many cases all three methods of inactivation are used. Some also use surrounding cells called astrocytes, to inactivate these neurotransmitters. Astrocytes are not nerve cells but play a vital role in the metabolic support of neurons. In fact glia cells, as they are called, outnumber neurons ten to one. In the case of the neurotransmitter glutamate, it is the astrocyte that both manufactures glutamate and inactivates it when the impulse has passed to the next neuron.

The number of neurotransmitters found in the brain has grown by leaps and bounds, and more are being discovered. Thus far there are over 50 known and suspected neurotransmitter substances operating in the brain and spinal cord. Some of these chemicals are not actually transmitters of information between cells but rather modulate these signals, possibly cutting out background noise so as to sharpen the signal. Some transmitters activate neurons and some inhibit them. For example, the neurotransmitter GABA is an inhibitory transmitter. We know that some neurons have both inhibitory and excitatory synapses connected to them. This further fine tunes the signal. Interestingly, some of the newest neurotransmitters to make the list, cholecystokinin and vasopeptide, actually were first found to be involved in intestinal and gall bladder function.

PUTTING IT ALL TOGETHER

How the brain puts all this together into speech, hearing, sight, mentation, emotions, and supportive bodily functions remains a mystery. But we have some clues. We know that one neuron may interconnect to thousands of other neurons and that this vast array of interconnections roughly resembles the circuits of some of our most complicated computers. With each event, such as moving our little finger, there occurs an incredibly complicated series of interactions between the cerebellum, the sensorimotor cortex, the parietal lobes, and a maze of circuits in the nuclei deep within the brain.

The brain is much more resilient than most people think. I have had people ask me, once they find out that I am a neurosurgeon, if a person will die if you touch the brain. Boxers pound their brains repeatedly and continue to function rather normally. I can remember back in my residency training the case of a child of six who had been shot through the brain, the bullet passing in one side and out the other, without a single neurological deficiency being evident. But some areas of the brain, such as the hypothalamus, are very sensitive. Even slight damage to this vital structure can lead to death.

THE BLOOD BRAIN BARRIER: PROTECTING THE BRAIN

As we have seen, the brain is a chemical factory which depends on careful quality control for its operation. The amounts of these chemicals used to transmit signals is infinitesimal. Even small fluctuations in these concentrations can result in dramatic disruptions of brain function, and even death of certain cells. (For example, there is considerable evidence that schizophrenia is caused by an overabundance of a neurotransmitter called dopamine. Injecting dopamine into the ventricles of humans can precipitate an acute psychotic episode, including hallucinations.)

The brain receives the same blood that flows through the body. Therefore, it is exposed to high concentrations of chemicals in the blood, both from metabolism and from the diet. Some of these chemicals are quite toxic to the brain. For example, glutamate can cause widespread destruction of certain brain cells in concentrations normally found in the diet. This is especially so when we consider the enormous amounts of glutamate added to our food in the form of the taste enhancer, monosodium glutamate or MSG. Without the blood brain barrier this glutamate would do serious damage to the brain and spinal cord. But, this protection has certain limitations which will be discussed later in the book.

The blood-brain barrier excludes some substances and allows others free passage. (FIG 1-8) In general, the amino acids are carefully regulated, because so many also serve as neurotransmitters, or transmitter precursors. For example, the amino acids, glutamate, aspartate, and glycine are all neurotransmitters. Tryptophan and tyrosine are precursors, which are converted into neurotransmitters within the brain itself. Tryptophan is converted into serotonin, and tyrosine is converted into norepinephrine and dopamine. Without careful control of these substances, each time we ate

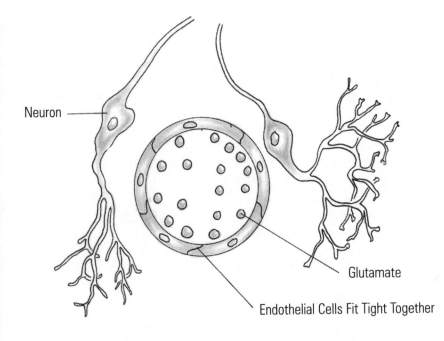

Neuron

Glutamate

Endothelial Cells Fit Tight Together

1-8 *The Blood-Brain Barrier: The barrier exists between the blood vessels (capillaries) that course throughout the brain tissue and the extracellular space within the brain. It prevents certain molecules in the blood from entering the tissue space of the brain itself. It is thought that the major portion of the "barrier" lies in the tight junction between the cells (endothelial cells) that line the capillary walls. Blood vessels in other parts of the body have relatively large spaces between the cells that allow passage of even large molecules.*

a meal our brains would go berserk.

However, the barrier is not perfect. In fact, some parts of the brain never develop a barrier system at all. For example, the hypothalamus, the circumventricular organs, the pineal, and a small nucleus in the brain stem called the locus ceruleus, are without barrier protection.

There is also evidence that the barrier is broken down or at least partially malfunctioning under certain conditions. For instance, strokes temporarily break down the barrier, resulting in swelling of the brain. Brain tumors also cause the barrier to break, and may, in fact, cause it to break down at some distance from the tumor. Head injury, degenerative diseases, infections, and a multitude of other injuries can also cause this protective system to fail.

In some cases we want the barrier to break down. It is this barrier which keeps many of the anticancer chemotherapy drugs from entering the area of a brain tumor. By using special techniques, neurosurgeons can temporally cause the barrier to fail, allowing these drugs to enter the area of the tumor in high concentrations. But this is dangerous, since other harmful agents can also enter.

One of the most important questions yet to be answered is whether the blood-brain barrier breaks down with aging. Studies thus far are conflicting. Some studies indicate that there is at least a partial breakdown of the barrier system while other studies have found no correlation with aging.

CONCLUSION

This three-pound universe, as it has been called, is as amazing and wondrous as the cosmic universe itself. The repertoire of actions available to the brain is mind-boggling. We are just now discovering some of its most closely held secrets. But what we do know is that its proper functioning requires a careful balance of nutrients. Too much or too little of certain critical nutrients can adversely effect this wondrous organ.

It is also obvious that the brain can be a very resilient organ. Its capacity to recover from some injuries is almost miraculous. But at other times it can be quite sensitive and even delicate. This is especially so during development, when all of these intricate circuits are being formed. As we will see, it is especially important that the brain be protected during this critical stage of development, for injuries during the formation period can result in devastating effects years later, as the child grows and matures.

·2·

Very Special Amino Acids

The human body is one of the most complex, intricate, and mysterious creations that we know of, even when compared to the most sophisticated technological creation of man. Much of its complexity centers around the chemistry of the life process itself. Every second of every day thousands of chemical reactions are taking place throughout every cell and in every tissue of the body. The primary purpose of eating is to support these chemical reactions. Some may argue with this, claiming that they eat because it gives gastronomic pleasure. But even this hedonistic reaction to eating involves a host of chemical reactions designed to encourage us to eat, so that we will supply the machinery with the chemicals it needs. Many of the substances absorbed from our food play a vital role in the overall metabolic process of life. We should always keep this in mind.

What frightens most beginners in biochemistry are the names, such as phosphofructokinase, alpha ketoglutarate, and glutathione reductase. It is like a foreign language. But once you understand a few basics, it all starts to make sense. Most biochemical reactions involve building something from smaller molecules, breaking down larger molecules into smaller ones, or converting one compound into another one. The body is like a giant chemistry set.

One of the two basic reactions occurring in biochemistry involves breaking down compounds in our food so as to release energy. But it doesn't do this by simply burning food. Rather it is a step by step process. If the body simply burned the food to a crisp in one sudden flash, the heat generated would boil our brains. So the process, called catabolism, has to take place in many gradual steps. Carbohydrates, for example, are broken down in the gut into simpler sugars (called disaccharides) such as sucrose, maltose, and lactose. These in turn are broken down into even simpler sugars called glucose, fructose and galactose. Eventually, all sugars absorbed from the diet are converted into glucose in the liver.

While glucose is the main "sugar" in the blood, it still cannot be used by the cells for energy. First, the glucose must enter the cell where it can be used. This occurs only if insulin is available to escort the glucose inside the cell. Fortunately, the brain doesn't need insulin to push its glucose into the neurons. Otherwise diabetics, who lack insulin, would die very rapidly. Once the glucose is inside the cell, it is broken down piece by piece in a series of chemical reactions involving many enzyme catalysts. Enzymes are chemicals which facilitate chemical reactions, so that they can occur rapidly and with ease.

Once glucose enters the cell it is broken down by a series of enzymatic steps into various compounds. Initially this is done without the use of

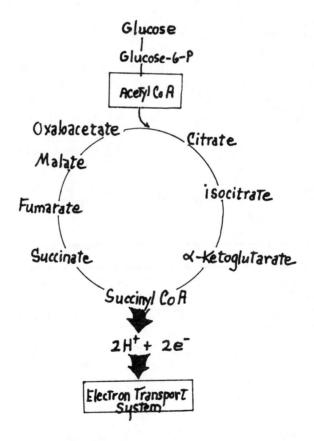

2-1 *Electron Transport System*

oxygen, hence the name anaerobic glycolysis. If oxygen is not eventually supplied to the cell, the reaction will end by producing large amounts of lactic acid, the substance that causes muscles to fatigue and ache with strenuous exercise. But should oxygen be supplied, the reaction enters a new phase. Here the end product of glycolysis spins through a cycle of biochemical reactions known as the Kreb's cycle with the resulting release of enormous amounts of energy. (FIG 2-1)

As glucose is progressively broken down in the Kreb's cycle, electrons are given off and captured by special molecules that propel them through another series of reactions, transferring the electrons from one compound to the next. At critical points in this reaction energy is produced. This series of reactions is called the electron transport system. (FIG 2-2) It should be noted that all of the energy released from these reactions must be in a form that the cell can use, and that can be stored for later use. Therefore, most of this energy is stored in the form of a special molecule called ATP, which stands for adenosine triphosphate. Another storage form of this energy is in a molecule called phosphocreatine. When one molecule of glucose passes completely through all of the reactions it will generate 36 ATPs. In terms of cellular energy that is a lot of stored energy. So basically, when we burn calories we are in reality using ATPs.

This series of reactions needed to break down glucose also depends on an adequate supply of vitamins, minerals and trace elements being present.

These act as co-factors and co-enzymes (helpers) that help spur the reactions along. These vital supplements should be supplied by the diet because when deficient, serious disease can occur. Far too many physicians, because of a neglect of nutritional courses in medical training, do not appreciate the critical nature of these nutrients in human health.

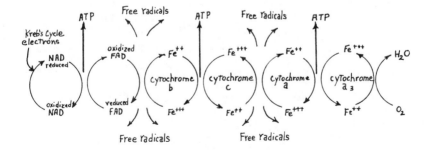

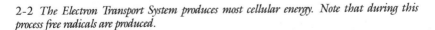

2-2 *The Electron Transport System produces most cellular energy. Note that during this process free radicals are produced.*

WHAT IS AN AMINO ACID?

Because most excitotoxins are amino acids, you will need to know something about amino acids in general. Basically, amino acids are nothing more than chemical building blocks used to create proteins. They are made of nitrogen and carbon units bonded together in various shapes and sizes. (Some amino acids contain other elements such as sulfur.) Humans possess about twenty different types of naturally occurring amino acids, which are supplied from either plant or animal proteins. (TABLE 2-1) The cells build proteins by linking these amino acids in various combinations, much like tinker toys are used to build things. (Each protein can use these amino acids multiple times within its structure.) Some proteins are small, consisting of no more than five to ten amino acids linked together. Others, are enormous, highly complex configurations containing over a thousand amino acids. Collagen, the largest protein in the body, contains some 1500 amino acids in its structure. Insulin contains 86 amino acids.

The structure and shape (configuration) of these protein molecules is very important. Short proteins are essentially arranged in a straight line, whereas, the giant protein molecules are folded upon themselves in a complex, three dimensional configuration. These three dimensional structures play an important part in the function of the protein, since the folds and electromagnetic forces that hold them together, must be exact for the molecule to operate properly. For example, the hemoglobin molecule has a particular shape that is necessary for it to function as an exchange molecule carrying carbon dioxide to the lungs to be expelled and oxygen to the tissues to support metabolism.

TABLE 2-1
CLASSIFICATION OF AMINO ACIDS

Aliphatic Amino Acids	**Aromatic Amino Acids**
Glycine	Phenylalanine
Alanine	Tyrosine
Valine	Tryptophan
Leucine	**Basic Amino Acids**
Isoleucine	Histidine
Serine	Lysine
Threonine	Arginine
Cysteine	**Acidic Amino Acids**
Cystine	Glutamate
Methionine	Aspartate
	Glutamine

The neurotransmitters used by the neurons for communication also depend on a particular shape for their function, just like a protein molecule. In fact, their configuration is so critical that pharmacologists, by manipulating the shape of certain transmitter molecules, can cause them to have an opposite effect. For example, just by changing the shape of neurotransmitters that function to elevate the blood pressure, a "false transmitter" can be created that will block blood pressure centers in the brain thus lowering the blood pressure.

Proteins are used by the body for a variety of functions. Some form part of the membrane structure of the cell itself, while others may be used to form enzymes, hormones, and components of various tissues. Hemoglobin is one of a unique class of complex proteins that combines with a metal (in this case iron). A similar protein that is very important in energy production in the cell, cytochrome C, contains copper. As you can see, proteins play critical roles in the body.

The process whereby proteins are constructed within the cell is called anabolism, a building process that goes on all the time. It is because proteins are constantly being broken down that they must be replaced. And it is for this reason that a certain amount of protein must be supplied in our diet. These proteins can be provided by plant and animal proteins. Other amino acids are utilized as they exist, without being made into complex proteins. For example, the brain uses some of the unaltered amino acids as neurotransmitters. Glutamate, aspartate, and glycine are three such amino acids.

Some amino acids are slightly altered before being used as neurotransmitters. The amino acid tyrosine, found in high concentrations in cheese, is converted by specific reactions into at least two neurotransmitters— norepinephrine and dopamine. The amino acid tryptophan, found in high concentrations in milk and turkey, is converted into serotonin, another neurotransmitter. Interestingly, it has been found that diets high in these two amino acids can, in fact, increase the brain levels of the respective neurotransmitters and thereby affect behavior. Tyrosine, by increasing the brain's level of norepinephrine, can elevate the mood and stimulate a sense of well being, whereas foods high in tryptophan can produce a tranquilizing effect and help bring on sleep at night, by increasing brain serotonin levels.

Types of Amino Acids

Biochemists classify amino acids in several different ways. Sometimes they group them according to their basic chemical structure. For example, the aromatic amino acids all have a ring-like structure attached to their basic carbon unit. These include the amino acids tyrosine, tryptophan, and phenylalanine. Others have short, straight chains and are called aliphatic amino acids.

Some amino acids contain sulphur which plays a vital part in cell function. Included in this group are cysteine, cystine, and methionine. These amino acids are of interest to radiation biologists since they appear to provide animals with considerable protection from radiation by stabilizing DNA. Because its tissues contain large concentrations of cysteine, the lowly cockroach is virtually immune to high doses of radiation. And methionine is important in protecting the liver from the effects of alcoholism and certain toxins or poisons. However, some of the sulphur-containing amino acids also play an important role in causing certain degenerative brain diseases.

Another way to classify amino acids is by their acidity or alkalinity. The acidic amino acids contain two special "acid" sub-units attached to the primary carbon skeleton. The amino acids glutamate and aspartate belong to this group. Others have more than one nitrogen atom attached per molecule making them alkaline or basic. The basic amino acids include histidine, lysine, and arginine. All of the other amino acids found in humans are considered neutral. This classification system is important because we now know that all the amino acids within a particular group compete with one another for absorption from the gut and into the brain by way of the blood-brain barrier.

When you eat a food high in tyrosine, such as cheese, tryptophan absorption is inhibited. Both being neutral amino acids, they compete for the same site of absorption in the gut. And once in the blood stream, they similarly compete for passage into the brain. But since only one can enter at a time, this can have profound effects on behavior. The old adage, "You are what you eat" is being found to be scientifically correct in some instances. By eating foods high in tyrosine, one could aggravate one form of depression by interfering with the brain's supply of tryptophan. The reverse is also possible, since tyrosine is concentrated in the brain into a transmitter which elevates our mood.

A final classification system is based on the ability of the body to synthesize certain of the amino acids. Sometimes particular amino acids can actually be synthesized from other substances found in the cell. These are referred to as non-essential amino acids because they do not need to be supplied in the diet. The amino acid serine can be manufactured in the body from aspartate and glucose. Most of these non-essential amino acids are formed from the breakdown products of glucose as it travels through the

Kreb's cycle. The essential amino acids, on the other hand, cannot be synthesized from other substances and must be supplied in the diet.

EXCITING AMINO ACIDS

In the early 1950's a neuroscientist by the name of Dr. T. Hayaski, found that when monosodium glutamate (MSG) was injected into the grey matter of a dog's brain, the dog would fall down in its cage and begin to convulse wildly.[1] Based on this observation, he concluded that glutamate was causing the dog's brain cells to become overexcited and fire uncontrollably. Despite this important observation the report was largely ignored. The Japanese continued to use large amounts of MSG in their cooking and food preparation. Likewise, it had no effect on American use of MSG.

Then in 1959 two other researchers, working in a different laboratory, found that when glutamate was placed on the muscle tissue of invertebrate crustaceans, it caused the muscle to contract vigorously.[2] From these two observations it was concluded that glutamate, by some then as yet unknown mechanism, caused neurons to fire spontaneously and repeatedly. Another acidic amino acid, aspartate, caused a similar effect.[3] They named this remarkable group of molecules excitatory amino acids because they caused nerve cells to become excited. Thus far, over seventy such excitatory amino acids have been discovered.[4]

While some suggested at the time that glutamate, and possibly aspartate, could be a neurotransmitter in the nervous system, most brain scientists rejected the idea, even though it was know that the brain contained relatively high levels of glutamate. Previous experiments had shown that the brain used glutamate as a source of energy and to manufacture other molecules. It was therefore assumed that it was merely a brain fuel.

By 1973 a group of neuroscientists demonstrated that glutamate, indeed, met all of the characteristics necessary to be considered a neuro-transmitter—it was found within the nerve terminal, was released by the electrical discharge of the nerve, and it was removed by the normal mechanism seen for other neurotransmitters.[5] The next step was to demonstrate a specific receptor for glutamate.

A LOCK AND KEY

In order to understand how glutamate works in the nervous system we must first understand the concept of receptors.[6] I said earlier, during the crash course on how the brain works, that neurotransmitters are released from the terminal ends of nerve axons, where they seep into the tiny cleft between the nerves (the synapse), attach themselves to the membrane of the next nerve in line, and cause it to fire. But how does the transmitter actually cause the nerve cell to discharge and why does it cause only specific neurons to react? This is a beautiful process that is still not fully understood.

Simply put, the transmitter molecule attaches to a receptor on the membrane of the nerve fiber (dendrite) and causes the molecule in the membrane to undergo a change in their conformation, or shape. (FIG 2-3) This in turn opens a microscopic hole or pore in the membrane. When this pore opens, sodium and/or calcium pours inside the axon and triggers the cell to fire thereby transmitting a signal down its axon fiber. This process takes place very rapidly, in a fraction of a second. But how the transmitter molecule attaches to the receptor is what makes this all so amazing. The receptor and its neurotransmitter can be thought of as a lock and key. The receptor on the membrane is the lock that requires a specific key to be opened. The transmitter is the key. This makes the whole process very specific, so that the lock cannot be opened by just any key.

But the story of this specialty gets even more complicated in the case of glutamate receptors. While glutamate was the key and the glutamate receptor on the membrane the lock, it was soon discovered that there were at least three types of glutamate receptors.[7] (It is now believed that there may be more than twenty subtypes of glutamate receptors.) This discovery was based on the use of glutamate analogues, or look-a-like molecules.[8] It was found that the substance N-methyl-D-aspartate (more conveniently

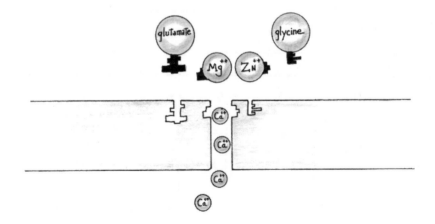

2-3 *The Lock and Key Theory: Molecules of specific shape (keys) fit within similarly shaped receptors on membrane (locks).*

called by its initials NMDA) stimulated only certain classes of glutamate receptors and not others. A second substance, called quisqualate, was then found to stimulate another completely different set of glutamate receptors but not the NMDA receptors. You would think that this would be complicated enough, but nature is never that simple. Yet a third receptor subtype was discovered that responded only to the chemical kainate. So now we have three subtypes of glutamate receptors on nerve cell membranes, each named after the chemical that stimulates them: called NMDA, quisqualate, and kainate receptors. Glutamate (MSG) can stimulate all three types of receptors, as can aspartate.

THE NMDA RECEPTOR: A COMPLEX RECEPTOR

The NMDA receptor is the most common of the three types of glutamate receptors found on neuron membranes in the brain. Consequently, we know the most about this type of receptor or lock. Essentially, it acts as the gate keeper of a special cell membrane pore called a calcium channel.[9] This channel, or pore, regulates the entry of calcium into the inside of the neuron. The channel is opened when the neuron is activated by the neurotransmitter glutamate, the specific key. Aspartate can also open this calcium channel.

So far we have learned that receptors and transmitters act like locks and keys. (FIG 2-4) But in the case of the NMDA receptor more than one key is required. It is sort of like a door in a New York apartment, as it takes a lot

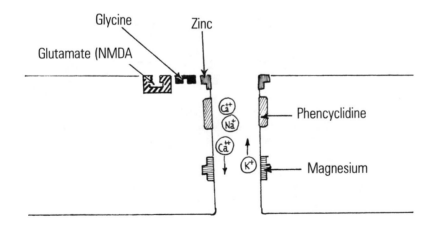

2-4 *The Lock and Key Theory as applied to the glutamate receptor; this causes the calcium channel to open, allowing calcium to enter the cell.*

of keys to open. The other locks on the membrane include a zinc receptor, a magnesium receptor, and a glycine receptor.[10] Zinc can only lock the door—it closes the calcium channel tight. Magnesium also locks the door, but there is an important difference between the two. The zinc blockade of the calcium channel remains even if the neuron is fired, whereas the magnesium blockade is automatically released when the neuron fires. On the other hand, glycine, another amino acid, is absolutely necessary for the calcium channel to open. Experimentally when glycine is removed from a culture of nerve cells, no concentration of glutamate can make the nerve cell fire.[11] But when glycine is added, the neurons become much more sensitive to excitotoxin activation and if unrelieved they are eventually destroyed.

Once the neurotransmitter glutamate comes into contact with the receptor, it slides into the lock (the glutamate receptor) like a perfectly fitting key. Then glycine is inserted into its lock close by. When normal levels of magnesium and low levels of zinc are present near the neuron, the channel will then open wide, and calcium and sodium will pour into the neuron, causing it to fire. It's much like the fail safe system for the launch of

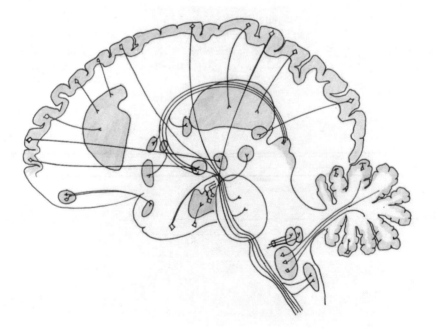

2-5 *Distribution of glutamate neuron fibers in the brain, demonstrating their wide distribution throughout the brain.*

nuclear missiles, it takes more than one key to activate the system and these keys must be inserted and turned simultaneously.

GLUTAMATE RECEPTORS IN THE BRAIN

Neuroscientists have discovered that glutamate is one of the most common neurotransmitters in the brain. Its role is primarily that of an excitatory substance, that is it causes the brain to be stimulated, much the way cocaine does. Using biochemical mapping techniques, we now know that many areas of the brain (such as the cortex, striatum, hippocampus, hypothalamus, thalamus, cerebellum, and the visual and auditory system) all contain an extensive network of glutamate type neurons.[12] (FIG 2-5) This

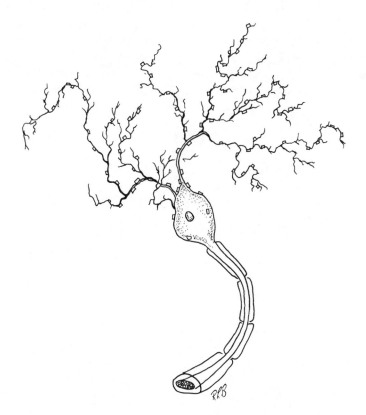

2-6 *Extensive Glutamatergic Nerve Pathways Within the Brain. These are neurons that use glutamate as a neurotransmitter. A far larger number of brain neurons contain glutamate receptors even though they primarily use another chemical for a neurotransmitter.*

means that glutamate is involved in a wide variety of brain functions. It has also been demonstrated that activation of cortical glutamate neurons can in turn activate other neurons within the nuclei located deep within the brain, even those not using glutamate as a neurotransmitter. The importance of these connections will become obvious when we examine excitatory amino acids and neurological diseases.

After studying a number of brains specifically stained for these special receptors, scientists determined that the glutamate receptor is located on the cell body of the neuron and its dendrite—on the fibers emanating from the neuron cell body like the branches of a tree. (FIG 2-6) (Most are located on the dendrite.) Being excitatory transmitters, glutamate and aspartate both are involved in activating a number of brain systems concerned with sensory perception, memory, orientation in time and space, cognition, and motor skills. It is important to appreciate that the brain is an organ that depends on a delicate balance of excitatory and inhibitory systems, that is, positive and negative impulses. Disruptions of this balance can lead to anything from a minor tremor of the hands to an uncontrollable writhing motion of the body, or even the violent explosion of a full blown seizure. In the living organism, a balance of positive and negative systems is all important.

·3·

Exciting Cells to Death

In 1908 Dr. Kikunae Ikeda, a chemist working in a laboratory at the Imperial University of Tokyo, made a most remarkable discovery that would eventually lead to a multibillion dollar industry.[13] He was trying to isolate the chemical that was responsible for the taste enhancing properties of the seaweed known as Kombu or "sea tangle". The Japanese had used this seaweed based flavor-enhancer in their recipes for thousands of years. It had the uncanny ability to greatly enhance the flavor of almost any food to which it was added.

Fortunately, Dr. Ikeda had received training in Germany under the tutelage of a famous chemist, Dr. Wolff, who had perfected the technique for isolating glutamate from proteins. To his surprise, Dr. Ikeda found that the mysterious flavor-enhancing ingredient of the seaweed was glutamate. In 1909 Professor Ikeda joined with his friend, Dr. Saburosuke Suzuki, in forming a company which would manufacture this incredible taste-enhancer in the form of monosodium glutamate. They named their company Ajinomoto, which translates to "the essence of taste" in English.

By 1933 Japanese cooks were using over ten million pounds of this taste enhancer every year. They found that it made even the most bland recipes taste scrumptious. During the war, the Japanese government added MSG to their soldier's rations. Unlike American rations, theirs tasted delicious. American soldiers, having obtained some of the rations from their Japanese prisoners, returned with stories of this delicious tasting military food. This then led to an investigation by the American military.

In 1948 a meeting was held by the Quartermasters of the Armed Forces in conjunction with most of the major food manufacturing giants in America. The list of names of those attending this meeting reads like as who's-who of American food manufacturing, including such names as Pillsbury, Oscar Mayer, Libby, Stokley, Campbell Soups, Continental,

General Foods, and Bordens. During these discussions it was concluded that this Japanese taste-enhancer did indeed have some remarkable properties. It suppressed undesirable flavors, gave "zest" to food, removed the "tinny" taste of canned foods, and turned bland foods into gourmet meals. In short, it held the possibility of a financial boom for the food industry.

Following this remarkable discovery the American food industry drastically increased the amount of MSG being added to prepared foods, which has since *doubled* every decade since the late 1940's. Today MSG is added to most soups, chips, fast foods, frozen foods, ready-made dinners, and canned goods. And it has been a heaven send for the diet food industry, since so many of the low-fat foods are practically tasteless.

As Dr. George Schwartz has pointed out in his remarkable book *In Bad Taste: The MSG Syndrome*, often MSG and related toxins are added to foods in disguised forms. For example, among the food manufacturers favorite disguises are "hydrolyzed vegetable protein", "vegetable protein", "natural flavorings", and "spices". Each of these may contain from 12% to 40% MSG. (See Appendix I for more information about hidden sources of MSG.)

Hydrolyzed vegetable protein is a special case and deserves a closer look. If you will recall, the manufacturing process (as described in the introduction) is a series of chemical processes; first boiling vegetables in sulfuric acid for several hours, then neutralizing the acid with a caustic soda (an alkalizing agent often used to make soap), and then drying the resulting brown sludge. Additional MSG may be added as well to the fine brown powder. The result is marketed as hydrolyzed vegetable protein. When particular amino acids are combined with the basic hydrolyzed vegetable protein they can bring out a "beefy" taste that makes it useful in barbecue sauces and fast foods. Other protein combinations bring out a "creamy" taste that is frequently used in canned and instant soups, salad dressings and sauces.

Analysis of this taste enhancing substance reveals some interesting findings. Not only does it contain three very powerful brain cell toxins—glutamate, aspartate, and cysteic acid—but it also contains several known carcinogens (cancer causing substances). Incredibly, the FDA does not regulate the amount of carcinogens allowed in hydrolyzed vegetable protein, or the amount of hydrolyzed vegetable protein allowed to be added to food products. As we shall see later, this substance poses an even greater danger than MSG itself.

EXCITOTOXINS: TOO MUCH OF A GOOD THING

By the early forties it was known that the human brain normally contained relatively large concentrations of the amino acid glutamate, which at that time, was thought to act primarily as a brain fuel. Based on this idea, in 1949 Dr. Weil-Malherbe tested a group of mentally retarded children to see if glutamate would improve their mental capacity.[14] Fortunately, as it turned out, the experiment was a failure. I say this because had the experiments continued, greater injury to these children's brains would have eventually occurred.

Then, in 1957 two ophthalmology residents, Lucas and Newhouse, tested monosodium glutamate and aspartate on infant (suckling) and adult mice while studying a particular eye disorder.[15] What they found came as a complete surprise. After completing the experiment they sacrificed the animals and examined their tissues under the microscope. Of the animals that had been tested with monosodium glutamate, virtually all of the nerve cells in the inner layer of the animals' retinas had been destroyed. The worst damage occurred in the newborn mice, but even the adults showed significant injury. They also found that the amino acid aspartate caused similar, though less severe, damage. Keep in mind that aspartate is one of the main ingredients in NutraSweet®, the artificial sweetener.

Unfortunately this important finding went virtually unnoticed by the medical world, and especially by the food industry, which at the time was adding tons of MSG to foods, including baby foods. It wasn't until ten years later that someone saw the importance of this discovery. That person was a neuroscientist, Dr. John W. Olney.

In 1968 Dr. Olney, working out of the Department of Psychiatry at Washington University in St. Louis, repeated Dr. Lucas and Newhouse's experiment using the same kind of animals and the same doses of MSG.[16] But what Dr. Olney found was even more shocking. He discovered that not only did MSG cause severe damage to the neurons in the retina of the eye, but that it also caused widespread destruction of neurons in the hypothalamus and other areas of the brain adjacent to the ventricular system, called the circumventricular organs. (FIG 3-1) Again, this damage was most severe in the immature or newborn animals. He hypothesized that this area of the brain was affected most because it did not have a blood brain barrier system to protect it from toxic substances circulating in the blood.

Despite the fact that his findings were confirmed in a number of animal studies using a wide variety of species, few paid attention to this critical discovery. The medical journals read by most practicing doctors, especially those caring for newborn babies, neglected to publish his findings. Private practicing physicians, at the time of this discovery, rarely read the basic science research literature and were therefore unaware of the immediate dangers to their patients—especially to newborns and developing babies.

Without a public or professional outcry, the food industry continued

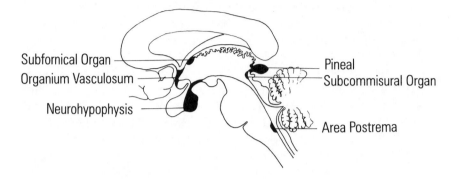

Subfornical Organ

Organium Vasculosum

Neurohypophysis

Pineal

Subcommisural Organ

Area Postrema

3-1 *Circumventricular Organs of the Brain. These areas lack a blood-brain barrier.*

to add more and more monosodium glutamate and hydrolyzed vegetable protein to foods. And at the time of Dr. Olney's report, even baby foods contained relatively large doses of MSG. Mothers, unaware of the danger to their children, were delighted to see their little ones eating so well. Because MSG and hydrolyzed protein are such powerful taste enhancers, they make most foods, even the bland ones, taste scrumptious.

The discovery by Dr. Olney was particularly important because the hypothalamus plays such an important role in controlling so many areas of the body. This little piece of brain, no larger than the fingernail of your little finger, controls a multitude of systems: regulating growth, the onset of puberty, most of the endocrine glands, appetite, sleep cycles and waking patterns, the biological clock, and even consciousness itself. Dr. Olney's studies on various species of test animals disclosed that MSG, when fed in doses similar to those found in human diets, destroys hypothalamic neurons. This type of hypothalamic damage produces a particular syndrome in animals which caused them to be short in stature, obese, and to have reproductive problems. Later experiments demonstrated that MSG could cause the hypothalamus to secrete excessive amounts of a reproductive hormone (called luteinizing hormone) which is associated with an early onset of puberty.[17] Many of these endocrine effects did not appear until the animal was much older. This will be covered in greater detail in chapter 4.

EXCITOTOXINS AND THE DEVELOPING BRAIN

Recognizing the immediate danger to the public, especially to the unborn child, Dr. Olney and others testified before Congress concerning these dangers. As a result of their vigilance, MSG was voluntarily removed from baby foods in 1969.

But no one had warned pregnant women of the danger to their developing babies caused by the MSG found within their own food. This danger would exist if the glutamate from the mother's blood entered the blood of their unborn baby. In 1974 Dr. Olney demonstrated that MSG, when fed to pregnant Rhesus monkeys, could cause brain damage to their offspring.[18] Other researchers found similar results when pregnant rats were fed MSG.[19] Yet millions of pregnant women continued to eat foods laced with MSG and other equally potent excitotoxins while the FDA remained silent. And gynecologists and pediatricians were not told to warn their patients of this real danger.

After birth and following weaning from bottled or breast milk, most mothers begin feeding their babies food from the table. These foods frequently contain large amounts of MSG and hydrolyzed vegetable protein. Dr. Olney found that these children were receiving doses of MSG from the table food that equaled the dose used experimentally to produce severe brain cell destruction in animal experiments. By that I mean proportionally equal. Often, critics of this observation claim that humans rarely receive such high doses. This is just not true. Incredibly, humans develop higher blood levels of glutamate following ingestion of MSG than does any other animal species known.[20] Dr. Olney noted that:

> The amount of MSG in a single bowl of commercially available soup is probably enough to cause blood glutamate levels to rise higher in a human child than levels that predictably cause brain damage in immature animals.[21]

When adult humans are fed 100 to 150 milligrams per kilogram of body weight of MSG their blood levels rise twenty times higher than normal as compared to a four-fold rise seen in experimental mice fed a comparable dose. Monkeys develop a zero-fold rise in blood glutamate after similar doses of glutamate. We know that children are frequently exposed to doses of MSG and other related excitotoxins in their food in extremely high doses. But the fact that humans concentrate glutamate in their blood to a greater degree than other animal species means that the parts of the human infant's brain not protected by the blood-brain barrier is exposed to even higher doses following MSG or hydrolyzed vegetable protein ingestion than is used experimentally to produce brain damage in animals.

And, it should be noted, the child's brain is four times more sensitive than is the adult brain to these toxins.[22] A survey of children's diets indicated that they often consume the same amounts of MSG as adults. This is especially true with the large number of junk foods and fast foods containing massive amounts of MSG and other excitotoxin taste enhancers, such as chips, frozen dinners, canned pasta, and diet drinks (containing aspartate).

When my own children were small toddlers, my wife and I were amazed at how much they loved a special canned pasta dish called *ABCs and 1-2-3s* by Chef Boyardee. These are little pasta alphabet letters and numbers in a mixture of tomato sauce. Our children wanted it for every meal. Once I became aware of the danger of MSG, I discovered that this delicious meal-in-a-can contained both MSG and hydrolyzed vegetable protein. No wonder they loved it! We began to examine our children's food and discovered that many foods specifically advertised for children contained large doses of such excitotoxin taste enhancers.

Dr. Olney astutely pointed out the irony of this food industry practice:

> Thus, today we are witnessing an ironic situation; while knowledgeable neuroscientists are fervently attempting to develop methods for protecting CNS [brain] neurons against neurotoxic potential of endogenous Glu [glutamate] and Asp [aspartate], other elements of society are vigorously promoting the unlimited use of exogenous Glu and Asp as food additives.[23]

Today the experimental evidence demonstrating the neurotoxic potential of these excitotoxins is so overwhelming, as can be seen from the scientific citations in this book, that it can no longer be ignored.

HOW EXCITOTOXINS WORK

The studies showing how excitotoxins work have greatly increased our understanding, not only of brain function, but also of the very basis of the degenerative brain disease process itself. In this discussion you must keep in mind that the excitotoxins added to food are the exact same ones that produce experimental brain damage in animals. And the glutamate in our discussion is the same substance and active ingredient found in MSG. The neurotoxin aspartate is a major component in the artificial sweetener aspartame (actually a mixture of two amino acids, phenylalanine and aspartate, and methanol or wood alcohol).

As I said earlier, glutamate and aspartate are neurotransmitters (the keys) found normally in the brain and spinal cord. And even though they are two of the most common transmitter chemicals in the brain and spinal cord, when their concentrations rise above a critical level they can become deadly toxins to the neurons containing glutamate receptors (the locks) and to the nerve cells connected to these neurons. This latter point is especially important. What it means is that excessive glutamate will not only kill the neurons with the receptors for glutamate but it will also kill any neurons that happen to be connected to it, even if that neuron uses another type of receptor. This will become important when we discuss Alzheimer's disease and Parkinson's disease.

Both glutamate and aspartame can cause neurons to become extremely excited and, if given in large enough doses, they can cause these cells to degenerate and die. It is for this reason that the nervous system carefully controls the concentration of these two amino acids in the fluid surrounding the neurons (called the extracellular space). It does this by several methods, the most important of which is a system designed to remove any excess glutamate from this extracellular space. This is accomplished by a special pumping system that transfers the excess glutamate back into surrounding glial cells. (FIG 3-2) Glial cells surround the neurons and supply them with energy. This pump acts like a bilge pump on a ship. If the pump fails the ship fills up with water and sinks. Normally, the glutamate clearing system is very efficient. This is one possible reason why experimentally it takes higher doses of MSG to fatally damage the neurons of adult animals than infant animals—the adult glutamate system may be more competent. But remember, even small doses can damage these neurons without actually killing them.

While this pumping system is very effective, it requires an enormous amount of cellular energy (in the form of the energy molecule ATP, or adenosine triphosphate) for its operation. It is sort of like the old-time fire brigade, where a line of people hoisted buckets down a human chain to put out a fire. It required a lot of energy on the part of the people making up the bucket brigade. If they ran out of energy the fire would rage out of control. The same thing happens when energy production is reduced in the brain: the protective pumps begin to fail and glutamate begins to accumulate in the space around the neuron, including in the area of the synapse. If the energy is not restored the neurons, in essence, will burn up—they are literally excited to death.

A DOUBLE WHAMMY

Within fifteen to thirty minutes after being exposed to high doses of MSG, neurons suspended in tissue culture are seen to swell like balloons. (FIG 3-3) Under the microscope you can see degeneration of the small structures within the cell, called organelles, and also clumping of the chromatin of the

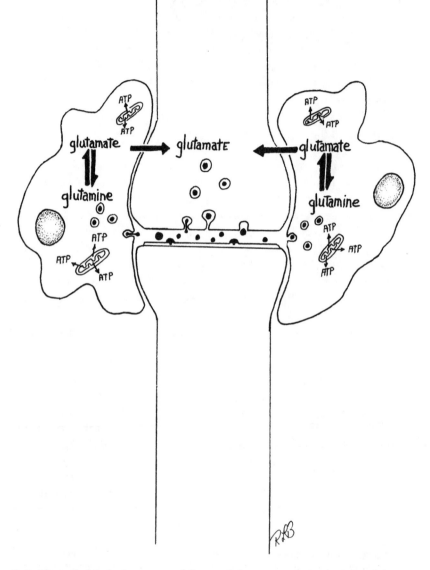

3-2 *The method the brain uses to carefully control glutamate concentrations around the neuron. Glutamate appears to dissipate both by diffusion and by means of a special carrier molecule (the glia) that transports glutamate to the astrocyte. When this carrier molecule is deficient, as in ALS, glutamate can accumulate in dangerously high concentrations around the neurons. This process requires enormous amounts of energy in the form of ATP.*

High Concentration MSG　　　　# Lower Concentration MSG

Immediate

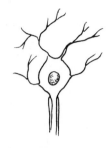

One hour

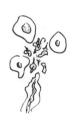

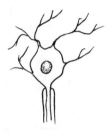

Two hours

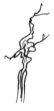

3-3 *When a neuron is exposed to a massive dose of MSG, the cell immediately begins to swell and dies within one hour. At two hours the macrophages begin to clear the remains of the dead neuron away. When a lower dose of MSG is used, nothing appears to happen immediately. But after the second hour the neuron suddenly undergoes rapid death. This delayed death of neurons is characteristic of MSG, aspartate and other excitotoxins. There is some evidence that subtoxic doses of excitotoxins can alter the cells physiology.*

nucleus. Within three hours these neurons are not only dead, but the body's defense mechanisms begin to haul away the debris. Under experimental conditions using animals, this degenerative reaction is seen when MSG is either ingested in the diet, injected into the abdominal cavity, or applied directly to the neurons in tissue culture or into the brain by way of cannula or tube.[24][25]

But when lower doses of MSG were used, scientists discovered something very strange and different. Most of the neurons after thirty minutes appeared to be not only unharmed, but perfectly normal in every way. Then, suddenly, two hours following the exposure, long after the MSG had been removed, the neurons began to die. It was as if a clock had been set so that the neurons would all commit suicide at the same time. Within 18 to 24 hours after exposure to MSG all of the neurons were dead. But during that initial two hour period the cells appeared to be perfectly healthy.

It became obvious to scientists that these two reactions, the acute and the delayed, must have different mechanisms of action. The acute reaction closely resembled neuron injuries caused by a sudden influx of sodium to the inside of the cell. This rapid movement of salt into the cell's interior would literally suck water inside and cause it to balloon and die. To test this hypothesis, scientists added MSG to a culture of sensitive neurons, but they removed the sodium from the bath medium. They found that no matter what concentration of MSG they used, the cells would not die during that critical two hour period. It was concluded that MSG kills neurons acutely by allowing excess sodium, and thus water, to enter the cell.

Yet removing the sodium had no effect on the delayed reaction. After two hours the neurons still died. From earlier studies, scientists knew that sodium entered cells by a special microscopic channel or pore that was controlled by special triggering chemicals. Apparently glutamate acted as a trigger that opened the sodium channel on the cell membrane. This led them to consider another channel that might explain the delayed reaction. They repeated the experiment, but this time they removed calcium from the tissue medium. Anxiously they waited. Two hours passed and the neurons still appeared healthy. Twenty-four hours later they were still perfectly normal. Calcium, it appeared, was the culprit. Apparently glutamate opened a special channel designed to allow calcium to enter the neuron, and it was calcium that triggered the cell to die. But how?

CALCIUM AND CELL DEATH

It has been known for some time that many cells, especially neurons, contain special pores or channels that regulate the entry of calcium into the cell. These special pores are named calcium channels. These channels play an important role in the normal functioning of the neurons. In fact, it is thought that the calcium channels play a vital role in activation of neurons and transmission of their impulses. When a neurotransmitter (the chemical messenger or key) comes into contact with the receptor (the lock) on the neuron fiber's membrane, the calcium channel opens and the in-flowing calcium triggers the neuron to fire or be activated.

Normally this opening and closing of the calcium channel is carefully regulated. When stimulated this channel opens for only a fraction of a second, allowing minute amounts of calcium to enter the neuron. Like glutamate concentrations outside the cell, calcium concentrations inside the cell are carefully controlled by special protective mechanisms. Should too much calcium enter the cell, special calcium pumps drive the excess back out of the neuron. Some of the calcium is also captured and stored within the endoplasmic reticulum of the cell, a long wavy structure within the cytoplasm.

It appears that several of the excitotoxins, including glutamate and aspartate, work by opening calcium channels, at least on certain subtypes of receptors. When these neurotransmitters are allowed to come into contact with the receptor in too high a concentration or for too long a period of time, the calcium channel gets stuck in the open position, allowing calcium to pour into the cell in large amounts.

When this happens the protective mechanisms are triggered. But, as with the glutamate pumps, the calcium pumps also require large amounts of energy as ATP. This energy must be supplied continuously, especially if the calcium continues to enter in large amounts and for a prolonged period of time. Again, it is like bailing out a boat that has a large hole in the bottom. To keep from sinking you must bail the water out faster than it flows into the boat. If you have ever been in this position, you know that it takes a lot of energy to do this.

So how does calcium actually kill the cell? This is an area of intense research and interest because these calcium channels appear to play an important part in a multitude of seemingly unrelated diseases, such as strokes, heart attacks, arthritis, brain injury, migraine headaches, and cancer.

INTRACELLULAR RELAY GAMES

In order for the nervous system to function properly, not only must information be passed from neuron to neuron, but there must also be a system whereby information can be transferred into the cells and among the various parts inside the cell. As with communication in the brain, this language is spoken in chemical linguistics.[26] Special chemicals are used to carry messages around the inside of the cell. This is called the second messenger system. (FIG 3-4) (Actually there are third and even fourth messengers.) You can think of these chemicals as runners in a relay race, passing the baton from one runner to the next.

Once calcium enters the cell it activates one of these messengers called protein kinase C. This runner in turn causes more calcium to be released from a special calcium storage site within the cell, called the endoplasmic reticulum. As a result, even more calcium pours into the cytoplasm of the cell. There is also evidence that protein kinase C alters the membrane calcium channel causing it to be stuck in the open position.[27] As a result calcium continues to pour into the interior of the cell.

All of this excess calcium then triggers a special enzyme within the cell called phospholipase C. This enzyme breaks down some of the fatty acids that make up the cell membrane. Fats are made up of building blocks (called fatty acids) much like proteins are made of amino acids. One of these fat building blocks, called arachidonic acid, is released during this reaction. Arachidonic acid can cause great harm to the cell's interior when it accumulates in high concentrations. (FIG 3-5) Things get really complicated at this

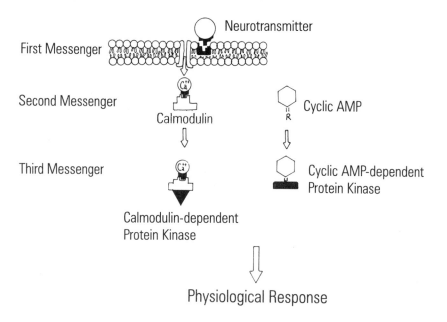

3-4 Second messenger system of the brain. The neurotransmitter reacts with its receptor, opens the calcium channel and the calcium reacts with the second messenger—calmodulin. This in turn reacts with an enzyme (protein kinase) which acts as a third messenger. This final link triggers the response of the neuron.

point. You are now, no doubt getting some idea as to the complexity of the brain.

The newly released arachidonic acid then is attacked by two different enzymes (called lipoxygenase and cyclo-oxygenase). Once this occurs a series of destructive reactions take place that resemble falling dominos. Some of the chemical products produced by these reactions can bring about rapid cell death.[28]

A Cascade of Destruction: The Free Radicals

Once this cascade of destruction is triggered by the influx of calcium, the whole process proceeds with the explosiveness of a nuclear chain reaction. As the reaction proceeds, a particular breed of nasty particles, called free radicals, are produced. To the biochemist, free radicals consist of any atom, molecule, or group of atoms with an unpaired electron in its outer orbit. A better way to visualize this is to think of them as a shower of red hot particles that can damage anything they touch. Once released they bounce all over the inside of the cell burning holes in everything, even the genes. (Actually, they destroy the cell by reacting with other chemicals within the

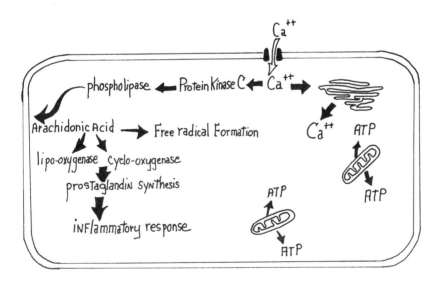

3-5 *How calcium activates destructive reactions within the neuron by triggering prostaglandin synthesis and free radical formation.*

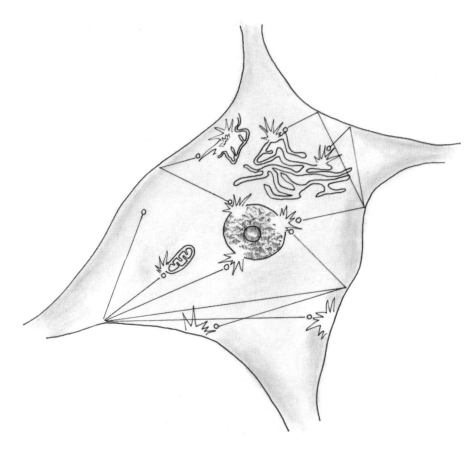

3-6 *Schematic demonstration of free radical damage to the neuron.*

cell.) (FIG 3-6)

It is important to understand free radicals because they play such a central role in almost every injury and disease known; from arthritis, to cancer, and even aging itself.[29] [30] But free radicals are produced not only during disease or injury, but also during every minute of the day in the course of normal cellular metabolism. Energy is normally produced in the cells by a complicated breakdown of the simple sugar glucose. During this breakdown process, called metabolism, free radicals are inadvertently produced. They are in tiny quantities, but they are there nonetheless.

Two of the most important free radicals are the superoxide radical and the hydroxyl radical. Of these two, the hydroxyl radical is the most potent. Also present in abundant amounts is a substance you might recognize called hydrogen peroxide. That's right, it is the same stuff some people bleach their hair with, or use for cuts and scrapes. While hydrogen peroxide is not a free radical itself, it can generate the extremely destructive hydroxyl radical.

Normally these free radicals are produced in minute quantities during energy metabolism by the cells. If nothing is done about them, they would eventually accumulate in high concentrations and begin destroying cells. This is why the cells must have a way to protect themselves.

NATURE'S SPONGES

Fortunately, the body has a method of neutralizing these nasty particles. This system uses a set of compounds called free radical scavengers or antioxidants. Essentially, they are like little sponges that can soak up these harmful chemicals. The most important antioxidants are alpha-tocopherol or vitamin E, and ascorbic acid, also known as vitamin C. The brain normally contains one of the highest concentrations of vitamin C in the body.[31] Unfortunately, it has lower levels of vitamin E.

The advantage of these antioxidants is that they can easily enter the blood brain barrier and reach the brain cells where they are needed most. This means that you can increase the level of these antioxidants in your brain through your diet or by taking vitamin supplements. There is another system the brain uses to guard against free radicals. This involves three enzymes called catalase, superoxide dismutase and glutathione peroxidase. The bad news is that the brain contains only small quantities of these protective enzymes. This leaves the brain quite vulnerable to free radicals produced by disease, toxins, and injury.

As a result, the brain depends on vitamin E and C for its protection. There are also other antioxidants normally supplied by the diet. Most are vitamins, but some are minerals. Beta carotene is a very powerful antioxidant. Others include vitamins K, D, A, and the minerals, magnesium, chromium, zinc, and selenium.

THE COMMON LINK

One of the age old quests of science has been to find the unifying principle that will explain all phenomena. For physics, this is represented by the unified field theory which was supposed to explain all forces in nature. Thus far, no such unifying principle has been found for biology and medicine. But we are moving closer. One of the most interesting discoveries is the central role calcium channels play in disease, injury, and aging.[32]

For a multitude of human disorders (cancer, arthritis, inflammation, injury, strokes, heart attacks, kidney diseases, and even the aging process) calcium channels appear to play a central role. Even many poisons appear to act via calcium channels.[33] Drugs that block calcium channels can often neutralize certain poisons that attack the liver.

It used to be thought that when the brain was injured, say from a blow on the head, all of the damage to the brain occurred at the moment of impact. But we now know that much of the ultimate brain damage that will result occurs hours after the accident—it is delayed. All of these changes I have discussed so far occur in the injured brain: glutamate accumulates in the brain, calcium channels are opened, and calcium pours into the brain cells.[34] This, in turn, sets up the chain reactions involving destructive enzymes and free radicals. As a result, millions of brain cells will eventually die that might have survived otherwise. All of this occurs during the ambulance ride to the hospital and during the first few days of hospitalization. This is referred to as secondary damage.

Experimentally it has been shown that following a brain injury, the ascorbic acid (vitamin C) levels in the brain begin to fall rapidly.[35] It is hypothesized that this occurs because, as an antioxidant, vitamin C is being used up fighting free radicals that develop as a result of the initial brain injury.[36] Within twenty-four hours the brain's level of ascorbic acid falls to barely detectable levels. This leaves the brain vulnerable to further free radical attack.

Once the brain has exhausted its supply of antioxidants, it can no longer protect itself from the enormous amounts of free radicals being generated. We know that following an injury to the brain, the metabolism of the entire body speeds up rapidly. This acts as a continuous generator of free radicals. As a result, the brain's supply of antioxidants is quickly exhausted, creating a condition where the body has a critical need for more antioxidants. The same is true of any injury to the nervous system whether it is a stroke, infection, or chronic degenerative disease. Such patients should be given extra doses of vitamin C, E, and the other antioxidant vitamins and minerals.

CHEMICAL HIT MEN

The excitotoxins do not kill all brain cells—they are very selective. They can totally destroy some brain cells and leave other cells adjacent to them completely unharmed.[37] This selective killing is based on the presence of special receptors for glutamate on some neurons and not on others. That is, the cells that will be killed have been marked for death. We know that almost all excitotoxins act by attaching to the glutamate receptors on the membranes. For example, aspartate, as well as glutamate, stimulates neurons by attaching to this receptor.

Thus far, we have learned that there are three types of glutamate receptors, called NMDA, quisqualate, and kainate receptors. The most common is the NMDA receptor. Overall, the mammalian brain utilizes glutamate as a neurotransmitter in about 50% of the forebrain synapses.[38] They play a very important excitatory role in brain function. That is, they activate the brain and prepare it for action. Because these receptors are concentrated in specific brain areas known to be affected in certain chronic brain diseases such as Alzheimer's disease, ALS, Huntington's disease, etc., it has been proposed that excitotoxins may play a central role in these disorders as we shall see in chapters 5 and 6.[39 40 41 42 43]

In general, we would expect a brain toxin to affect all brain cells equally. But now that we have identified toxins that can act only on specific cells, a whole new understanding of these brain diseases has presented itself. Based on this new knowledge, we may, for the first time, be able to treat diseases that before were considered incurable. But even more exciting, this opens up a whole new field of treatments designed to prevent disease.

EXCITOTOXINS AND BRAIN CELL ENERGY

In 1989 Dr. R.C. Henneberry and coworkers demonstrated that when neurons were deficient in energy they became much more sensitive to the toxic effect of glutamate and other excitotoxins.[44] Using neurons from the cerebellum of the brain they found that when magnesium and glucose were present in a tissue culture medium (that is, brain cells suspended in a glass container) even high levels of glutamate (levels as high as 5 millimoles) did not cause cell death. But if the glucose was removed, doses a fraction of this (as low as 0.02 millimole) could cause cell destruction. When magnesium was also removed from the tissue bath, even small doses of glutamate could kill the cells. Remember, magnesium helps keep the calcium channel closed so as to protect the cells. In this experiment, it didn't matter what caused the cell's energy failure, lack of oxygen, low glucose, or metabolic poisons, the effect was the same—the neurons were made extremely sensitive to the toxic effects of glutamate merely because energy was in short supply.

Later, Henneberry found that low cell energy reserves by itself could cause the neuron to fire spontaneously, which then relieved the magnesium blockade of the calcium channel, thus allowing calcium to pour into the neuron. It is important to remember that magnesium only blocks the calcium channel in NMDA type of receptors and not the quisqualate and kainate type receptors. (The calcium channel activation appears to be directly linked only to the NMDA type receptor and not the quisqualate and kainate type glutamate receptors.)

It is now known that anything that can make the neuron fire will remove the magnesium blockage of the calcium channel. (This is why the channel is called a voltage sensitive calcium channel, or VSCC.[45]) One condition which can cause neurons to fire spontaneously is hypoglycemia or low blood sugar. In fact, you might have experienced this if you suffer from this condition. The anxiety that you feel as the intense hunger grips you is caused by the hyperactivity of the excitatory neurons in your brain. It is possible that this has survival value in primitive conditions since it heightens one's senses. In such a primitive setting this would make it easier to catch wild game. It also intensifies one's courage and anger, as most hypoglycemics know. Again, this makes for a ferocious hunter.

So, while magnesium offers considerable protection against overloads of excitotoxins acting on NMDA type receptor neurons, this protection is reduced when brain energy levels are low, no matter the cause.

Earlier I said that the brain protects itself from excessive glutamate accumulation by actively pumping it into special storage sites. This process requires a considerable amount of cellular energy. Should the energy production system fail, these protective mechanisms can no longer operate causing glutamate to accumulate outside the neuron.

It is also known that glutamate causes neurons to become very excited and fire repetitively. This hyperactivity burns up considerable amounts of energy, further depleting ATP stores, thereby causing the cells to die even faster. Once the calcium flows into the neurons, other protective mechanisms that capture calcium within a special structure within the cells (called the endoplasmic reticulum) are thrown into operation in an effort to save the cell.[46] (FIG 3-7) But this intracellular pumping mechanism also requires energy, and lots of it. If the cell is already energy depleted, as with hypoglycemia or with enzyme defects in the energy production system, this protective mechanism cannot work. The energy exhausted cells then die.

All of this has been demonstrated experimentally in animals and in tissue cultures. For example, when kainate, a substance that stimulates one of the subtypes of glutamate receptors or locks, is injected into the brain in microscopic amounts, there is a rapid depletion of brain energy molecules, primarily phosphocreatinine and ATP.[47] Utilizing a special scanning technique, called PET scanning (that allows scientists to actually watch the brain metabolize energy) similar increases in brain energy utilization have been demonstrated when kainate is injected into special areas of the brain. As we shall see later, this connection between deficiency in brain energy and heightened sensitivity to excitotoxins may play a vital role in human neuro-

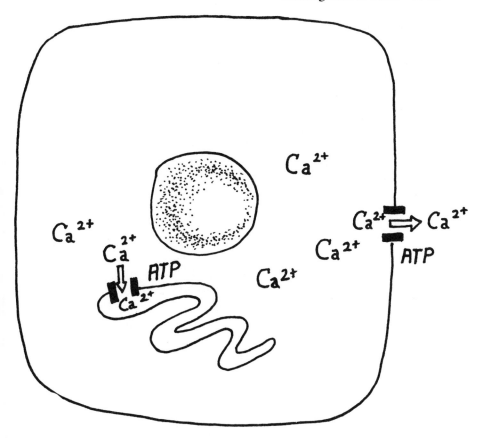

3-7 *To prevent excess calcium buildup within the cell, a special system is used as a pump. There is also a second backup system that drives intracellular calcium into the endoplasmic reticulum. These protective pumps require large amounts of cellular energy in the form of ATP.*

degenerative diseases, in which there is a slow deterioration of brain function. This will also help you to understand how excitotoxins in our food may produce this very same damage, especially during periods of hypoglycemia.

ANALYZING RESEARCH DATA

Since much of what we know about excitotoxins comes from animal research and tissue culture models, it is important that we understand the limitations of this research. Most important, we should also recognize the nature of experimental research in general. The idea that research is always a noble search for truth is naive at best. One need only read Thomas S. Kuhn's, *The Structure of Scientific Revolutions*, to appreciate this statement.[48] As he points out, scientists often acquire the same prejudices of their mentors. They are taught a certain way of looking at the world and of interpreting data that interjects a certain degree of bias. As John Lubbock has said, "What we see depends mainly on what we look for."

It takes almost a superhuman will to resist the temptation to alter one's data to fit a proposed theory. It is particularly difficult to admit one has been pursuing a false notion after having spent one's life in the pursuit of that idea. Can you imagine dedicating twenty or thirty years studying a phenomenon that is later shown not to even exist? Einstein suffered these pains of denial when the theory of an expanding universe was supported by the finding of background microwave radiation. It was only after he was figuratively clubbed over the head with undeniable evidence, that Einstein finally admitted that his static universe model was false. Scientists suffer from the same personality flaws as the rest of us. For the most part scientists are honest, hard-working, and dedicated professionals who are in search of answers. But many of their weaknesses are subconscious and unintentional.

When interpreting experimental studies it is important to know how the study was done. Sometimes experiments are performed using living animals. These studies are called *in vivo* studies. More often, especially in neuroscience, small bits of nervous tissue are used instead. This may consist of slices of whole brain, or cells separated and maintained in a special culture medium. Sometimes layers of neurons are grown in special incubators called tissue cultures. These types of studies are called *in vitro* tests.

Both methods have their advantages. While whole animal testing is closer to real life, the *in vitro* or isolation studies allow us to examine individual phenomenon without the problem of interfering factors. Using special microtechniques, scientists can now study isolated events inside of cells. For example, cell membranes, mitochondria, and other organelles can be isolated and studied. This is how much of our knowledge of the function of calcium channels came about.

But when applying what we have learned, we still must understand how the system works in the whole living organism. For example, when neurons are exposed to glutamate without astrocytes (special glial cells) being present, they are found to be one hundred times more sensitive to the toxic effects of this compound.[49] So in this instance an experiment conducted to test the sensitivity of neurons to glutamate using tissue cultures containing only neurons would give us a false picture of the sensitivity of these neurons to glutamate in a whole brain by a factor of one hundred.

Yet, man is a very unique species. On some occasions humans react to certain drugs and chemicals as no other animal. This may be the case with excitotoxins. We know, for example, that the rhesus monkey is more resistant to the toxic effects of excitotoxins than is either man or mouse. This is because of the poor absorption of glutamate in monkeys. And as we have seen, humans concentrate glutamate in their blood following a dose of MSG in higher concentrations than any other species of animal and are more sensitive to the toxic effects of this glutamate than are experimental animals.

Thus far, over seventy types of excitotoxins have been discovered. Each of these toxins differ in some unique way. This must be taken into account when interpreting data from experiments. Kainate type toxins, for example, behave in an entirely different way than NMDA toxins. They affect different types of neurons and do so in entirely unique ways. Kainate is not normally found in the brain.

The route of administration of the excitotoxin is also important in interpreting data. Excitotoxins are given in a multitude of ways. It may be injected directly into specific areas of the brain in microscopic amounts, ingested with food or water, injected into the abdomen, or even painted on the surface of the brain. When given by injection into the abdomen kainate will cause seizures and destruction of the limbic parts of the brain. But microinjections into specific areas of the brain can produce discrete lesions, often used as functional probes to study brain function.

There seems to be some difference in the sensitivity of some animal to these excitotoxins, even within the same species. For example, some animals require several times the dose of glutamate to produce the same brain cell destruction as in another animal of the exact species, sex, and weight. But then, all living things differ in their sensitivity to toxins. This may be because some cells are naturally stronger than others, or they may have more efficient protective mechanisms, such as the glutamate and calcium channel pumps. We know that the absorption of glutamate from the gut varies considerably from species to species. Humans concentrate ingested glutamate in their plasma in higher concentrations than any known species of animal. Monkeys absorb glutamate very poorly.[50] Mice, while being closer to monkeys in this regard, will concentrate significantly more glutamate following oral feeding of MSG than monkeys. The number of variables are quite numerous.

These differences in all animal species, as well as humans, are why some people can smoke three packs of cigarettes a day for thirty years and never develop lung cancer while another person develops cancer after only ten years of lighter smoking. We are all unique individuals created by God.

The effect produced also depends on the concentration of the excitotoxin, and the duration of exposure. High doses of glutamate can cause rapid cell death whereas low concentrations may not kill the neurons outright but can severely injure them. Of considerable interest is the possibility that these low concentrations slowly bring about brain cell death in neurodegenerative diseases of humans.

An animal's age is also important. Dr. Olney found that immature animals were four times more sensitive to the toxic effects of glutamate than older animals. The opposite may be true of the excitotoxin kainate. When given to seven-day-old mice little happens. But when given to 21-day-old mice, there was a widespread destruction of neurons. Kainate is also unusual in that it appears to kill neurons some distance from where it is injected.

All of these factors must be taken into consideration when comparing experiments and extrapolating or transferring these results to humans. This is especially so where one study seems to contradict another. Often the majority opinion is wrong. Scientific truth is not found by democratic methods or a show of hands. Frequently the lone iconoclast is found to be correct. Scientific history is replete with such examples.

BIAS IN SCIENCE

Scientists are human, just like the rest of us. Too often we envision them almost as religious figures, dedicated to a quest for truth and wisdom that is pure and logical. But a closer examination reveals that sometimes they have a weakness for short cuts to success—dishonesty, distortion of results, faked data, and other forms of deceit. One only needs to survey William Broad and Nicholas Wade's book, *Betrayers of the Truth: Fraud and Deceit in the Halls of Science*[51], or Dixy Lee Ray's book, *Trashing the Planet*[52], to realize the truth of this statement.

In the case of excitotoxins there is a more pertinent example. When Dr. John Olney discovered the harmful effects of food borne MSG on the brains of developing animals he attempted to alert the FDA concerning this danger. He assumed that they would welcome his information with open arms and open minds. But he was soon to learn that government protected industries can be formidable foes. Dr. Olney stated that soon after he had published the results of his experimental findings on the toxicity of MSG in 1969 he came under tremendous fire from various directions. A multitude of papers were published attacking his data, claiming that when his experiments were repeated in their labs no toxicity was found.

But he found that these distractors all had one thing in common, in that "they were all affiliated in one way or another with the Glu [glutamate] and/or food industries." Further, he noted, one group of food industry apologists wrote an indignant letter to the scientific publication *Science* claiming that Dr. Olney's experiments were invalid because he had used baby animals and baby animals were inappropriate subjects for the study because they had immature enzyme systems that made them especially vulnerable to glutamate toxicity. Incredibly, this was at a time when the food industry was adding large amounts of MSG to baby foods. Their logic escapes the rational mind, unless it is motivated by industrial profits.

Dr. Olney, realizing the terrible implications for the health of millions of babies, continued his fight to alert the public and the FDA concerning this danger. The FDA referred this tough issue to a government-sponsored "Food Protection Committee" in an effort to resolve the MSG/baby food controversy. Along with the food and glutamate industry spokesmen, Dr. Olney testified before this committee. Incredibly, the members of this committee seemed more interested in what the food industry spokesman had to say than what a highly respected neuroscientist had to contribute.

One spokesman for the food and glutamate industries stated that even if MSG did indeed destroy the arcuate nucleus in the hypothalamus, it didn't matter because it was not known to have any functional significance. Yet it was well known at the time that the arcuate nucleus of the hypothalamus played a vital role in the regulation and release of important hormones from the pituitary. The committee continued to declare MSG safe as a food additive even in baby foods. Dr. Olney states that at this point he began to look into the backgrounds of the members of the "independent" FDA committee and discovered that "it was founded by, funded by, and totally controlled by the food industry and that most of the members of the subcommittee appointed to investigate the Glu [glutamate]/baby food issue had strong financial ties with the glu [glutamate] and/or food industry. The committee chairman was receiving money from both industries at the time of the committee deliberations."

After Dr. Olney described these events to a Senate committee, pressure was exerted upon the FDA to use more objective reviews. But there is little evidence that the FDA has really changed its ways. Dr. George Schwartz discovered that a pamphlet put out by the FDA outlining the consumer "facts" concerning the safety of MSG as a food additive had in truth been compiled and published by The Glutamate Association, which describes itself as an "organization of manufacturers, national marketers, and processed food users of glutamic acid and its salts, including monosodium glutamate."[53] When Dr. Schwartz pointed this out to the FDA authorities they quietly removed the pamphlet from circulation.

But the deception doesn't stop there. Dr. Olney points out that another method used by the industry is to fund numerous studies that purportedly demonstrate the safety of MSG. These studies appear to be carefully designed to avoid finding such neurotoxicity. Interestingly, these studies were published in Toxicology journals that are "editorially controlled by the very authors of the studies (or their cronies)". When challenged in public forums about the safety of MSG in the food, Dr. Olney says, these fellow-travellers of the industry merely produce a tall stack of such deceptive studies, and as a result, the more important studies by experienced and highly respected neuroscientists are numerically overwhelmed. Industry spokesmen typically say, "The overwhelming number of studies demonstrate no such toxicity." That is, the evidence is "weighed by the pound" and not by quality of the work done. Olney notes that over the past fifteen years the FDA has accepted such tainted studies uncritically.

It is obvious that the FDA has been captured by the chief MSG manufacturer, the Ajinomoto company, the food industries and their public relations organization, The Glutamate Association. By producing a multitude of spurious studies purportedly showing that MSG is safe as a food additive they can say with impunity, "The weight of the scientific evidence demonstrates that MSG is safe for human consumption."

The public has the perception that the FDA, being a government organization designed and dedicated to quality assurance and safety, would never allow an unsafe product to be used by the food industry. In fact, most of us assume that the FDA is, if anything, too cautious. This has been the case with their rulings on carcinogenic compounds in the food. They have come under increasing criticism from a number of groups and scientists for using too stringent criteria in such determinations.

But in this instance, we have seen that powerful industrial giants have been able to capture a government agency and use it to promote an unsafe product.

The following story will help give the reader some idea as to the obstacles that are being faced by those who wish to expose the safety issues involved with MSG and other excitotoxins.

In 1971 Dr. W.A. Reynolds and coworkers reported that they were unable to confirm Dr. Olney's previous findings that MSG fed to infant monkeys consistently resulted in injuries to specific areas of the hypothalamus. That is, they found that large doses of MSG fed to newborn monkeys had no toxic effect on infant monkeys' brains.

Dr. Olney became suspicious of the study when he realized that they were feeding massive doses of MSG to these infant animals. In his experience, such doses almost always caused the animals to vomit. But if the monkeys did indeed vomit, Dr. Reynold's data would be completely invalid since little of the MSG would have actually been absorbed.

Later, at a public hearing, Dr. Olney asked Dr. Reynolds if their monkeys vomited. In front of a large audience she admitted that they had. Yet, a few months later, when the report appeared in *Science* magazine, no mention was made of vomiting, a critical omission.

Dr. Olney wrote *Science* magazine a letter asking why this vital data was omitted. They referred his letter to Dr. Reynolds. This time she denied that the animals had ever vomited.

Four years later Reynolds and others published another paper admitting that the monkeys had vomited after feeding them large doses of MSG. But of even greater importance, for the first time they admitted that their monkeys were under anesthesia throughout the entire experiment, using a drug called phencyclidine. This powerful anesthetic agent is also one of the most potent antagonists of glutamate receptors known. (It is related to MK-801.) This drug is known to totally prevent MSG lesions of the hypothalamus. Therefore, their entire experiment was invalid from the beginning. It is hard to believe that they were unaware of this protective effect of phencyclidine.

Finally, Dr. Olney pointed out that the photomicrographs of the animals' hypothalamus submitted with the articles were taken from areas of the hypothalamus known not to be affected by MSG. That they knew this was proven by the fact that Dr. Olney invited one of their researchers to observe the MSG damaged area in his laboratory. The researcher admitted that MSG was indeed causing the lesions. Yet, according to Dr. Olney, Dr. Reynolds used this same "negative" photomicrograph in a subsequent article to "prove" that MSG was safe.

Dr. Olney concluded, "How does one defend the fact that instead of investigating this laboriously, FDA has uncritically accepted, cited, promoted, and relied heavily on the Reynolds, et al. monkey data as basis for continuing to classify glutamate as GRAS (generally recognized as safe)?"[54]

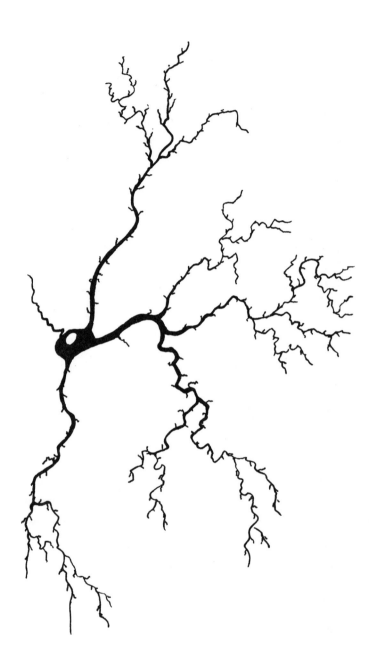

4-1 *A Typical Neuron and its Extensive Dendrite Tree.*

· 4 ·

Effect of Excitotoxins on the Developing Brain

There are over one hundred billion neurons within the fully developed brain. While this is an enormous number of nerve cells, it is dwarfed by the trillions of fiber connections between these cells. (FIG 4-1) It is these connections that make the brain operate as the wondrous organ that it is. What has puzzled scientists for years is how these connections can come together so flawlessly during embryonic development. After all, most of these trillions of connections must be exact in their location for the brain to function properly. With a hundred billion nerve cells we soon see that there are almost an unlimited number of possible patterns in wiring these cells together. When the brain is miswired we can see the results in human terms, with such disorders as cerebral palsy, epilepsy, autism, learning disorders, and Down's syndrome.

Recent experiments have shown that stimulation of the brain is one event that is critical to the development and proper wiring of this organ. This stimulation can occur by way of touch, speech, or vision.[55] For example, it has been shown that babies who spend most of the first year of their life lying in a crib undisturbed will develop much slower than babies who are held, cuddled and talked to.[56] Some of the unstimulated babies could not sit up at age twenty-one months, and less than fifteen percent could walk by age three.

Experimental studies on the development of the nervous system have shown that the neuron fibers must "feel" their way along until they find and connect with their target area. (FIG 4-2) For example, the nerve fibers from the eye must migrate along the optic nerve and connect ultimately to the back part of the brain (called the visual cortex). But how can these nerve fibers find their way among so many other fibers and neurons to arrive at the exact neurons controlling vision?

Apparently they use a method very similar to that used by ants. When

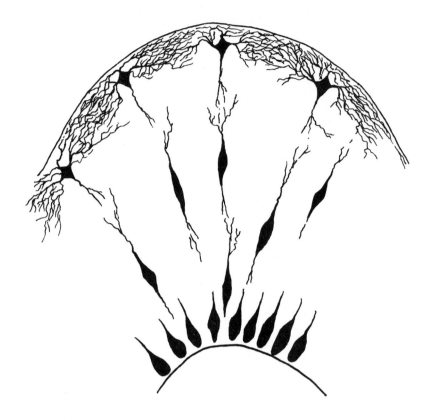

4-2 *Microscopic view of the migration of neurons from the inner germinal layer to the cortex during embryonic development. Glutamate excess may interfere with this delicate process.*

ants search for food, they first send out a scout. After the scout finds the food he makes his way back to the nest. On his way back he will leave a chemical trail for the other ants to follow. It appears that within the brain there are special cells that also secrete a molecular "trail" for the axon fiber of the neuron to follow. The neuron's dendrite has specialized "growth cones" at the tips of its spines that act as a sensor used in following this trail. These growth cones are critical to the normal development and ultimate wiring of the brain.

Often the neuron's first attempt at wiring its pathways is rather crude and inaccurate. To correct this the growth cone will continuously fine tune the process. This fine tuning depends on just the proper amount of stimulation of the neurons. It is known that timing of these events is critical, that the stimulation must occur at just the right moment. Recently researchers have found that glutamate receptors play a critical role in this development process.[57] In fact, these experiments have clearly shown that glutamate can affect the growth cone itself.[58]

In one critical experiment, it was shown that glutamate, in concentrations that were not toxic, could selectively cause the dendrite to shrink, even though the axon (nerve fiber) continued to grow.[59] When the concentration of glutamate was increased to levels known to be lethal to the neuron, even the axon stopped growing. What this means is that glutamate, even in doses not known to be lethal to neurons, can cause this critical brain development mechanism to fail. As a result, this "pruning" of dendrites can cause the brain to be miswired. This has been shown to occur in the hippocampus as well as other parts of the brain.[60]

The process by which the brain is "wired" and even "rewired" is referred to as plasticity. (FIG 4-3) This means that the brain is always changing and repairing itself. It is the plasticity of the brain that is critical to learning. We now know that even the brains of adults are constantly changing and being rewired. The main stimuli for this plasticity appears to be by way of neurotransmitters and electrical activity of the neurons themselves. Of all the neurotransmitters playing a role in brain development in the fetus and plasticity in the adult, the most important is glutamate.[61]

We know, for instance, that when drugs that block glutamate are placed on the developing visual cortex of animals their visual system will not develop.[62] But, of equal importance, is the finding that too much glutamate can cause the same area to be miswired. This could mean that excitotoxin additives used in the food eaten by pregnant women, such as MSG and aspartate (NutraSweet®), could cause miswiring of the developing brain of their babies, should these excitotoxins pass through the placenta.

It must also be appreciated that the brain at birth is still in a primitive stage of development and that much of the rewiring process is still going on. In fact, it is suspected that brain development continues even into adulthood.[63] As a result, newborns and toddlers are at a very high risk when exposed to excitotoxic food additives. This exposure does not depend on passage of the glutamate through the placenta.

Dr. Stanislav Reinis and Jerome M. Goldman recognized this potential danger in their book, *The Development of the Brain*[64], when they stated: ". . . It is still a bit unsettling to realize that in the past monosodium glutamate had been added to commercially prepared infant foods."

The excitotoxin food additives not only damage the "growth cones" of the developing neurons, but also affect development of the brain by acting as powerful stimulants.[65] Previously I stated that the two most potent

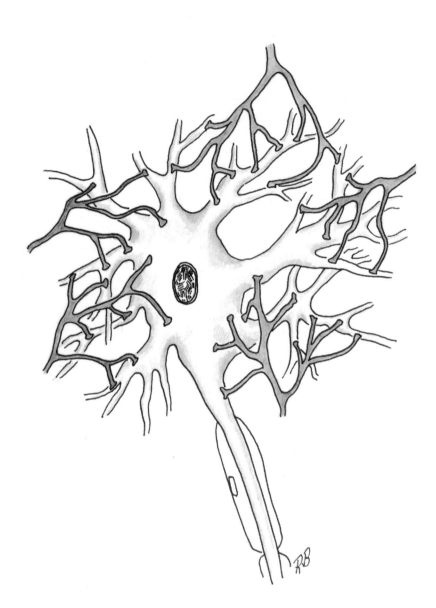

4-3 *Extensive Connections of Nerve Fibers to a Single Neuron. It is the development and alter-ation of these connections that make up what scientists call the ''plasticity'' of the brain. Scientists also know that excess glutamate and aspartate can alter this process.*

stimuli for brain "wiring" were neurotransmitters (primarily glutamate) and electrical activity or stimulation of the brain. This electrical activity must be present for the brain to develop, but too much activity can cause the development to be misdirected. Excitotoxins, as we have seen, can cause excessive electrical activity of the brain and can even cause seizures.

It is clear that brain development is a very delicate process involving many specialized events. The timing of these events is also known to be critical, in that there is a specific sequence of events that occurs during development that requires brain stimulation by way of neurotransmitters and electrical activation. Excessive stimulation, as seen with excitotoxins, can severely interfere with this delicate process and possibly lead to learning disorders, emotional illness, or even major psychological disease later in life.

CHEMICAL DEVELOPMENT OF THE BRAIN

When we consider the biochemical complexity of the brain, the picture becomes almost too difficult to comprehend. Often laymen look at the brain as if it were a static structure—an organ formed before birth that never really changes thereafter. But this is not true. As simple as it may sound, the brain is a living, growing, and expanding organ. All of its parts are alive and nothing in the brain stays the same. Over a lifetime the nervous system is replaced biochemically hundreds of times.

This means that every part of the brain—the membranes, the genes, the transmitters, the receptors—literally everything that makes up the nervous system is constantly being replaced. There is a continuous turnover of all the chemicals that make up this intricate organ. This is why humans must eat, to provide nutrients to replace these vital substances, including vitamins, minerals and trace elements.

The number of chemical reactions taking place in the nervous system at any given time number in the hundreds of thousands. Everything that is broken down in the brain, all of the transmitters generated, every energy reaction, all of the structural proteins and lipids, and the process of interconversions of substances to create other substances, occurs via complex biochemical reactions. Anything that upsets this delicate balance can disrupt how the brain develops, and, therefore, how it will eventually function. So we must also consider the biochemical development of the brain as well as its structural development.

THE MALLEABLE BRAIN: PLASTICITY

What makes the brain basically different from a computer is that the brain can change its circuits so that it forms new pathways, develops new circuits, and bypasses injured areas. If we examine the dendrites of a neuron (input fibers) we see that they contain hundreds, or in some cases thousands, of tiny spines or bulbs, giving them a hairy appearance under the microscope. These bulbs are contact points between various neuron fibers. The more contact points the better the circuit works. By comparing the number of dendritic bulbs, scientists have been able to differentiate between smart animals and dumb animals.[66] Naturally, smart animals have a lot more bulbs or connection points. (FIG 4-4)

We also know that the nervous system can repair itself, in a limited way, by sprouting new nerve filaments. We see this in cases of spinal cord injuries and, to a more limited extent, in brain injuries.[67] [68] Under the microscope we can see evidence of extensive sprouting by the cut neurons and axons in an attempt to repair themselves. Unfortunately, humans are able to do so only to a limited extent.

On a biochemical level, we also see growth and repair mechanisms at work in the nervous system. Most biochemical pathways have alternative methods to achieve the same effect. This double layering of the nervous system adds protection to the system. If, for example, the glucose supply is cut off from the brain, it has a limited capacity to burn fats for energy. In fact, under proper conditions, fats can supply up to fifty percent of the brain's energy needs. Also the brain can produce non-essential amino acids and other biochemical raw materials simply by utilizing special emergency biochemical pathways.

Neurons are adaptable themselves. For example, they can often secrete more than one type of neurotransmitter, and at times, even change transmitters as required. Also the number of active receptors on the neuron's membrane can change depending on the temperature and the presence of additional calcium.[69] What this means is that when the animal's brain temperature rises or if more calcium bathes the brain the neurons adapt by producing more transmitter receptors (locks) so as to improve signal conduction. The brain is a very versatile organ, with a multitude of protective mechanisms. This versatility and ability to mold and adapt itself to changing conditions is also a part of the nervous system's plasticity.

We know that plasticity of the brain plays a major role in learning. Even while a baby is still within its mother's womb, its brain is being stimulated by sounds, touch, and even light causing it to change its structure in important ways. Babies move, play with their toes, suck their thumb, and react to noise after only six weeks of development. All of this stimulation induces the pathways in the brain to change and develop. When a calf is first born, its mother licks it thoroughly, as do cats and other mammals. This is done not only to remove the amniotic fluid, but also plays a vital role in the

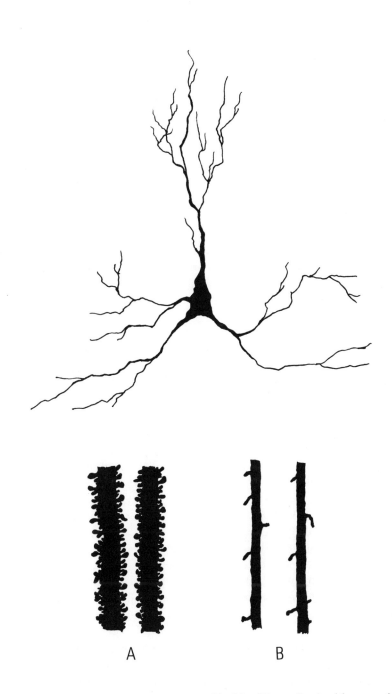

4-4 *A Typical Neuron. a) Microscopic close-up of dendrite of "smart" animal demonstrating extensive synaptic "buttons". b) Fibers from animal deprived of learning stimulation during early development. Notice that there are few synaptic "buttons".*

development of the newborn's brain. The stimulation of the skin triggers important stimuli within the brain causing it to develop more fully.

This process of molding the brain continues all through life, even into the advanced years. But the majority of this restructuring occurs from the first week after conception to a period as long as six or seven years after birth.[70] This is a critical period. Over stimulation can result in devastating effects on this development.[71] Some neuroscientists feel that excitotoxins added to foods and fed to newborns and young children can result in this type of over stimulation.[72] [73] Sometimes the effects might be subtle, such as a slight case of dyslexia, or more severe such as frequent outbursts of uncontrollable anger. In fact, injection of minute amounts of glutamate into the hypothalamus of animals has been shown to produce sudden rage.[74] Even more severe cases could result in conditions such as autism, schizophrenia, seizures, and cerebral palsy. There is a possibility that early exposure to excitotoxins could cause a tendency for episodic violence and criminal behavior in later years. While there is no proof that excitotoxin exposure early in life can result in these conditions in humans, there is experimental evidence in animals that such exposure can result in behavioral changes.

In one carefully controlled study twenty-two rats were given a daily low dose of MSG by injection beneath their skin.[75] The injections began on the first day after birth and continued for eleven days. When the rats were examined they were found to be shorter and fatter than control animals fed a normal diet. But more importantly, the rats exhibited hyperactive behavior. At first this would imply that the animals were brighter. But when they were tested in mazes it was found that they had considerable difficulty escaping from even the simplest maze, whereas all of the control rats were able to escape the mazes in the usual amount of time.

In one test where the rats had to escape an electric shock by jumping up onto a rod suspended over the maze, the MSG treated rats were never able to learn how to escape. When tested for their ability to discriminate between different types of stimuli, the MSG treated rats showed significantly more difficulty than the control rats. They concluded that the "MSG treated rats behaved like animals with lower intelligence." It is important to remember that humans concentrate glutamate in their blood to a much greater degree than rats and they are equally susceptible to its toxic effects once it enters the brain.

In an earlier study Dr. John Olney and Dr. Lawrence Sharpe treated a single newborn rhesus monkey with MSG, again given subcutaneously (beneath the skin) by injection. They carefully observed the animal for signs of behavioral problems, but found none—the animal appeared normal.

The monkey was then killed and its brain examined. To their surprise they discovered evidence of significant damage to the animal's hypothalamus (primarily in the area of the arcuate nucleus). This study was important because it demonstrated that brain cells can be destroyed by MSG when given during critical periods of brain development without there being overt signs of brain damage to an outside observer. However, after the animal matures, this damage manifests itself not only in abnormal behavioral functions, but also in problems with other areas of the brain, including endocrine function. Olney and colleagues repeated this experiment on nine additional rhesus monkeys with identical results.[76]

One of the reasons why it is so difficult to convince the FDA bureaucrats of the connection between MSG and delayed brain damage in humans is because it may take years before clinical signs of neurological damage show up. This damage is slow and cumulative, with each dose of MSG or aspartate damaging a number of important brain areas. While a baby exposed to large doses of MSG or other excitotoxins may not show signs of brain damage at birth, they may do so many years later.

We know, for example, that a simple concussion, in which a person is only briefly knocked out, kills a relatively small number of brain cells. But these individuals usually recover completely without any signs of neurological damage. They are completely normal in all ways. Imagine, however, that they were to get knocked out on a regular basis, as happens to some professional boxers—the damage would then begin to accumulate. The result can be a "punch drunk" individual who speaks slowly and has difficulty thinking and remembering.[77] But this may take many years to manifest. The same may be true with repeated excitotoxin exposure from food. Each exposure may kill some brain cells—and over many years a point is reached where the effects of the loss becomes obvious.

It is known that early damage to the frontal lobes of the brain can lead to arrested moral and social development. Our moral development occurs during the early stages of behavioral development and allows us to be able to concentrate and retain what we are taught. It also requires an ability to restrain our desires and emotions, otherwise known as self-control. One study of two adults who had suffered damage in early life to both of their frontal lobes, demonstrated arrested development and learning disabilities in the realms of insight, foresight, social judgement, empathy, and complex reasoning.[78] It is important to realize that the obvious signs of injury to the frontal lobes of the brain may not become apparent until the child begins to interact with others on a more advanced social level, such as upon entering into school.

The end result of exposure to dietary excitotoxins would depend on the severity and duration of the exposure, the age during which exposure occurred, and the child's individual inborn self-control mechanisms. Yet early, even subtle, damage to the brain of a developing baby, while silent at the time, could possibly cause severe changes in their personality several decades later. Because of this delayed effect, proving a direct connection to early exposure to excitotoxins in the food would be very difficult.

PROTECTING THE DEVELOPING BRAIN

THE PLACENTAL BARRIER

It is well recognized that humans, including pregnant women, develop sharp rises in plasma glutamate levels following oral ingestion of MSG. An important question is whether this glutamate can pass through the placenta and enter the baby's circulation. If it can, we know that at certain toxic levels it can damage the baby's immature brain. One study seems to indicate that certain amino acids not only pass through the placenta, but also concentrate on the fetal side of the circulation.[79] This means that the baby is exposed to a higher concentration of the amino acid than the mother. (FIG 4-5)

Unfortunately, this study was primarily concerned with the study of the amino acid phenylalanine. But the study did find that all amino acids, including glutamate and glutamine (a precursor of glutamate) were higher in the baby's blood than in the mother's. The highest fetal levels were seen early in the pregnancy, and especially in prematurity. This differential was attributed to lower maternal levels of amino acids than actual elevations of fetal levels.

Steglink and coworkers did a more detailed study of glutamate passage across placental barriers and concluded that passage was very unlikely.[80] But upon examination of their results it becomes obvious that the placenta is not an absolute barrier to glutamate. Yet in this study, when pregnant rhesus monkeys were infused with glutamate in a concentration of 0.4 grams per kilogram body weight the fetal levels of glutamate rose ten fold above normal. It is also important to note that their study was conducted using monkeys in the last trimester of their pregnancy. Previous studies have shown that the most sensitive time for amino acid transfer across the placenta was earlier in the pregnancy.[81] Others have found that the placental barrier can be overcome simply by giving a large enough dose of glutamate or aspartate, and that this can indeed damage the brain of the fetus.[82] Still other studies have shown that MSG fed to pregnant animals can damage the brains of their offspring.

It appears that the placental barrier, like the blood-brain barrier, is not

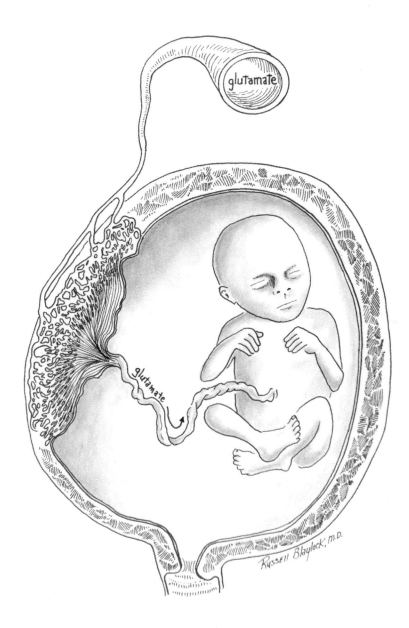

4-5 *Maternal glutamate and aspartate blood levels can reach very high concentrations follow-ing a meal high in these excitotoxins. If these levels are high enough, significant amounts can enter the baby's brain. Lower levels may enter the baby's brain if defects in the placental barrier exist.*

an absolute barrier to the passage of excitotoxins. It should also be remembered that some of the excitotoxins, such as cysteine, can easily pass through the placental barrier and damage the developing brain of the baby. (Cysteine compounds are present in hydrolyzed vegetable protein and are being added to some bread doughs.)

Other factors must also be considered. There are several conditions during which the placental barrier could possibly become incompetent. For example, during periods of fever or viral infections other barrier systems such as the blood-brain barrier can temporarily lose competence. The same must be true of the placental barrier. At times the placenta becomes partially separated from the uterine wall, again possibly disrupting the barrier.

One of the most common lesions affecting the placenta of humans is infarcts.[83] Quite simply this means strokes of the placenta—areas where the blood supply to parts of the placenta have been occluded. This could interrupt any existing barrier mechanism, especially at the margins of the infarct. The placental barrier consists of a single layer of cells, which makes it very delicate and prone to injury.

These areas of infarction can vary from small single infarcts (which are seen in virtually all placentas) to multiple infarcts of large size. The number and severity of these infarcts depends on several medical conditions, such as hypertension or diabetes in the mother.

There are also conditions in which a person's blood level of glutamate can rise to extremely high levels for prolonged periods of time following MSG ingestion. This could create a situation in which the placental barrier would be breached, thereby exposing the baby to toxic doses of glutamate or aspartate.

The Developing Blood Brain Barrier

Many substances considered harmless to the body and found normally in the blood are quite toxic to the brain. This is why the environment of the brain is carefully controlled by a multitude of specially designed protective mechanisms. One of these mechanisms is the blood-brain barrier, whose job it is to exclude harmful substances in the blood from entering the brain. We have learned that several of the amino acids can harm the nervous system, especially the excitotoxic amino acids such as glutamate, aspartate, and cysteine. Under normal conditions, two of these are carefully regulated by the blood-brain barrier. That is, they are excluded from the brain (but not totally).

But like the rest of the nervous system, the blood-brain barrier must also be constructed during development. We are not born with an intact and functional blood-brain barrier system. It is known that this protective barrier is incompletely formed in the newborn, and when it reaches a state of full maturity is unknown.[84] There is some evidence that it may not reach complete maturity until adolescence. During this period of growth and development the nervous system is particularly vulnerable to the damaging effects of a multitude of excitotoxic compounds.[85]

INTERNAL DEVELOPMENT OF THE BRAIN

Right after birth, a baby's brain is metabolically homogenous—the biochemical reactions occur evenly throughout the brain. Yet soon after birth the brain undergoes a period of rapid growth and development during which time biochemical reactions are separated into special compartments within the brain.[86] During this period the level of glutamine, a precursor of glutamate, rises very rapidly in some of these compartments. As the brain matures, glutamate levels also rise. And, as we have seen, glutamate plays a vital role in brain development by regulating the wiring of its various components.

During this rapid growth phase, the brain grows from 300 grams (two-thirds of a pound) at birth to 1250 to 1500 grams (about three pounds) at maturity. By the age of four, the brain has reached eighty percent of its adult weight, and by eight years of age, ninety percent. At age sixteen the brain is full size. But this does not mean that the teenager's brain is fully developed. We know that the organization, reprogramming of circuits, and development of new connections continues for a much longer period, making the teenager potentially vulnerable to the effects of food-borne excitotoxins. As all parents know, it is during these formative years that our children crave "junk food", the very type of processed food that contains the highest concentration of excitotoxin taste enhancers.

It has been proposed that exposure to excitotoxins (such as glutamate and aspartate) during fetal life may cause alterations in brain development that could later result in such serious brain disorders as autism, learning disorders, hyperactive behavior, and possibly schizophrenia.[87] We have seen that excess glutamate can trigger abnormal nervous system development by interfering with the establishment of proper nerve connections, that is, the wiring of the brain.[88] [89] I have stated earlier that the onset of these behavioral and learning disorders may not show up immediately but rather may be delayed for many years following birth because of the timing of the onset of specialized brain functions. Injury to the speech areas of the brain, for example, would not be evident in the newborn baby, but would be evident when the child began to learn to speak. Such injuries could result in delayed speech or stuttering. Likewise, damage to areas of the brain concerned with complex learning skills would not be evident until the child started school and was exposed to math and reading. Until that time, the child would be considered to be normal.

It is known from experiments that the final effect produced by exposure to excess excitotoxins depends on the timing of the exposure to the toxin. This is because the development of the nervous system goes through a normal sequence of developmental events. The final effect of the exposure depends on what part of the nervous system is undergoing development at the time of exposure. In the instance of other malformation-causing drugs we know that these drugs do so only if given during critical times of development. In general, the baby's brain is most vulnerable to gross malformations during the first eight weeks of embryonic development. For example, vitamin A in megadoses can cause serious malformations of the developing brain when given to pregnant mothers during this critical period.

It is entirely possible that the blood-brain barrier does not develop and mature at the same rate throughout the brain. Some areas are more likely to mature later than others. There is some experimental evidence that this is true, at least with regard to the hypothalamus.[90] This would mean that the areas with a more immature barrier would be infinitely more susceptible to the effects of excitotoxins in the food since they could easily enter that portion of the brain. In the case of the hypothalamus, this could result in severe derangements of the endocrine control mechanisms. Indeed this is what has been seen in a multitude of animal studies.[91]

Another protecting mechanism that undergoes gradual development in the embryo is the various cellular pumps that regulate ions and glutamate levels around the neurons. The development of these systems occur on a microscopic and even a molecular level. These pumps, as we have seen in chapter 2, are very complex and depend on exact anatomical construction. They are also heavily dependent on energy supplies, primarily from ATP and phosphocreatine. Experimentally, it has been shown that these protective membrane pumps are not fully developed until well after birth. The exact time when they reach full maturity has not been worked out as yet. But it is evident that some of the key enzymes needed to protect the neurons from excess glutamate and aspartate are absent in the immature brain.[92] This is one reason why experimentally the dose of MSG needed to damage the developing nervous system in baby animals is only one-fourth that needed to do damage in adults.[93] Once these protective systems become fully operational, they are very efficient in providing this protection.

It is also known that some animals and humans lack these critical enzymes altogether needed for protection against excitotoxins in the diet. One such enzyme (glutamate dehydrogenase) functions to convert gluta- mate into a harmless compound. This enzyme has been found to be defec- tive in some human neurodegenerative disorders.[94] Interestingly, when these individuals eat diets containing MSG their blood levels of glutamate rise much higher than normal persons, and remain high for prolonged periods of time. It appears that the defect in this critical enzyme is present from birth. It is also known that others may not lack the enzyme com- pletely, but rather have less of it than other people. Most such individuals would be unaware of their biochemical defect. This would make them more susceptible to food additive excitotoxin exposure as well.

EXCITOTOXINS IN FOOD AND THE PREGNANT WOMAN

Thus far, we have learned that the brain gradually develops important pro- tective mechanism to guard against the effects of harmful levels of excito- toxic amino acids, and that should these toxic substances get past the brain's protective systems, they can alter the development of the nervous system in important and destructive ways. From experiments we know that the infant's brain is four times more sensitive to excitotoxins than is the adult brain.[95] But what do these excitotoxins actually do to the develop- ing nervous system?

Recently it was found that glutamate can actually activate certain genes.[96] Further, this capacity to activate genes may play an important part in the plasticity of the nervous system, that is, the ability of the nervous system to adapt and change in response to the stimuli of learning and observing the outside world. This is very important, not only in the ini- tial development of the nervous system (while the baby is in the uterus) but also much later during childhood and adolescence. This is how the various mental and motor skills develop. Learning is a process of absorbing, storing, and analyzing the events about us. This requires a multitude of incredibly complex brain circuits that are much more complex than the most sophisti- cated computer ever built. But unlike a computer, especially during these early formative years, our brain is constantly growing, reorganizing, and rewiring itself to adapt to new conditions and a flood of incoming data. Glutamate, as we have seen, is one of the more important chemicals playing a role in this developmental rewiring of the brain.[97]

That excess glutamate may adversely effect the formation of the brain was shown in 1987 by Doctor Klingberg and coworkers, who studied the behavioral effects of glutamate on brain development.[98] This study indicated that MSG, when given soon after birth, could cause not only significant growth problems, but could also severely affect intellectual development. At about this same time, in another laboratory, other workers found that MSG given to pregnant rats during their last week of pregnancy could damage vital areas of their offsprings' brains.[99] Dr. Olney had shown in 1972 that large doses of glutamate given to pregnant rhesus monkeys late in gestation also resulted in damage to the fetus' brain.[100]

Adults, including pregnant women, frequently ingest large concentrations of MSG and other excitotoxins in their food. In one study it was found that some restaurants add as much as 9.9 grams of MSG to a single dish, enough to produce brain damage in experimental animals.[101] Liquids containing MSG, such as soups, are absorbed faster and more completely than solid foods. Experiments have shown that MSG in a liquid form is much more toxic to the brain than when included in solid food. Also, humans have been found to have higher blood levels of glutamate following ingestion of MSG than does any other animal species.[102]

Remember, the protective enzymes in the baby's brain are still immature, and therefore are unable to detoxify the excitotoxins that enter its brain. This would mean that in the case of pregnant women eating diets high in excitotoxin taste enhancers, the baby could possibly be exposed to these high glutamate levels for many hours. It is not unreasonable to assume that mothers will eat several meals and snacks containing various forms of excitotoxins such as MSG, hydrolyzed vegetable protein, and aspartame. This could produce a high concentration of glutamate exposure in the baby's brain several times a day.

A question frequently asked is whether or not the glutamate enters the baby's brain. While there is no direct evidence in humans (it would be unethical for scientists to conduct such experiments in pregnant women) we do have experimental evidence that it does in animals. Researchers J.H. Thurston and S.K. Warren found that when they treated newborn mice with MSG their brain glutamate, as well as blood glutamate, was significantly elevated.[103]

Dr. Inouye, in a later experiment, found similar results.[104] In this experiment he labeled MSG with a radioactive tracer and injected it into newborn mice to study its distribution in the animal's tissues. (He used MSG at a dose of 1 mg/gram, a dose known to produce brain lesions in mice.) He found that the MSG reached very high plasma levels within fifty minutes following injection and then rapidly fell to low levels. But, surprisingly, the brain then began to accumulate the MSG, reaching a peak concentration three hours after the injection, after which it slowly decreased. He observed an earlier high concentration of the labeled glutamate in the hypothalamus, the hippocampus, the ventricles, and the thalamus. These areas retained the radioactive labeled MSG for twenty-four hours. It is interesting to note that these are the same areas of the brain known to be damaged by MSG exposure in experimental animals. What this experiment means is that the MSG passes through the immature blood-brain barrier of the mouse and accumulates in certain vulnerable brain regions over a three hour period, so that these neurons are exposed to the excitotoxins at a high concentration over a prolonged time. In fact, the labeled MSG remained in these brain areas for twenty-four hours. If the same is true for humans, and it should be, this would mean that the brain could contain high concentrations of glutamate throughout extreme periods of brain hypersensitivity, such as hypoglycemia, fever, or high energy demand. This would throw into question studies that claimed the safety of food borne excitotoxins based on the idea that blood levels of glutamate fall rapidly following oral ingestion of MSG, since brain levels would continue to rise long after blood levels had returned to normal.

A third study done by Toth and Lajtha confirmed these findings and the principle that the length of exposure to excitotoxic amino acids is very important.[105] Using mice and rats they found that when given aspartate and glutamate, either as single amino acids or as liquid diets, over a prolonged period of time (from several hours to days) they could significantly elevate brain levels of these supposedly excluded excitotoxins. Aspartic acid (a principle ingredient in aspartame) levels rose as high as 61% and glutamate rose as high as 35% in brain tissue during prolonged feeding. They concluded that while these excitotoxic amino acids cannot be taken up by the brain rapidly they can, over a longer period of time, enter the brain in increasing concentrations. Humans are exposed to high concentrations of excitotoxin food additives throughout the day by consuming a variety of processed foods and diet drinks.

When the brain tissue of experimental animals exposed to excitotoxins is examined under the microscope one sees extensive rearrangement of the synapses.[106] The dendrites undergo sprouting and may develop abnormal connections. There is also evidence that immature brain cells exposed to excitotoxins can show a time dependent loss of the cellular antioxidant glutathione.[107] Remember, it is the anti-oxidants that protect the cells once the sequence of destructive events is triggered by the excitotoxins. In fact, the antioxidant vitamin E has been shown to significantly block the toxic effect of glutamate in brain cell cultures.[108]

While it has not been shown that glutamate and aspartate can penetrate the placental barrier except at high concentrations, we know that there are conditions under which this barrier may be faulty. Besides, until the issues are adequately studied by independent scientists, why risk permanently injuring your baby's brain? Should the developing infant's brain be further assaulted by high levels of glutamate or aspartate, as could occur when its mother consumes foods and drinks high in MSG, aspartate (NutraSweet®), and other excitotoxic food additives, these protective mechanism can be overwhelmed, leaving the brain vulnerable to toxic attack.

Newborns: A Difficult Beginning

Entering the world can be a very traumatic event for a newborn infant, not just because of all the lights, sounds, and occasional pains that come with birth, but rather because for the first time the baby is cut loose from its mother and, at least metabolically, must go it alone. This transition between dependence on its mother's blood supply to independence is especially dangerous because the newborn must supply its own brain with adequate amounts of glucose and oxygen, and must be able to remove waste products by way of the blood.

This newborn's survivability depends on a strong heart, good lungs, normal red blood cells, and an adequate supply of glucose from the diet. Far too often, one or more of these vital substances are inadequate or even missing. One attempt by doctors to guage how well the newborn baby was adapting to its new environment was the development of the Apgar score. This score was graded from one to ten, with 8 to 10 indicating the best condition and four or less signaling severe problems. In between scores indicate reason for some concern.

When not enough oxygen is getting to the brain for prolonged periods of time, severe damage can occur to the nervous system. In fact, oxygen supply must be restored within five to six minutes to prevent permanent damage under most conditions. Most people are aware that oxygen is vital to the brain, but they are not aware of just how much oxygen the brain consumes. When at rest the brain uses 20% of all the oxygen in the blood.[109] And when you consider that the brain makes up only 2% of the weight of the body, that's an enormous amount of oxygen.

This oxygen is delivered to the brain and spinal cord through miles of blood vessels. Every minute almost a quart of blood rushes through the brain carrying oxygen and glucose. Should the blood-flow to the newborn's brain be stopped, say by a cardiac arrest, within one minute the amount of ATP (the energy molecule) in the brain falls by 80%. Remember, ATP is the primary energy molecule in the brain. After two minutes ATP is only barely detectable.

Another condition that robs the brain of its energy is hypoglycemia, or low blood glucose. Normally the amount of glucose in the blood is fairly constant. But all too often, newborns will suffer from a fall in the amount of glucose in their blood. There are a multitude of reasons for this fall, such as diarrhea, poor food intake, leucine (an amino acid) sensitivity, viral infections, enzyme defects, and even some drugs taken by their mothers that can cause hypoglycemia. We often see hypoglycemic babies of diabetic mothers taking anti-diabetic medications. Aspirin can also induce severe, even fatal, hypoglycemia in some infants.

As with oxygen, the brain consumes enormous amounts of glucose all the time, even when you are in a deep sleep. In fact, the average three pound brain consumes about 25% of all the blood's glucose. Unlike other parts of the body which can use other substances such as fats and amino acids, the nervous system is dependent on glucose for its energy. (It can burn some fats, but not enough to sustain life.) All of this energy is used to maintain the various functions of the brain such as neurotransmitter synthesis and packaging, operation of the various electrolyte pumps (calcium and sodium), intracellular transport of chemicals, and the synthesis of special lipids and other complex molecules used by the brain. But, as we have seen, most important is the use of energy to protect the brain from toxic amino acids such as glutamate and aspartate—the excitotoxins.

Interestingly, the type of neuronal destruction seen when the brain is deprived of oxygen or glucose is very much like that seen when large doses of MSG are fed to experimental animals.[110] But why would a lack of oxygen or glucose cause the same pattern of selective destruction of brain tissue as is seen with a toxin? By the same pattern, I mean the same pattern of cell destruction, with the glutamate receptor neurons being killed and other non-glutamate type neurons right next to them being unaffected.

The answer to this puzzle lies in the protective glutamate and calcium channel pumps that we discussed earlier. Both of these protective membrane pumps are heavily dependent on energy and when the brain's energy supply is lost, for whatever reason, large amounts of glutamate will begin to rapidly accumulate around the neurons. So where does this glutamate come from? Most of it pours out of the astrocyte (the glia cells surrounding the neurons), which manufactures glutamate from glutamine. But glutamate can also enter the brain from the diet, especially in the infant whose blood-brain barrier is still immature and is being fed foods containing large concentrations of excitotoxin taste enhancers such as MSG.

To prove that glutamate accumulation is the cause of brain damage in cases of oxygen deficits and hypoglycemia, neuroscientists next gave such animals a drug known to block the toxic effect of MSG, called MK-801.[111] And as they suspected, when these treated animals were exposed to hypoxia or hypoglycemia, little brain damage occurred. This means that the brain cells were not dying because they were starving to death, but because glutamate and aspartate were building up in the energy-deprived brain and killing the cells. More and more neurological conditions are being found to be related to excessive excitotoxin exposure, such as hypoglycemia,[112] head injury,[113] migraine headache,[114] seizures,[115] and possibly the neurodegenerative diseases.[116]

What all of this means is that newborns often develop periods of hypoglycemia (low blood sugar) and occasionally hypoxia (low blood oxygen), which makes them especially vulnerable to excitotoxins from whatever source. Dr. Vincent Marks and Clifford Rose's monumental book on hypoglycemia lists forty-four causes for hypoglycemia in children,[117] some of which frequently go undiagnosed for many years.

Prior to the late 1960's the food industry was regularly adding MSG to baby foods. Based on the growing evidence of MSG toxicity on the brain prior to this period, this exposed these infants to a significant risk of brain damage. The extent of this damage depended on the timing of the exposure as well as the dose, that is the amount of MSG it was exposed to. Also of importance is the circumstance under which the child was exposed to these brain toxins.

Let's say, for example, a baby is given aspirin for a fever. The baby hasn't been feeling well for several days and as a result has eaten poorly. Mom tries to help by feeding the child prepared baby foods. In this case the aspirin and poor diet will have made the child hypoglycemic. As a result, the baby's brain becomes especially vulnerable to the damaging effects of excitotoxins. The baby food contains MSG which significantly raises the child's blood level of glutamate. But the child's brain is unable to counteract the high glutamate levels because the energy-dependent protective systems have failed. Remember also, the immature brain is four times more sensitive to the damaging effects of excitotoxins as is the adult brain and that following a dose of MSG, the baby's blood level of glutamate may remain high for many hours.

Often this damage is subtle and not detected initially. But as the child matures and begins its learning process, these subtle injuries may become more evident. This process may even explain autism and hyperactive behavior[118] since early excitotoxin exposure may have resulted in a faulty wiring of the developing brain. The extent of this faulting wiring would, again, depend on the timing of the exposure and the dose. If the child is not hypoglycemic or hypoxic at the time of the exposure, the toxic effects would be much less. It would also depend on the status of the child's natural free radical scavengers. For instance, the child might have high vitamin

E levels or abundant protective enzymes at the time of MSG exposure. This would greatly reduce the toxic effect. We are all individuals and some will naturally have more efficient protective mechanisms than others. The problem is, we have no way of knowing who possesses abundant natural protective mechanisms and who does not.

There are a multitude of variables that determine one's individual sensitivity to excitotoxins, such as age, genetic susceptibility, the total amount of the excitotoxin you are exposed to, frequency of exposure, and the timing of exposure. Even temperature, such as with fever, can activate more receptors on the glutamate type neurons making them more susceptible to excitotoxin damage.

We also know that excitotoxins have a compounding effect when given together. For example, MSG, aspartate, and hydrolyzed vegetable protein given together in a single meal is much more toxic than when given individually.[119] Many foods contain two or more of these excitotoxins. I have seen single frozen diet food dinners that contain MSG, hydrolyzed vegetable protein, and natural flavoring together. Add a diet drink sweetened with NutraSweet® and you have a single meal with four known excitotoxins. (Remember that hydrolyzed vegetable protein contains very high concentrations of two excitotoxins—glutamate and aspartate.)

ENDOCRINE EFFECTS OF EXCITOTOXINS: HORMONES

In 1969 Dr. John W. Olney demonstrated that newborn mice exposed to high levels of glutamate developed extensive destruction of important groups of neurons in their hypothalamus.[120] The worst damage was seen in the arcuate nucleus of the hypothalamus.[121] This nucleus controls important endocrine functions by regulating the amount of hormone-releasing factors secreted by the hypothalamus and the pituitary. It is also known to control the release of the hormone (GHRH) that controls the secretion of growth hormone by the pituitary. Growth hormone is critical in producing growth of the skeleton and other tissues and organs in the developing child. Too little hormone results in dwarfism, and too much in gigantism.

When these animals were further studied, it was found that MSG could stimulate a wide range of abnormal endocrine responses from the hypothalamus. The release of these hormones by the hypothalamus and pituitary controls the release of hormones from the endocrine glands throughout the body—such as the thyroid gland, the adrenal glands, and the gonads. Researchers found decreased levels of growth hormone, prolactin, and luteinizing hormone in animals exposed to MSG.[122] Normally, even in humans, growth hormone is secreted by the hypothalamus in intermittent pulses. Following MSG exposure, these mice were found to have this pulsatile flow markedly diminished. This phenomenon has now been shown in a multitude of independent studies.[123] Prolactin levels were also found to be decreased following MSG exposure and appeared to be caused by blockage of the normal release mechanisms in the hypothalamus.[124] Prolactin plays an important part in the production of breast milk following birth.

Most of these experiments were conducted in newborn animals. But Dr. Shimicu and coworkers demonstrated that when MSG is given to pregnant mice their offspring also have similar injuries to their hypothalamus.[125] (FIG 4-6, Series of four photographs) Again, this confirms that glutamate passes across the barrier of the placenta and enters the fetus' bloodstream.

With all of these endocrine malfunctions you would expect these mice to develop abnormally, and they do. Consistently, the animals exposed to MSG were found to be short, grossly obese, and had difficulty with sexual reproduction. One can only wonder if the large number of people having difficulty with obesity in the United States is related to early exposure to food additive excitotoxins since this obesity is one of the most consistent features of the syndrome. One characteristic of the obesity induced by excitotoxins is that it doesn't appear to depend on food intake.[126] This could explain why some people cannot diet away their obesity. It is ironic that so many people drink soft drinks sweetened with NutraSweet® when aspartate can produce the exact same lesions as glutamate, resulting in gross obesity. The actual extent of MSG induced obesity in the human population is unknown.

It is also possible that many of today's reproductive problems, such as infertility and menstrual disorders, are similarly related to excitotoxin exposure in early life. It has been shown, at least experimentally, that excitotoxins such as MSG and aspartate can cause an early onset of puberty in female rats.[127] [128] This is consistent with the observation that smaller doses of MSG can stimulate the hypothalamus to secrete large amounts of luteinizing hormone, which controls reproduction and onset of puberty.[129] It appears that MSG causes the immature neurons within the hypothalamus to become reorganized so as to disrupt the production and release of these critical reproductive hormones.[130] This again emphasizes that the excitotoxins can adversely effect the development and wiring of the brain in newborns.

This adverse effect on reproduction is not limited to females. Researchers have demonstrated a marked reduction of fertility in male rats treated with MSG as well.[131] [132] This does not appear immediately, but rather the effect

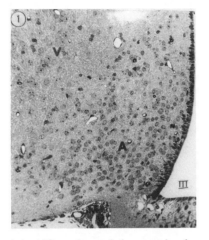

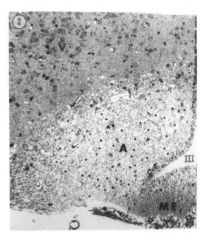

4-6 *a) Photomicrograph demonstrating the normal hypothalamus in the region of the arcuate nucleus of a ten-day-old mouse.*

b) The same area seen in a ten-day-old mouse six hours after receiving a dose of three grams per kilogram of glutamate. Notice that the neurons in the area of the arcuate nucleus are now greatly swollen and distorted.

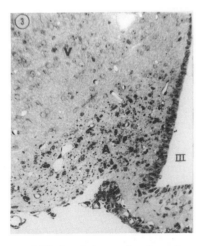

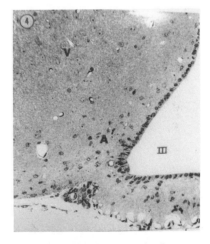

c) The hypothalamus of an eleven-day-old mouse twenty-four hours after a three gram per kilogram dose of glutamate. Notice that the cells are now degenerating and being cleared away by phagocytic cells.

d) The hypothalamus of a fourteen-day-old mouse four days after receiving a three gram per kilogram dose of glutamate. Observe that the area of the arcuate nucleus is now devoid of most of its neurons. What cells are left are mostly astrocytes. The arcuate nucleus plays a vital role in the regulation of growth hormone.

is delayed until the rats develop sexual maturity. If the same effect occurs in humans, this would mean that with exposure to MSG during the neo-natal period (soon after birth) one would not see the adverse reproductive effects of this exposure (such as infertility) until the child also reaches puberty. Pizzi and coworkers found that both male and female mice exposed to MSG early in life developed severe delayed abnormalities of reproduction in adulthood.[133] The females had fewer pregnancies and smaller litters and the males were significantly less fertile than normal mice. Again, they found that the mice exposed to MSG were obese and had shrunken pituitaries and gonads (testes and ovaries). Similar findings have

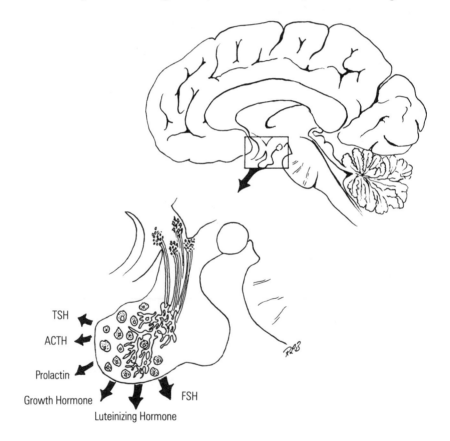

4-7 *The Neurons in the hypothalamus that secrete special hormones, that in turn, cause the pituitary gland to release its hormones. Glutamate appease to be a major neurotransmitter for this control system.*

been seen in all other species of animals tested, which means that the toxic effect of MSG on reproduction is not a peculiarity of mice or rats.[134]

So how would MSG in lower doses cause these devastating endocrine problems? We know that at birth the arcuate nucleus of the hypothalamus is in a very immature developmental state, in that its circuits are still being wired.[135] It is these same centers that control the normal release of the hormones that control the reproductive system in both males and females. (FIG 4-7)

Based on careful studies conducted in experimental animals, researchers are convinced that MSG, by causing abnormal development of the hypothalamus and damage to specialized neurons, causes the ovaries to become atrophied (shrunken) thus leading to severe problems with the reproductive cycle in females.[136] So it appears that MSG has both direct toxic effects on the nerve cells in the hypothalamus and can cause the organization of the developing brain centers to be miswired. Both of these effects can lead to severe endocrine problems later in life. This is why it is critical that you avoid MSG, aspartate and other excitotoxic food additives in both your food (especially if you are pregnant) and in your children's food.

It has also been found that animals fed large doses of glutamate have lower thyroid hormone levels and higher cortisone levels than normal.[137] Another interesting finding is that glutamate can unmask diabetes in mice that are genetically susceptible to the disease.[138] That is, these mice might never develop full blown diabetes unless exposed to glutamate. This might explain the high incidence of diabetes in the elderly, since many have had a lifetime exposure to high levels of glutamate. It could, as well, act as a trigger for early onset diabetes of childhood, which is also hereditary. It certainly is an area that needs further study. We know that children who develop diabetes do inherit a gene for the disorder, but that some, as yet unidentified, environmental event triggers the actual onset of clinical diabetes. While most authorities have assumed the trigger was a virus, it could be an excitotoxin.

DO CHILDREN GET ENOUGH EXCITOTOXINS IN THEIR DIETS TO CAUSE PROBLEMS?

One of the big controversies involved in this debate over safety is whether babies and children are exposed to enough excitotoxins in their food and beverages to cause damage to their brains. It is important to remember several things before we begin this discussion. The animal closest to man in glutamate and aspartate sensitivity is the mouse. But even then, man is five times more sensitive to these excitotoxins than is the mouse. (FIG 4-8) Humans accumulate glutamate in their blood streams following ingestion in much higher levels than do other animals and it remains at a higher level for a much longer period of time.[139] Together, these two factors, higher blood concentrations and longer duration of brain exposure, make humans much more sensitive to excitotoxin damage than the animals upon which sensitivity studies were originally done.

We know that mice will begin to develop brain damage when they are fed monosodium glutamate in a concentration of 500 milligrams per kilogram of body weight.[140] This represents a plasma concentration of 60 to 100 micromoles per deciliter. In adult humans ingesting 200 milligrams per kilogram of MSG their blood levels reach around 80 micromoles per deciliter, which puts them in the toxic range of known brain damage.[141] One neuroscientists has done a hypothetical dose curve for excitotoxin exposure (glutamate plus aspartate) in a two-year-old child taking in 200 milligrams per kilogram of these excitotoxins in known food/beverage mixtures.[142] (This is based on consuming a reasonable helping of soup and an aspartame-sweetened drink.) (FIG 4-9) In this instance the child would receive an excitotoxin dose of 500 micromoles per deciliter which is six times the plasma concentration needed to cause neuron destruction in the hypothalamus of experimental animals.

Even using the data from one of the leading defenders of the safety of food additive excitotoxins, Dr. Lewis D. Steglink, we see that even when modestly low amounts of MSG and aspartame are consumed the plasma glutamate rises 5 to 6 fold. This, Dr. Steglink admits, is enough to destroy neurons in the hypothalamus of a mouse.[143]

Steglink's data was done on adult humans—we know that the same dose in a two-year-old child represents an even higher concentration in the plasma. It is not uncommon for adults to consume ten grams of glutamate per day, with at least one gram being free glutamate.[144] Added MSG, aspartate, and other taste enhancing excitotoxins can drastically increase the levels of free excitotoxins in the average person. If you feed your children off of your plate or let them drink beverages and other foods sweetened with NutraSweet® you may be exposing them to dangerously high concentrations of excitotoxins.

The younger the child the greater the danger. Babies exposed to excess glutamate and aspartate are at particularly high risk. We know that infant animals fed MSG have higher blood levels of glutamate and these levels stay higher longer than in adults.[145] It has been pointed out that for twenty years prior to 1969, the amount of glutamate added to a single 4½ ounce jar of baby food contained up to 25 times more free glutamate than could be

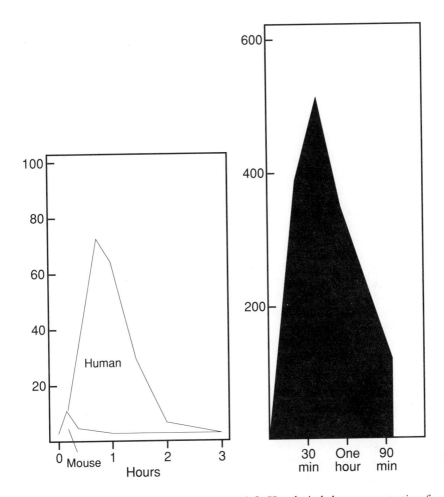

4-8 *Comparative levels of plasma glutamate in mice and in humans.*

4-9 *Hypothetical plasma concentration of glutamate plus aspartate if a child consumed a soup and beverage meal containing a total excitotoxin load of 200mg/kg based on other experimental data. The plasma concentration of glutamate required to destroy neurons in the hypothalamus in immature mice is approximately sixty to one hundred mmole/dl. With such a food/beverage challenge one might reasonably see plasma values as high as 400-500 mmole/dl in a child.*

found in the same amount of mother's milk.[146] This same jar of baby food contained approximately one-fourth the amount of glutamate needed to cause hypothalamic destruction in an infant animal brain.[147] But remember, the human infant is five times more sensitive to the same concentration as a mouse. This would mean that human infants could have been damaged by a single jar of this baby food.

TRUTH IN THE SCIENCES

Not all researchers have confirmed these findings. Soon after this phenomenon was described some disputed the idea that MSG can cause hypothalamic lesions at all. Dr. Charles B. Nemeroff, who is a primary researcher in this field, has done an extensive review of the scientific literature and concludes that most reliable evidence indicates that MSG consistently produces significant injuries to the hypothalamus of a wide variety of animal species and causes disruption of many endocrine hormones.[148] As to the reports that deny such damage, he notes that when he attempted to get samples of MSG-treated animals from these investigators who reported no histological lesions, "unfortunately, all such requests have been denied."

But there is even more direct evidence that disrupts these negative claims. Most such negative studies are based on older studies that have relied on light microscopic examination of the hypothalamic tissues of the animals exposed to MSG. The problem with such studies is that they are only able to detect actual death of the neurons within the hypothalamus and cannot detect less than lethal injury. For example, we know that in some of these negative studies doses of MSG were used that will damage the functioning of the cells but will not actually kill them (called a sublethal injury). This cannot be seen through a light microscope.

So how can sublethal damage be detected? One way is to examine the neurons with the electron microscope so that you can see the minute structures deep inside the cells. Another way is to use radioactive isotopes that will selectively demonstrate damaged neurons, called autoradiography. Dr. W.K. Paull used this technique and found that when MSG was given to newborn animals, it tended to accumulate in the arcuate nucleus of the hypothalamus, which contained the largest population of MSG-sensitive cells.[149]

Another method of detecting subtle damage to brain cells is to use special stains that demonstrate enzymes within the tissues, such as peroxidase. Using this method, Dr. W.J. Rietvelt and his coworkers observed decreased activity in the cells of the arcuate nucleus in rats treated with MSG.[150] It is thought that this particular enzyme plays an important role in the release of the reproductive hormone LHRH from the hypothalamus. In a separate laboratory researchers demonstrated a marked loss of cells specifically staining for the hormone ACTH in the hypothalamus of newborn rats exposed to MSG.[151]

A more direct method of measuring damage to the neurons secreting these vital hormones in the hypothalamus is to measure the specific levels of the hormone by special assays of the tissues. When this was done it was found that even in MSG-treated adult animals there was significantly less of the hormone oxytocin within the nuclei of the hypothalamus than is seen in normal animals. Oxytocin is responsible for the secretion of milk from the breast of females after the birth of their newborns.

Some critics of these studies charge that MSG does not enter the brain because of the blood-brain barrier. There are two problems with this argument. First, in the newborn the blood-brain barrier is incompletely formed and will allow MSG to enter the brain. And second, the hypothalamus, even in the adult, does not have a barrier. That MSG can enter the brain of newborn animals given MSG was shown by two researchers who demonstrated not only high blood levels but significant elevations of brain glutamate lasting up to three hours after the dose was given.[152] This has been confirmed by Dr. Inouye, who demonstrated the passage of radioactively labeled MSG into the neonatal brain following MSG injections.

One of the problems in proving that MSG could cause major injuries to the hypothalamus was in explaining how it could injure neurons in this area when so few neurons of the glutamate receptor type were know to exist in the this tissue. But then it was only recently that glutamate was found to be the primary neurotransmitter in the hypothalamus.[153] Using various staining methods, neuroscientists found that glutamate neurons connect to every major nucleus in the hypothalamus. Interestingly, these neurons were found to be sensitive to all glutamate-like compounds, such as NMDA, quisqualate, and kainate as well as aspartate and MSG. This indicates that a wide range of excitotoxins can destroy and affect these vital neurons in the hypothalamus.

What this means is that glutamate type-neurons control every neuroendocrine function of the hypothalamus. This neuroendocrine function is designed to control the thyroid gland, adrenal glands, reproductive functions, gonadal function, body growth, and certain aspects of metabolism. But in addition, glutamate controls all the other functions of the hypothalamus, such as the biological clock, the autonomic nervous system, sleep-wake cycles, hunger and satiety, the emotions of anger and rage, and even consciousness itself.

So we see that anything that disrupts or impairs the normal functioning of the hypothalamus can have devastating effects on the organism as a whole. Early exposure in life to high doses of glutamate, or the other excitotoxins, could theoretically produce a whole array of disorders much later in life, such as obesity, impaired growth, endocrine problems, sleep difficulties, emotional problems including episodic anger, and sexual psychopathology.

Whether such changes would be reversible or not depends on the dose of excitotoxin given, the timing of the dose, and how long the child was exposed to high doses of excitotoxins. As for timing, we know that for glutamate, the earlier the exposure to the toxin, the more likely is permanent damage. If exposure is delayed until several years after birth, the injury may be less severe. It is also possible that some neurons are injured but not killed. We know that subtoxic concentrations of glutamate can alter the function of hypothalamic neurons without destroying them.[154] Also, earlier exposure would increase the likelihood of abnormal wiring of the circuits within the hypothalamus. **So parents, it is important to stop your child's exposure to excitotoxins now!**

It is important to emphasize that there is ample experimental evidence that glutamate and aspartate both effect the neurological development of the hypothalamus. That is, it alters the way the cells and pathways in the hypothalamus develop. This can result in permanent alteration of the anatomy, as well as the function, of this most important brain organ.[155] There is also evidence that MSG acts as a growth factor, as a chemical directly stimulating the growth and maturation of brain cells, thereby acting to alter the development of the brain itself.[156]

You should remember, aspartate is also toxic to the hypothalamus.[157] This is probably one of the most common types of exposure see in pregnant women. Most pregnant women are trying to avoid too great a weight gain so they figure, "I'll cut down on the sugar." That sugar is a major cause of fat gain is a common misconception today. Nonetheless, dieters frequently switch to diet colas and other foods sweetened with NutraSweet®. NutraSweet®, or aspartame, is a sweetener made from two amino acids, phenylalanine and the excitotoxin aspartate. It should be avoided at all cost.

Interestingly, the manufacturer of aspartame warns those with the metabolic disorder phenylketonuria, not to drink NutraSweet®. In this disorder there is an abnormal metabolism of the amino acid phenylalanine so that when it is ingested in the diet dangerously high blood levels, and hence brain levels, of this toxic amino acid develop. But there is no warning to pregnant women to avoid the aspartate in NutraSweet®. When a pregnant woman drinks liquid aspartate, for example in a diet cola, the aspartate enters her blood stream rapidly, potentially passing through the placenta where it would flood the developing brain of her baby. Now that we are aware that the hypothalamus is extremely sensitive to these substances, avoiding excitotoxins such as NutraSweet®, MSG, and hydrolyzed vegetable protein, is especially critical.

One reason the FDA has not issued a warning is that babies exposed to MSG and NutraSweet® are not born obviously deformed, as were those exposed, for example, to the drug Thalidomide. (The otherwise safe drug Thalidomide caused severe deformities of the arms and legs in the offspring of mothers using the drug early in their pregnancy.) Instead, many of these hypothalamic-endocrine disorders are subtle and difficult to connect directly to excitotoxin hypothalamic damage; primarily because no one has measured the function of the hypothalamus in children of mothers who were heavy users of excitotoxins during pregnancy. Also, the effects of hypothalamic damage usually do not show up until many years later, even during adulthood, as has been shown experimentally on several occasions. Therefore, a scientifically stringent connection is difficult to make.

CONCLUSION

Thus far we have reviewed extensive and compelling evidence that excitotoxins can severely effect the development of the brain in experimental animals of all species tested. This sensitivity of the brain varies with the age of the animal at the time of exposure, with the greatest sensitivity occurring while the baby is still in its mother's uterus. At this stage the brain is very immature and many of the enzymes and mechanism that protect the adult brain from high concentrations of excitotoxins have not yet developed. Thus the baby's brain has no way to protect itself.

The transition from a high degree of sensitivity to excitotoxin damage seen in the newborn to a low susceptibility in the adult occurs very gradually over many years. That is, the animal doesn't suddenly at a particular age develop all of the protective mechanism that guard against neuron toxicity. Since this slow transition to full brain protection is seen in all animal species tested, it can be safely assumed to be true in humans as well. This would mean that your child's sensitivity to food borne excitotoxins would continue for several years after birth, possibly even into adolescence. This has never been tested so we don't know the exact length of this hypersensitive period.

Based on experimental studies in animals we can reasonably assume that when the pregnant woman eats or drinks foods containing high doses of excitotoxins, such as MSG, hydrolyzed vegetable protein, and NutraSweet®, her baby's brain is at potential risk of being exposed to these excitotoxins. This, especially if the exposure continues day after day for nine months, could lead to significant damage to the child's hypothalamus as well as other areas of the brain. We have seen that the hypothalamus plays a vital role in controlling a multitude of endocrine systems and physiological functions and that this damage can either be quite subtle or, at times, devastating. In either case, the onset is often delayed years or even decades.

We have also seen that excitotoxins can potentially lead to severe mis-development of other parts of the brain, possibly leading to learning disorders, autism, and serious psychological problems. This has been suggested in experimental studies, but as yet there is no firm proof of the connection in humans.

You must keep in mind that all of these excitotoxin food additives serve only one purpose: they enhance the taste of food. They are not preserva-tives that keep food from spoiling, and they have no nutritional value. Potato chips, frozen foods, diet foods, soups, and gravies almost all depend on excitotoxic taste enhancers.

· 5 ·

Creeping Death:
The Neurodegenerative diseases

NEUROLOGICAL TIME BOMBS

Most of us are at least familiar with some of the diseases that affect the brain and spinal cord. For example, you can understand how a virus might invade the brain and cause it to become inflamed (called encephalitis), or when a bacteria infects the linings of the brain and spinal cord to produce meningitis. Likewise, it is easy to understand, at least in a basic way, how the brain is injured by a stroke.

But sometimes the brain is injured in more subtle and mysterious ways. For example, with Huntington's disease a specialized group of brain cells may begin to die and shrivel up, causing uncontrollable writhing movements and dementia. In another instance with Parkinson's disease, different brain cells in another location may begin to die producing a fine tremor of the hands and rigid, plastic-like movements of the body parts. When the loss of these specialized cells is more widespread, such as in Alzheimer's disease, it may lead to severe dementia and disorientation.

What characterizes all of these diseases is that they develop in previously normal brains and progress, in most instances, very slowly, causing the brain and/or spinal cord to eventually degenerate. A multitude of these degenerative diseases are known to exist, including amyotrophic lateral sclerosis, olivopontocerebellar degeneration, Alzheimer's disease, Huntington's disease, and Pick's disease.

What is so unusual about these diseases is that most of the people who are affected by them have lived perfectly healthy lives up until the time the disease strikes, which is usually late in life. After the onset of symptoms the signs and symptoms of the disease inexorably progress over the ensuing years, or even decades, until the individual is crippled.

The puzzle of what causes these particular neurons to start dying after decades of normal function has intrigued neuroscientists for many years. Until recently, one of the more interesting theories was based on the idea that these neurons age faster than normal neurons, and that this premature aging is programmed in the genetic structure of the cells. This means that some neurons would be programmed to live only fifty-five years rather than the normal one hundred plus years. This idea was popularized by a famous neurologist, W. R. Gowers, at the turn of the century. He called this process abiotrophy.

But then evidence began to appear indicating that even though the symptoms do not appear until the later years, the pathological destruction of the neurons begins much earlier, even decades earlier. As we shall see later, the symptoms of Parkinson's disease do not manifest themselves until over 80 to 90% of the neurons in the involved nuclei (called the substantia nigra) have died.[158] The neurons didn't all suddenly die at the same time, rather they slowly and silently deteriorated over many years. The same is true for Alzheimer's disease. This is why prevention is so important.

What is causing these neurons to slowly die? Why are only certain neurons susceptible to this death while neighboring neurons remain perfectly healthy? We know that some viruses can cause neurons to die slowly. Scientists have renamed these slow viruses ''prions''. But so far an intensive search for these prions has failed to make the connection with the major neurodegenerative diseases.[159] Also, most of the prion diseases have much shorter durations.

Other scientists are of the opinion that malfunctions of the immune system are the cause of many of these diseases.[160] This is particularly so with Alzheimer's disease. This theory is based on the idea that occasionally the immune system gets confused and accidently attacks the nervous system, or parts of it. There are diseases where this happens, for example, allergic encephalomyelitis, a disease in which the immune system mistakenly attacks the nervous system. Yet, thus far, the results of extensive studies of such a connection to the neurodegenerative diseases are not that impressive.

The most impressive line of investigation is the possibility of an environmental toxin as the causative factor. While most attention has been directed toward the metal aluminum, there are problems with this theory as we shall see. But first let us explore other possibilities, namely plant toxins.

THE ENVIRONMENTAL CONNECTION: THE MYSTERY OF THE CHAMORRO INDIANS

As American troops invaded the islands of Guam following World War II, the military doctors were astounded to find that large numbers of the

Chamorros Indians, living on the Mariana Islands, were dying of a mysterious disease that left the Indians too weak to stand or even swallow their food.[161] Their bodies were horribly wasted. Later, when other research doctors returned to the islands, they discovered that the mysterious disorder closely resembled another disease seen in the West called amyotrophic lateral sclerosis or ALS. What made this finding so incredible was that the incidence of the disease on these islands was 50 to 100 times higher than ALS seen in the developed countries. Obviously, something very strange was going on.

Scientists who came to study this mysterious disease knew that the people had suffered terrible hardships and famine during the war. But famine and stress were common in all wars, yet this clustering of such a rare disease had never before been seen. In the United States and Europe ALS has a frequency of one or two cases per 100,000. Clinically, the disease is identical to that seen in Guam, with progressive weakness, usually beginning in the hands, spreading up to the shoulders, and finally involving all four limbs. Death usually follows three to five years of an inexorable progression of severe weakness and wasting of the muscles. The mind stays perfectly lucid throughout the entire course of the disease.

The National Institutes of Health has been studying the cause of this clustering of ALS in Guam for the past thirty years. In fact, they set up a field office in Guam specifically for this purpose. Initially, they felt that the high incidence was caused by a genetic defect that was being compounded by tribal intermarriage within this isolated group of natives. But further study discounted this hypothesis. Others investigated a viral cause, but this too was disproven.

In 1954, epidemiologists studying the disease discovered that the natives frequently consumed large amounts of a particular plant called *cycas circinalis*, or cycad, during the war years.[162] Actually cycad, made from the false sago palm, had been eaten by the natives for centuries. In fact, the Indians knew the plant was poisonous and for that reason they developed a ritual to render it safe for eating. This process consisted of soaking the sliced seeds in water for several hours. This was repeated several times, each time using fresh water. After the last soaking, a chicken was fed some of the wash water. If it lived, the seed was deemed safe to eat.

Once made safe, the seeds were then ground into a flour, or sometimes it was used to make a medicinal poultice. During the war years, because of the famine, cycad flour made up a large portion of the natives' diet. Unfortunately, fresh water was also in short supply. As a result, the natives often abbreviated the washing technique, and sometimes they abandoned the chicken test. Often the natives made the flour for barter rather than personal consumption, so they used shortcuts which often eliminated the washing altogether.

When the scientists analyzed the seed they found that it contained various glycoside compounds, the most important of which was cycasin, a known liver toxin.[163] Cycasin was also found to induce cancer in rats. But multiple attempts to induce the ALS disorder in experimental animals failed. Later, another toxic compound was found in smaller concentrations. This compound, called β-N-methylamino-L-alanine or L-BMAA for short, was found to cause seizures when fed to mice but was not shown to cause the muscle wasting seen in human cases.

The idea that cycad flour contained a toxin that was causing the disorder seemed obvious to early investigators. Over the years, between 1962-1972, a series of "cycad conferences" were set up by the National Institutes of Health. At one of these conferences evidence was presented demonstrating that L-BMAA did not cause the ALS disease when fed to rats in large doses for 78 days. This report almost killed further investigations of cycad for good.

But one researcher, Dr. George Spencer, found that L-BMAA had some properties that were similar to another compound he had been working with called L-BOAA, which caused a spinal cord disease in humans called lathyrism. Lathyrism is a disorder that is characterized by the sudden onset of weakness or paralysis in the legs following consumption of diets high in the chickling pea (*Lathyrus sativus*).

In the late 1970s Dr. Spencer met another researcher, Dr. Leonard Kurland, who was working on the Guam ALS disease and its connection to the cycad seed.[164] From this meeting they immediately recognized the distinct possibility that both diseases could be caused by a related plant toxin. One phenomenon they both noticed was that the Guam (ALS disease) disease was often delayed for many years following ingestion of the seed.[165] Spencer toyed with the idea that this might represent a chronic toxic effect.

Then in 1980, Dr. R.M. Garruto and his coworkers studied a group of immigrants from the high risk area of Guam who had moved to the United States as young men and women.[166] They found that even though these immigrants had been separated from the toxin for over thirty years, they still suffered from a high incidence of ALS. Somehow the toxin had a delayed effect. As the scientists and doctors continued to study the Indians living on these southern islands of Guam, they discovered that many also suffered from other neurological diseases that, strangely enough, had characteristics of two other degenerative neurological disorders occurring in the West, Parkinson's disease and Alzheimer's-like dementia. They named this new disease Parkinson's-dementia complex of Guam. Some patients had features of all three diseases combined—ALS, Parkinson's disease, and dementia.

Clinically, all of these diseases are exactly like those seen in the United States and Europe. But pathologically there were differences. Most important, all of the Guamian patients had extensive neuritic plaques and neurofibrillary tangles scattered throughout their brains and spinal cords. These are microscopic clumps of degenerating material, usually seen with Alzheimer's disease. In fact, they discovered that even the Indians that were free of symptoms had numerous plaques and tangles in their nervous systems.

Spencer, while searching the research literature on cycad, found a most interesting report that had apparently been overlooked, and since buried in the research literature. It was a report of a single monkey fed a concentrated solution of L-BMAA for several weeks.[167] The animal developed the same disease seen in the natives on Guam, as well as having the identical pathological changes in its spinal cord and brain. He repeated the experiment, this time using thirteen monkeys.[168] After two to twelve weeks of feeding the animals a concentrated solution of L-BMAA, they began to show signs of severe weakness in their limbs, and as with the human cases of ALS, it affected the hands first and then spread to involve all of the limbs. When he examined their spinal cords he found the characteristic degeneration of the anterior motor cells, which control motor movement in the extremities. This is the same microscopic picture observed in human cases of ALS throughout the world.

But then something strange happened which would forever change our thinking regarding toxins and neurological diseases. He found that if he continued feeding the animals the L-BMAA beyond thirteen weeks, they began to develop a shuffling gait, assumed a blank stare, and a mask-like expression on their face. It was the exact picture of Parkinson's disease as seen in humans cases. For the first time it was demonstrated that the final disease produced by exposure to a certain neurotoxin depended on the length of time an organism was exposed to that toxin. Spencer concluded that acute high dose exposure to L-BMAA resulted in ALS and that more chronic exposure produced Parkinson's disease and possibly dementia, at least in monkeys.

But why did the immigrants from Guam develop ALS after being away from the toxin for thirty years? (Actually the incidence, at ten to fifteen times the U.S. rate, was less than that seen in those who continued to eat cycad flour.) Did the toxin sit quietly in the neurons and then decades later suddenly become activated and kill these same neurons in the spinal cord?

Not necessarily. There is another possible explanation. Remember, I said that clinical symptoms of a degenerative neurological disease do not present until 80 to 90% of the specific cells involved are dead. It may be that the cycad exposure during their youth killed off, say 50% of the anterior horn cells, which would leave them clinically unaffected or minimally affected.

Once these immigrants moved to the United States, they were exposed to other food borne excitotoxins such as MSG, hydrolyzed vegetable protein, cysteine, and aspartate. These are less potent excitotoxins than L-BMAA, but chronic exposure of these already weakened neurons to excitotoxins could lead to a gradual lethal injury to the remaining cells. Once 80 to 90% of the motor neurons were killed, symptoms of ALS would appear. Then why wouldn't all of the Guamians develop ALS since they had all been exposed to the toxin in the flour? Because, as you will recall, everyone has a different sensitivity to these toxins. Some are extremely sensitive and others are quite resistant. There is a lot of individual variability in toxin sensitivity. Resistance can depend on the protective mechanisms within the brain: the blood-brain barrier, the ionic and gluta-mate pumps and the free radical scavengers. Those with strong protective mechanisms would be less likely to develop the disease.

Also, dietary exposure to excitotoxins varies considerably. Those people who eat many foods containing MSG and hydrolyzed vegetable protein would be at greatest risk. Another factor would be the efficiency of the energy metabolism in their neurons. Remember, essentially all of the pro-tective mechanisms depend heavily on energy availability in the brain and spinal cord. For example, those suffering from bouts of hypoglycemia or who frequently go on low calorie diets could possibly be at high risk for developing the disease. Excessive physical stress, such as hard physical labor or exercise, heat stroke, and illness, would also add to the pre-existing damage. There are a multitude of variables to explain why some develop the disease and others are spared.

MORE EVIDENCE

Actually, Guam is not the only place where high concentrations of these diseases have been found. In fact, there are three distinct geographical areas of unusually high incidence of these neurological disorders: the Chamorros of Guam, the Auyu and Jakai people of West New Guinea, and the Japa-nese of the Hobara and Kozagawa districts on the Kii Peninsula of the Honshu Island.[169]

The incidence of these diseases on the Kii peninsula is 25 to 100 times that of the rest of Japan. Both of these locations are in remote, moun-tainous regions essentially cut off from the rest of Japan. On the southern island of West Guinea we find a very high incidence of all three of these diseases among the Auyu and Jakai people. Interestingly, neither increased incidences of ALS nor Parkinsonism are found in the surrounding larger populations outside this region. Both high incidence groups live on diets consisting of large amounts of sago flour. The overall incidence of ALS among these people is 147 cases per 100,000 population. This is 150 times higher than that found in the United States or Europe. It is the highest incidence of these diseases in the entire world. In some villages the incidence is 1300 cases per 100,000 population.

Characteristic of all of these areas of high disease incidence is a diet consisting primarily of carbohydrates derived from cycad flour. The higher the intake, the higher the incidence and severity of the disease.

MAGNESIUM, CALCIUM, AND ALUMINUM

One of the prevailing theories of the cause of Alzheimer's disease is a chronic exposure to aluminum. This idea was given a boost when doctors observed a dementia-like illness in certain kidney dialysis patients. When these patients were studied, it was found that they had very high levels of aluminum in their tissues. Later, it was discovered that the water used to dialyze these patients also contained high concentrations of aluminum. The incidence of this disorder fell dramatically once the aluminum was removed from the dialysis medium.[170]

When the microscopic plaques taken from the brains of Alzheimer's patients are examined, they are found to contain rather high concentrations of aluminum. From this observation, it was hypothesized that aluminum directly damaged the neurons. Immediately, doctors began to examine foods for excess aluminum content. Many foods and condiments contain aluminum. Table salt contains aluminum, as do some flours. Usually these aluminum salts are more absorbable than metallic aluminum. Once this became general knowledge, a scare was launched among the public. Cooking ware, soda cans, and even roll-on deodorants became suspect. But there was a problem with this theory—aluminum does not selectively kill the same neurons destroyed in Alzheimer's disease.

When scientists studied the soil of the various regions with a high incidence of these neurological diseases, they found high levels of aluminum and low levels of magnesium and calcium.[171] Yet when the neurons from victims of the disease were also examined they found high levels of calcium and aluminum and low levels of magnesium.[172] The most consistent finding in all of these areas is a low magnesium level in the soil and water as well as in the neurons of victims of these diseases. On the island of Guam they found that areas with the lowest levels of calcium and magnesium were also the areas of highest incidence for all of the neurological diseases.

If we go back to what we learned about the glutamate receptor mechanism in chapter 3, we see that magnesium plays a vital role in protecting the neuron from the lethal effects of excitotoxins. Remember, the lethal mechanism with NMDA receptors involves the rapid influx of calcium into the cell—it is this rush of calcium into the cell that triggers the series of destructive reactions that cause the cell to be injured or killed. Experimentally, neurons are much more vulnerable to the effects of excitotoxins when magnesium is low.[173] This is because magnesium normally blocks the calcium channel.

In the cases of cycad toxicity, we see that the neuron contains low concentrations of magnesium and high concentrations of calcium within the cell.[174] Such a condition would leave the neuron maximally susceptible to the toxic effects of excitotoxins. When rats are placed on diets low in calcium and magnesium they develop swelling and calcium accumulation in the anterior motor neurons of the spinal cord, the same cells destroyed in cases of ALS.[175] But if dietary calcium is low, as was found in all of these areas, how can calcium accumulate inside the neuron? It is because the neuron always takes precedence over the body's use of calcium for other purposes. When the calcium channels are opened, calcium will pour in, no matter the blood's concentration of the element.

The other condition, causing extreme vulnerability to excitotoxins, met in each of these areas was a low availability of energy food stuffs; in this case caused by famine. Food was scarce during the war and this led to low energy (caloric) intake. We have seen that the mechanisms that protect the brain from excess excitotoxin accumulation are heavily dependent on cellular energy. Experimental studies have clearly shown that low energy levels greatly enhance the toxicity of all classes of excitotoxins.[176] When magnesium deficiency is combined with low energy levels, maximum vulnerability is seen.[177] Even small doses of excitotoxins can produce damage otherwise seen only with massive doses of the toxin.

It is known that low dietary calcium can cause the parathyroid glands to malfunction. These are small glands located in the neck, next to the thyroid gland, that control calcium metabolism in the body, including its absorption from the gut. When calcium levels are low, the parathyroid glands secrete more hormones, thereby increasing calcium absorption from the gut. But, unfortunately, it also increases the absorption of aluminum, which accumulates in certain regions of the brain.

It may be that aluminum acts as a co-toxin in these diseases, adding to the toxicity produced by excitotoxins. When monkeys are fed diets low in calcium and magnesium but high in aluminum lactate, they become very apathetic and begin to lose weight. When their spinal cords are examined under the microscope, they show swelling of the anterior motor cells, plus accumulation of calcium and aluminum in these cells.[178]

We can conclude from this that the two conditions which increase the sensitivity of the nervous system to food borne excitotoxins include low energy availability and low magnesium levels in the brain and spinal cord. Under such conditions maximum sensitivity and therefore vulnerability to excitotoxins exist.

DESIGNER DRUGS: THE BIG SURPRISE

In 1982 a bright young man, who we shall call Tom, with a taste for the bliss of heroin, decided that he could produce a similar drug in his own home laboratory for a lot less money than the cost of street drugs.[179] The drug he sought to make was a simple opiate-like compound called MPPP. After mixing a few basic chemicals in a beaker, he filled a syringe with his concoction and deftly slid the needle into a large vein in his forearm. The drug burned momentarily as it rushed into his blood stream.

As Tom sat on the side of the bed waiting for the drug to take effect, he noticed that his vision had begun to blur. He eased himself back down onto the bed. But nothing seemed to be happening. After another hour, he decided that somehow he had mixed the drug improperly. The next morning, Tom was awakened abruptly by an uncontrollable shaking of his body. A metallic taste stung his tongue. Then, without warning, his legs and arms began to jerk. He tried to raise up from the bed but his limbs felt as heavy as lead. Tom felt a rush of fear grip his heart. "Something is wrong," he told himself. He struggled out of the bed and made his way to the mirror. As he stared at his reflection, he tried to speak, but his lips moved in silence. He struggled harder. But he remained mute. Tom convinced himself that it would pass with time.

The next day he continued to feel the jerking and shaking of his limbs, and it was all he could do to speak. His mind raced with fear. "I just need more time," he reassured himself. "It will get better."

That afternoon a friend dropped by to see Tom. As he entered the darkened bedroom he found his friend lying in bed, staring straight at the ceiling. He shook his friend gently by the shoulder. "Tom", he called out. But Tom didn't move. His friend called an ambulance, which then rushed Tom to a local emergency room.

The doctors hovering around Tom were baffled. They had never seen anything like this. Nothing they knew of could leave a young man alert, yet unable to speak or move his limbs. His arms and legs were as stiff as boards. They called in a neurologist for help. The neurologist performed a thorough examination and then turned to his colleagues, and stated that Tom had all of the findings of a patient with advanced Parkinson's disease.

But no one had ever seen a case of "sudden" Parkinson's disease, especially in someone so young. Most such advanced cases occurred only after years or even decades of slow progression. But in Tom's case the disorder appeared suddenly and with a vengeance. For the next two weeks his condition continued to deteriorate. The only way he could communicate with his doctors was by blinking his eyes with a code for "yes" and "no". He drooled continuously. The neurologist, knowing that L-DOPA was the drug of choice for Parkinsonism, decided to try it on the unfortunate young man. After a week on the drug, there was a slight improvement. But soon Tom began to deteriorate again and remained severely crippled by his self-induced disease.

What is usually found at an autopsy in the typical Parkinson's patient is the destruction of a particular nucleus found in the brain stem called the substantia nigra. These darkly—stained nuclei contain high concentrations of a pigment known as melanin. In Parkinson's disease these cells die and release their pigment. But there is one critical difference between experimentally produced Parkinsonism produced by MPTP and that of the typical Parkinson's patient; there are no Lewy bodies. These are microscopic collections of debris seen in the dying neurons of the brain nucleus damaged in Parkinson's disease (the substantia nigra). But even without them, the clinical picture in Tom's case was typical of Parkinson's disease of the elderly. Apparently, Lewy bodies, like the tangles and plaques of Alzheimer's disease, do not cause the disease but merely reflect damage done by the disease.

When doctors analyzed the drug Tom had taken, they discovered that instead of the opiate-like drug he sought to create, he had inadvertently created another chemical called 1-methyl-4-phrenyl-1,2,3,6-tetrahydropyridine, or MPTP. When they injected this chemical into monkeys they found that it produced a sudden, profound onset of Parkinson's-like disease.[180] This was a first. Until then, no one had ever found a drug that would exactly reproduce Parkinson's disease in experimental animals.

These researchers knew that other conditions could produce clinical states similar to Parkinsonism, but they always had other clinical features that made them distinct. For example, manganese poisoning and certain forms of encephalitis can both produce a similar condition, but they have other psychiatric, motor and sensory findings not seen with pure Parkinson's disease.

Following this initial report, doctors in emergency rooms began to see more and more of these young drug-induced Parkinson's patients. The drug culture coined their own name for the condition—"the frozen addict".

Researchers, excited with their new discovery, began to extensively study this enigmatic compound.[181] They found that there was a wide variability in an animal's sensitivity to the toxic effects of the compound. Older monkeys appeared to be more sensitive to its toxic effects than were younger animals, and squirrel monkeys were more resistant than rhesus or marmoset monkeys. But in non-human primates, the delay in onset of the full blown syndrome was 8 to 12 weeks instead of the two to three days seen in man.

There is also some evidence that the Lewy bodies, seen in classic Parkinson's disease, are the result of normal aging of the brain. When MPTP is fed to elderly experimental animals, they also develop Lewy bodies, whereas younger animals do not. It may be that human cases of MPTP poisoning lack Lewy bodies because the majority of victims are so young.

Interestingly, when MPTP is given to rodents, very little happens. Most of the animals recover completely from the initial effects. This may be because their brains clear the substance very rapidly, whereas monkeys retain it for weeks. Beagle dogs and cats also recover after initial toxicity. There is considerable variability in the sensitivity of animals of the same species, age, and sex to the same dose of MPTP. Why, no one knows. In man exposure to MPTP produces advanced Parkinson's disease that is permanent.[182]

How MPTP Works

MPTP is a very fat soluble substance that passes through the blood-brain barrier easily and concentrates in the lipids of the brain. There is some evidence that MPTP itself does not directly kill the cells known to be damaged in Parkinson's disease.[183] Instead, MPTP is converted by an enzyme in the brain, called MAO-B, into another compound called MPP+.

There is some support for this theory based on the observation that drugs that inhibit the converting enzyme, MAO-B, can completely block the toxicity of MPTP in all animal species.[184] Recent studies have shown that the MAO-B enzyme is increased in patients with spontaneously occurring Parkinson's disease (Parkinsonism occurring without exposure to MPTP).[185] It may be that the MAO-B enzyme increases the neuron's vulnerability to a number of neurotoxins.

One of the most promising anti-Parkinson's drugs, Deprenyl, may act as a long lasting MAO-B inhibitor. It also acts as a free radical scavenger. In fact, this is the first drug that had been shown to actually slow down the progress of Parkinson's disease in humans.[186] The only other substance shown to slow the course of Parkinson's disease is vitamin E.[187] Remember, vitamin E is a very powerful anti-oxidant free radical scavenger. In experimental studies, vitamin E has been shown to completely block the effect of excitotoxins on neurons in tissue culture.[188] Unfortunately, it does not offer complete protection in the intact brain in living persons.

There is some evidence that MPP+ damages the neurons in the substantia nigra by generating free radicals.[189] It is also known that this toxin can interrupt complex I of the main energy-generating system in the neuron: the electron transport chain in the mitochondria. When it fails, the neurons become especially sensitive to excitotoxin damage. Blocking the complex I system can cause the cell to generate more free radicals and this can eventually kill the cell.

Others have found that MPP+ may act through the excitatory neural system itself.[190] Certain glutamate-blocking drugs (NMDA antagonists) can protect against this toxic effect if administered throughout the entire time MPP+ is within the brain.

A recent study done to determine the presence of free radical activation of antioxidant enzymes (enzymes that neutralize these harmful free radicals) was completed using a series of autopsied Parkinson's patients. They found that there was a pronounced increase in the superoxide dismutase-like enzyme activity (one of the main antioxidant enzymes in the brain) in the nucleus substantia nigra of Parkinson's patients.[191]

The MPTP is actually the active component of a herbicide known as Cyperquat, which is used to kill nutsedge. Fortunately, the manufacturing division that was to make this herbicide closed down before it went to market. Chemically it is related to the dangerous herbicide Paraquat, which has been shown to kill cells by producing enormous amounts of free radicals, which consume all of the cell's antioxidants. MPP+ forms far fewer free radicals.

What makes the MPTP story interesting is that there are many compounds found in nature that have a similar chemical structure. The part of the MPTP molecule that appears to be necessary for producing Parkinson's disease is also found in many plants. In fact, ordinary tea contains two such compounds. Thus far, tests have not implicated tea in Parkinson's disease, but the testing period may have been too short. However, there is no difference in the incidence of Parkinson's disease among the English, who regularly drink strong tea, and Americans. Scientists are now busy examining foods and plant derivatives for the presence of this compound or its relatives.

PARALYSIS AGITANS: PARKINSON'S DISEASE

In 1817 Dr. James Parkinson described a disease of the elderly in which there was a characteristic tremor during rest, stooped posture, and other neurological signs. Further experience disclosed other findings that were peculiar to the Parkinson's patient. For example, Parkinson's patients blink their eyes infrequently, have a mask-like expression, and develop movements that are rigid. It is as if they are struggling against their own muscles.

Another frequent finding is a loss of balance. Actually, this is an inability to stop a forward motion once it has begun. It is as if they are always trying to catch up with their center of gravity. A tremor of their fingers while at rest is characteristic. When you see an elderly person sitting on a park bench with their hands resting on their knees involuntarily rolling their fingers in an imaginary circle they may be victims of this disease. This is referred to as the "pill rolling tremor", because it looks like they are rolling an invisible pill between their thumb and first finger.

As the disease progresses, the person becomes more rigid and develops a stooped posture. Their walk is shuffling and unsteady. The disease also affects their handwriting and even their speech, causing their voice to lose much of its volume so that it sounds like they are always whispering. This was one of the saddest things about my father's illness. Because I lived so far away from my parents, one of my greatest pleasures was talking to my father on the phone. But as his condition worsened, I could barely understand him, so I had to relay messages through my mother or via letters.

Handwriting changes usually appear late in the disease, with the writing becoming small and almost illegible. This is called micrographia. I struggled through many of my father's letters trying to make out the tiny scrawled letters. Gradually the disease robs the victim of most of life's pleasures. Toward the end, my father could barely get from the bed to his favorite chair, where he would sit, almost immobile, for hours.

It wasn't until recently that doctors began to recognize that a significant number of Parkinson's patients become demented toward the end of their disease. Fortunately, my father was spared this indignity. In some series it has been found that as many as 32% of Parkinson's patients develop dementia as part of their illness.[192] The dementia is exactly like that seen with Alzheimer's disease. Some patients will also develop features of ALS as well. My father did, however, develop ALS symptoms. His hands became so weak that he could barely pick up even small objects. When you recall that all three diseases, Parkinson's disease, Alzheimer's dementia, and ALS, can be produced by the plant toxin in Guam, one cannot be but surprised that doctors did not recognize this association before. But for years, medical textbooks treated these as three entirely separate diseases. Now let us look at the role of excitotoxins in the causation of Parkinson's disease.

EXCITOTOXINS AND PARKINSON'S DISEASE

Interestingly, MPTP is not an excitotoxin. But there is another drug that is an excitotoxin that can result in premature Parkinson's disease. This drug, amphetamine (and its analogs), is known by the drug faithful as "uppers". It has been known for some time that amphetamines stimulate the nervous system, and that not infrequently, they can precipitate a seizure.

It is suspected that amphetamines produce brain damage by way of glutamate—type neural pathways. They not only excite certain brain cells, but also initiate calcium triggered destructive reactions within specific neurons by way of NMDA—type receptors.[193] By exciting the neurons, they speed up depletion of cellular energy molecules such as ATP and phosphocreatinine, thereby making the neurons even more vulnerable to all types of excitotoxins including MSG.

Amphetamines are known to cause specific destruction of a group of neurons that are concerned with controlling fine and coordinated movements of the arms and legs.[194] This collection of neurons and their connecting fibers are referred to as the nigrostriatal system, which is the same nerve system destroyed in Parkinson's disease.(FIG 5-1)

Exactly how amphetamines destroy these neurons is not completely understood. There is some evidence that they stimulate the production of free radicals in these neurons.[195] The nigrostriatal system also receives a large fiber input from the outer layer of cells of the brain called the cortex. These fibers arise primarily from glutamate—type neurons, and it is through this cortical system that glutamate and amphetamines act to destroy the nigrostriatal system.[196] Further proof comes from the observation that a powerful blocker of NMDA types of glutamate receptors can completely block amphetamine toxicity.[197] Therefore glutamate, amphetamines and other excitotoxins may produce Parkinsonism by overexciting the cortical glutamate cells that connect to the nigrostriatal neurons lying deep in the brain. It is sort of like lightning hitting the power line outside your house and burning up all of the appliances connected to that line. The powerline represents the cortical glutamate neurons and the appliances, the nigrostriatal system.

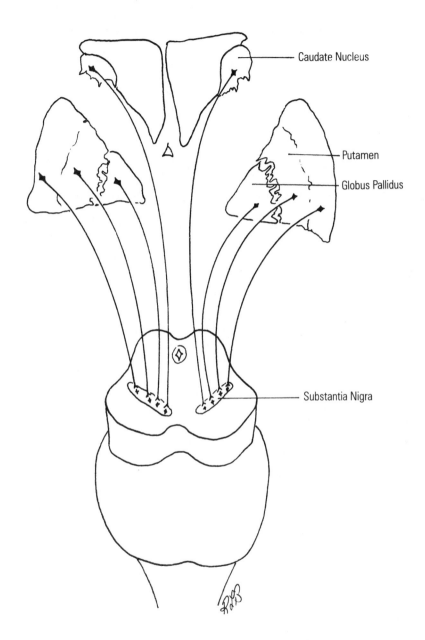

Caudate Nucleus

Putamen

Globus Pallidus

Substantia Nigra

5-1 *Nigrostriatal System: Some of the connections between the substantia nigra and the basal ganglion (corpus striatum).*

Further evidence comes from a recent observation involving one of the primary drugs used to treat Parkinson's disease L-DOPA. While this drug has done much to relieve the crippling symptoms of this terrible disease, and even to extend the lifespan of younger patients, there is some evidence that it may speed up the progress of the disease. Several studies have indicated that patients started early on L-DOPA therapy tend to deteriorate faster than those in which other drugs were used initially.

Part of the explanation of this phenomenon may lie in the findings of Dr. John Olney who demonstrated that L-DOPA is a mild excitotoxin.[198] It was found to be approximately half as potent as MSG. A metabolite of L-DOPA, called 6-hydroxy-DOPA is about six times more powerful than MSG. From this observation it would be reasonable to assume that high doses of the Parkinson drug L-DOPA could kill off already weakened neurons in the nigrostriatal system, thereby speeding up the progress of the disease. Dr. Olney suggests that L-DOPA does not act alone but rather acts with glutamate to produce the damage. This is one reason why persons with Parkinson's disease should avoid all foods and drinks containing excitotoxin additives such as MSG, hydrolyzed vegetable protein, cysteine, and aspartate (NutraSweet®). While there is no proof that these toxins penetrate these sensitive areas there is no proof that they do not. As we shall see, there is evidence that as we age our blood-brain barrier system tends to weaken, allowing previously excluded molecules to enter the brain. Throughout life, especially as we age, we are exposed to conditions and diseases that can disrupt the barrier. This would allow glutamate and aspartate in the diet to reach these already weakened neurons and speed up their destruction. It should also be recalled that cysteine can easily penetrate the intact blood-brain barrier and that hydrolyzed vegetable protein contains cysteine.

Ganging Up on Neurons

Critics of this hypothesis state that if food toxins and additives were the cause of Parkinson's disease why wouldn't all of us eventually develop the disease? That's a good question. (Of course I am not proposing that excitotoxin food additives are the primary cause of Parkinson's disease or any other neurodegenerative disease.) A closer examination will give us several explanations. It is a well recognized fact that there can be a considerable variation in sensitivity to a particular toxin even within the same species of the same size and sex. This may be because of differences in the concentration and competency of protective enzymes, the efficiency of cellular energy production, and differences in absorption from the digestive system. Some humans can take enormous amounts of arsenic without becoming sick, while others will die at a fraction of the dose.

There are also species differences in sensitivity to excitotoxins. For example, in the case of amphetamines, we know that the rat, which has been used as the model for amphetamine toxicity, is much more resistant to the effects of the drug than are humans. The lethal dose of amphetamines in humans is much lower than in the rat. (The lethal dose of amphetamine in humans is 7.5 mg/kg while in rats even a dose of 40mg/kg is not lethal.[199]) Also, you may recall that humans accumulate higher blood levels of glutamate after a similar dose of MSG than does any other animal species. And human neurons are just as sensitive at the same doses of MSG as are animals. In fact, humans are much more sensitive to the toxic effects of MSG than are monkeys.[200] There is a lot of individual variation in the vulnerability to these toxins between species of animals and even within the same species.

Part of the explanation as to why everyone does not develop these diseases after chronic exposure to excitotoxins lies in the competence of the various protective mechanisms used to prevent glutamate accumulation around the neuron. Remember, there is a pumping system that shunts excess glutamate into the surrounding astrocytes (see chapter 4). If this system is very efficient, it will take enormous amounts of glutamate to produce brain lesions.[201] But, also remember, this system is extremely energy dependent. If, for some reason, the energy supply is reduced, the protective pump will fail and toxic amounts of glutamate will accumulate around the neurons.

There is evidence that if we live long enough, a much larger percentage of us will indeed develop neurodegenerative diseases. In a recent survey of the incidence of Alzheimer's disease among the elderly, it was found that between the ages of 65 to 74 the incidence of the disease was 3%; between the ages of 75 to 84 the incidence rose to 18.7%; and after age 85 it soared to 47.2%.[202] The same may be true of ALS and Parkinson's disease.[203] This steep rise in the incidence of these diseases could represent a combination of factors: an increased vulnerability of aged neurons to a multitude of environmental hazards, the natural attrition of aged neurons, a gradual failure of the protective mechanism with aging, and the accumulated action of years of excitotoxin exposure on weakened neurons.

Other critics charge that even if large amounts of glutamate are consumed, the blood-brain barrier will keep the glutamate from entering the brain. Normally this is true. But there are several conditions under which the blood-brain barrier system will fail, such as head injuries, viral and bacterial infections of the brain and spinal cord, hypertension, exposure to some metals such as lead and tin, and an elevated core body temperature.[204]

One of the most common reasons for a breakdown in this barrier is stroke.

While major strokes (those that leave a person paralyzed on one side or with impaired speech) do occur frequently, much more often we see minor strokes. These may be so small that the person is not even aware that they have occurred. Usually they develop deep in the white matter of the brain and involve tiny blood vessels rather than major feeding arteries to the brain. We call these silent strokes. What makes them important is that they produce "holes" in the blood-brain barrier.[205] (FIG 5-2) These holes can act as leaks in the blood-brain barrier that allow normally excluded proteins and other potentially toxic substances to enter the brain.[206] Experimentally, we know that such leaks can allow normally excluded molecules, like glutamate, to seep in and eventually reach the entire brain.[207] The older you get, the more likely these silent strokes are to develop.

There is some evidence that as we age the blood-brain barrier begins to break down, at least for the passage of some molecules.[208] While it may still exclude the larger molecules, the smaller molecules, like the amino

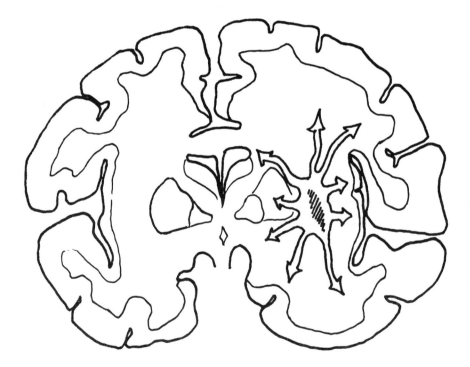

5-2 *This cross section of the brain demonstrates how a small silent stroke can act as a point of seepage for glutamate and other excitotoxins to by-pass the blood-brain barrier. In this way normally excluded excitotoxins from food can endanger the brain.*

acids aspartate and glutamate, may get through. There is also evidence that as we age the neurons within the nigrostriatal system slowly begin to die. In humans, by age sixty-five, 60% of the cells are dead. But is this a natural attrition of these cells? There is some evidence that it may not be. For instance, we know that rats lose only 20% of their neurons during a comparable period of time. As humans we eat a diet containing enormous amounts of excitotoxin food additives, and do so for decades, even a lifetime. Whereas, rats rarely have added excitotoxins, except in an experimental situation. It may be that this loss of neurons is the result of years of excitotoxin food additive exposure in humans, combined with other neurotoxic insults.

Yet we would also expect aged neurons to be more vulnerable to toxins.[209] There is evidence that aged monkeys are more susceptible to MPTP than younger animals.[210] The drug kainate (a powerful glutamate receptor excitotoxin) will not damage neurons in immature animals but will readily kill them in older animals. By the time we reach age sixty our neurons have undergone decades of trauma from a multitude of abuses, such as injuries, infections, stress, chemical toxins, drugs, heat, and of course, food borne excitotoxins.

But there is a logical connection. Low blood sugar precipitates cerebral symptoms of anxiety, confusion, and even anger because the brain is denied its supply of energy-giving glucose. Remember, the brain consumes 25% of the total body glucose. Its needs are great. When this need is not met, various systems begin to malfunction. And one of these systems is the protective pumps used to maintain a stable, low concentration of glutamate and aspartate around the neurons. As doctors have found in experiments, low energy levels greatly enhance the toxicity of glutamate and the other excitotoxins, so that even normally low doses of excitotoxins can become toxic. This toxicity can manifest itself as anxiety or confusion, and as episodes of anger.

RUNNING OUT OF FUEL

As I have pointed out throughout this discussion of glutamate toxicity, the brain is most sensitive when its energy supply is low. It does not seem to matter what causes the low energy supply—hypoglycemia, poor blood supply to portions of the brain, or a failure of energy production by the cells themselves.

There is some recent evidence that Parkinson's patients have a defect in their metabolism that leads to increased metabolism.[211] Such a defect would make them more vulnerable to the harmful effects of excitotoxins. In one study resting energy expenditure (the amount of energy being burned at rest) was measured in fourteen elderly patients with Parkinson's disease and compared to sixteen healthy control patients of similar ages. As a group, Parkinson's patients had metabolic rates significantly higher than the controls. This substantially increased energy requirement might explain the extreme weight loss frequently seen in Parkinson's patients.[212]

It is also common for the elderly to lose their appetite, especially with chronic debilitating diseases. As we age our taste buds lose some of their function, making food often seem tasteless. Since many elderly live alone and have difficulty preparing their meals, it may become difficult for them to eat enough calories.

With excitotoxin food additives being in virtually every manufactured food product, our brain is constantly being assaulted by excitotoxins. During a lifetime, many of us also experience many periods of hypoglycemia. Children frequently develop hypoglycemia during illness, because they usually lose their appetite. Some of the medications they take also can lower blood sugar. Adults, especially in today's fat conscious society, are constantly going on low calorie diets, and even "starvation" diets. Many of these diets call for foods low in carbohydrates, which may result in prolonged states of relative hypoglycemia.

There is another condition which may produce rather profound states of hypoglycemia—exercise. Intense, prolonged exercise, especially in the untrained person, has been shown to cause severe drops in blood glucose.[213] I remember when I first started going to the gym to exercise that after a hard workout I would have difficulty thinking clearly. I asked others and found out that they too suffered from this annoying problem. After research, I came upon several medical studies done on athletes which confirmed this post-exercise fall in blood sugar which explains the severe muscle weakness and trembling most of us experience following strenous exercise.

Later I came across an article in the newspaper on a marathon runner who was forced to quit the sport because of severe Parkinson's disease. He was totally incapacitated by his disease, and he admitted in the article that on several occasions he had suffered from heat exhaustion during marathon races. Under such conditions two events can occur that can enhance excitotoxic damage to neurons: elevated body core temperature and hypoglycemia. During prolonged running, such as occurs during marathons and triathalons, the body core temperature can rise sufficiently to cause (at least based on experimental studies) a temporary breakdown of the blood-brain barrier, which can result in leakage of glutamate and aspartate into the brain itself. Also, such physical stress can cause a prolonged fall in the blood glucose and hence in brain glucose, which results in greater vulnerability of the brain to excitotoxins both occuring naturally within the brain and those supplied by the diet. In addition, during extreme exercise a tremendous number of free radicals are formed within the tissues as a result of increased metabolism. This too will add to the damage.

In 1968 Dr. Kwock described a clinical condition caused by exposure to the MSG in Chinese food in which the victim developed headaches, sweating, nausea, weakness, thirst, burning and tightness of the face, neck and chest, abdominal pains, and sometimes diarrhea.[214] This reaction to MSG was given the name "the Chinese restaurant syndrome". But as Dr. Schwartz and others have shown, the syndrome is not limited to Chinese food—it is caused by exposure to high doses of MSG in *any food*.

The defenders of the MSG industry claimed that this reaction was rare and could be prevented by eating a diet containing carbohydrates. And, indeed, it was shown that people's response to MSG was highly variable. Some reacted to doses as low as 1 to 2 grams, while others required doses as high as 12 grams to produce the same reaction. Overall, about 10 to 25% of people eating a meal containing MSG developed these adverse physical reactions first described by Dr. Kwock.[215] Yet when human volunteers fasted overnight and then were fed MSG alone, virtually all developed full blown symptoms of the "Chinese restaurant syndrome".[216] So even moderate hypoglycemia plays a major role in magnifying the toxicity of these excitotoxins.[217]

One article defending MSG, written by the Glutamate Association in a popular magazine, claimed that MSG was not toxic, and then proceeded to state that toxicity was blocked by merely including the MSG in food.[218] Yet their statement that food "blocks MSG toxicity" must mean that MSG is toxic. As for the "blocking effect" of mixed diets, McLaughlan and coworkers demonstrated that tube-fed rats developed equally high levels whether MSG was given in a water solution or mixed with a meat suspension.[219] Another study found that MSG mixed with tomato juice produced a 20-fold rise in plasma glutamate in humans.[220] And Olney and coworkers were able to produce typical hypothalamic injuries using a mixture of MSG with cow's milk.[221]

Stegink and his coworkers later disclosed that very high concentrations of sugar could block glutamate aborption sufficiently to prevent brain injury.[222] In this study they used six average human volunteers who ate beef consumme containing 50 milligrams per kilogram body weight of MSG either with or without sucrose. They found that sucrose significantly reduced the amount of glutamate absorbed into the plasma. What I find interesting is that they used a dose that would be equal to ten of the packets of sugar that you use at your local diner. Is he suggesting that we eat ten packets of sugar each time we are exposed to foods containing MSG or aspartame? If we did, our problem wouldn't be brain damage, it would be diabetes.

In an earlier article Stegink suggested that you could dramatically reduce glutamate absorption simply by eating starches. In this experiment he found that you would have to eat an equivalent of 17 to 18 crackers to prevent significant plasma elevations of glutamate following a meal with 0.5 grams of MSG per kilogram of body weight. Who eats 18 crackers with every meal, snack, or before drinking a diet cola sweetened with aspartame? They found that when smaller amounts of starches were used **five out of eight subjects had no protective effect afforded by the carbohydrates**. It is obvious that sucrose or starches added to our diets do not afford adequate protection against excitotoxin food additives. **The only protection is to avoid them altogether.**

Parkinsonism: A Metabolic Error in Cellular Energy Production

One of the most exciting findings concerning this terrible disease is that patients with Parkinsonism seem to have an enzyme defect affecting only certain brain cells that prevents these neurons from producing adequate amounts of energy.[223] Within all cells, including neurons, energy is supplied by the mitochondria, which occurs via a series of reactions involving various enzymes and chemicals called the electron transport system. The first and most critical step in this energy producing process is called complex I.

TABLE 5-1
ELECTRON TRANSPORT CHAIN

Complex I-NADH	=	ubiquinone oxidoreductase
Complex II	=	succinate: ubiquinone oxidoreductase
Complex III	=	ubiquinonl: ferricytochrome c oxidoreductase
Complex IV	=	ferrocytochrome c: oxygen oxidoreductase
Complex V	=	ATP synthease

Should this step be defective, which is thought to occur in Parkinsonism, the neurons become severely depleted of energy and as a result become extremely sensitive to excitotoxins such as glutamate and aspartate.(FIG 5-3)

Dr. Schapira and his coworkers examined the brains of nine patients who died while suffering from Parkinson's disease and found that all demonstrated a marked reduction in the complex I enzymes. But interest-

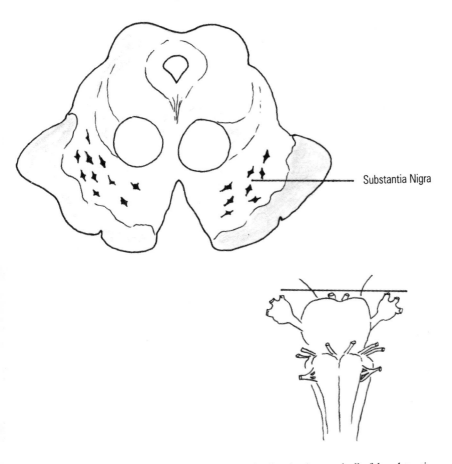

5-3 *A cross section of the midbrain of the brain stem showing the pigmented cells of the substantia nigra, one of the principle sites of injury seen in Parkinson's disease.*

ingly, these critical energy—supplying enzymes were deficient only in the neurons thought to be responsible for Parkinson's disease. Samples of neurons from other parts of the brain were normal. This indicated that for some unknown reason the cells in the substantia nigra have defective complex I enzymes. (In this study they compared similar neurons from normal controls matched for age and sex.)

A follow-up study of the brains of seven additional Parkinson patients demonstrated similar findings with a 42% reduction in complex I enzyme activity.[224]

This finding is important because it confirms earlier observations that glutamate toxicity is greatly magnified when cellular energy supplies are deficient.[225] In essence, persons destined to develop Parkinson's disease appear to have an inherited weakness in the energy-producing enzymes in the mitochondria of the neurons in their substantia nigra. This makes these neurons highly susceptable to the effects of excitotoxins such as glutamate and aspartate (both found normally within the brain and that supplied in the diet as taste enhancers). Yet other neurons in the brain, having normal energy-producing enzymes, are not affected. This makes the destruction very specific.

In the past, based on studies of identical twins, most authorities assumed that Parkinson's disease was not inherited. (Since identical twins share the same chromosome structure they should carry the same gene for Parkinson's disease.) It is now known that there is another kind of inheritance, one determined by genetic material within the mitochondria. We know that when glutamate overstimulates a neuron it can damage the mitochondrial genetic material, which would then pass on this altered gene to other cells. Such damaged mitochondrial genes could explain the unusual inheritance pattern of Parkinson's disease. Today we are finding more and more diseases having a mitochondrial inheritance rather than the usual chromosomal inheritance.[226]

If Parkinson's disease is caused by excitotoxin damage to specific cells in the brain, then blocking excitotoxins should help protect Parkinson's patients from progression of the disease. There is some experimental evidence that this occurs.[227] Doctors Thomas Klockgether and Lechoslaw Turski tested this hypothesis using a rat model of Parkinsonism and found that MK-801, a powerful drug that blocks the toxic effect of glutamate, did indeed offer significant improvement in symptoms as well as protection against the disease.[228] (They used low doses of the compound so as to prevent behavioral side effects such as learning difficulties and drowsiness.)

Some of the drugs used to treat Parkinson's disease may be beneficial because they act by blocking glutamate toxicity.[229] For example, the drug Memantine has been shown to be a rather powerful glutamate receptor blocking agent much like MK-801.[230] It may be that one of these excitotoxin-blocking drugs will hold great promise in combating this terrible disease.

As you have seen in the previous discussion, part of the damage caused by excitotoxins is secondary to the generation of free radicals within the neurons being stimulated. These free radicals are extremely reactive chemicals that injure many components within the cells, and if left unchecked can result in cell death. Dr. D.T. Dexter and his coworkers studied the brains of several patients dying with Parkinson's disease and found that all demonstrated significant degrees of free radical damage within the substantia nigra.[231] (All other brain areas were normal.) In fact, the level of MDA (a measure of free radical damage) was elevated 35% higher in Parkinsonism patients than normal controls matched for age.

There is also evidence that free radicals can stimulate further release of excitotoxic amino acids in the injured areas of the brain.[232] This produces a vicious cycle whereby excitotoxins stimulate free radical formation and the free radicals in turn stimulate further excitotoxin accumulation. Under such conditions it is the brain's natural antioxidant free radical scavengers that prevent the process from eventually killing the neurons. And there is some evidence that vitamins E and C (powerful free radical scavengers) can slow the progress of Parkinson's disease.[233] Some neurologists have even suggested the use of vitamin E for all Parkinsonism patients.[234]

Dexter and coworkers have demonstrated that patients dying with Parkinson's disease also have very high levels of iron within the neurons of the substantia nigra.[235] It has been shown that iron within tissues acts as a powerful stimulus for the production of free radicals. It appears that there is a direct connection between excitotoxin excess in the brain, low energy levels in the involved neurons, and a massive production of destructive free radicals. If left unchecked, the neurons within the substantia nigra nucleus will eventually die, causing all of the symptoms of Parkinson's disease to appear.

How Does Parkinson's Disease Develop?

As yet we do not know exactly how Parkinson's disease develops, but we are finding some important answers. We know that certain events occur in the Parkinson's patient. For example, we know that in Parkinson's patients the substantia nigra nucleus (a small black-pigmented clump of neurons located at the junction of the brain stem) contains more zinc, has higher levels of iron, impaired complex I function, evidence of severe free radical damage, and significantly lower levels of glutathione than in healthy brains.[236]

When we examine the brains of people dying of Parkinson's disease we cannot tell which of these events occured first. But a recent study has shed some light on this problem.[237] It was found that 8 to 10% of the average population at postmortem, despite having been entirely free of Parkinson's symptoms during life, will have changes suggesting the earliest stages of the disease. The amount of dopamine in these individuals is entirely normal, as are the zinc and iron levels. The complex I activity in this nucleus was found to be only slightly reduced. The surprising finding was that the level of reduced glutathione was drastically low. Normal levels were found in aged matched controls and in people dying from other neurodegenerative diseases.

So what is glutathione? It is a very important antioxidant enzyme that occurs in two forms: reduced and oxidized. It is by switching from the reduced form to the oxidized that this enzyme neutralizes free radicals. The level of reduced glutathione in this early, pre-clinical stage of Parkinson's was as severely depleted as the levels seen in the most advanced stages of the disease. Obviously this represents one of the earliest stages of the disorder. What makes this important is that neurons with low levels of glutathione are highly succeptable to free radical injury, which can be initiated by excitotoxin attack. As the free radicals begin to accumulate within the neurons they can further damage the complex I system, thereby severely impairing its energy generating capacity. This would create a situation of even higher vulnerability to excitotoxin injury.

PARKINSONISM AND THE DIETARY MSG CONNECTION

So, you may ask, what does all this have to do with MSG and other excito-toxins in my food? It appears that certain people are destined to develop Parkinsonism because of an inherited (via mitochondrial DNA) defect in critical energy producing enzymes within the mitochondria. As a result of this energy failure, the neurons become highly and selectively vulnerable to damage by excitotoxins occuring both naturally within the brain itself and from the diet.

But, you say, the brain should be protected from excitotoxins in the food by the blood-brain barrier. Normally this would be true. But, as I have pointed out, it appears that there are many conditions during which the blood-brain barrier can be temporarily broken down, such as with heat stroke, brain trauma, encephalitis, strokes, hypertension, and even severe hypoglycemia. Experimentally, it has been shown that special radioactively labeled MSG not only passes through the blood-brain barrier in neonatal animals but it also accumulates in high concentrations in areas known to be damaged by MSG and other excitotoxins, such as the hippocampus (which is vital to recent memory function.)[238] This study demonstrated that the MSG entered the brain slowly, bypassing the blood-brain barrier, and reached peak concentrations in the brain three hours after the MSG was given. Even more important was the finding that the high levels of MSG in the brain remained for twenty-four hours after the dose was given.

Disruptions of the blood-brain barrier could explain why most cases of Parkinson's disease occur in older age groups; that is, because they will have suffered a lifetime of insults to their blood-brain barrier. If these individuals are born with an energy deficit in the neurons of the substantia nigra the excess excitotoxin load from their diet could speed up their rate of clinical deterioration. It could also explain one other phenomenon seen with Parkinson's disease, which has only recently been recognized. That is the finding of cases of Parkinson's disease in combination with clinical features of ALS and dementia. It is now recognized that about one-third of cases of Parkinsonism will eventually develop dementia of some degree.

It may be that as these Parkinson's patients age and develop small strokes, hypertension, or other diseases of the brain, their blood-brain barrier becomes more porous, allowing excitotoxins in the blood to enter. By ingesting diets high in MSG, hydrolyzed vegetable protein, aspartame and other excitotoxins, these people would be exposing their brains to damaging levels of of this class of toxin. Eventually other neurons would be damaged, possibly leading to symptoms of Alzheimer's type dementia and ALS.

It is also possible that glutamate and aspartate can enter the brain without a breakdown in the blood-brain barrier. We know that certain areas of the adult brain have no, or incompetent, barriers. These areas are near the ventricular system (circumventricular organs) and can potentially act as points through which glutamate and aspartate in the plasma could slowly seep into the surrounding brain, thereby bypassing the blood-brain barrier. This would explain the delay in brain accumulation of radioactively labeled MSG following its injection in animals.

Many meals served in restaurants contain very high doses of MSG and other excitotoxic amino acids.[239] In fact, they equal or even exceed experimental doses that regularly produce brain lesions in animals. (Remember, humans concentrate glutamate in their blood following a meal containing MSG higher than any other known species of animal.) Even a single bowl of soup may contain several grams of MSG. Most salad dressings are loaded with MSG and hydrolyzed vegetable protein (also labeled as vegetable protein), as are croutons. If you use steak sauce, it frequently contains both, disguised as "natural flavoring" or "spices". Chips, creamy sauces, some gravies, rice dishes, and other gourmet foods can all be loaded with excitotoxic "taste enhancers".

I believe that there is enough research evidence demonstrating the harmful effects of excitotoxins in food additives that all persons having a history of sensitivity to MSG or a strong family history of one of the neurodegenerative diseases should avoid all foods and beverages containing these excitotoxin "taste" additives. Doing so could mean the difference between a normal life and one spent suffering from a crippling disease. I will repeat these warnings throughout the book because they are so important. We must reprogram our eating habits to include fresh foods and excitotoxin-free beverages, at least until the food industry takes a responsible position on this most important issue.

The role played by selective energy defects in nigrostriatal neurons is further emphasized by another observation seen in patients treated with certain tranquilizers (neuroleptics).[240] It has been known for many years that 20 to 40% of patients treated chronically with these tranquilizers will develop Parkinsonism. One of the worst offenders is a drug known as haloperidol. Chemically haloperidol closely resembles the neurotoxin MPTP, which can induce Parkinsonism in experimental animals and humans. MPTP is a powerful inhibitor of the complex I enzyme system in the mitochondria, which leads to severe energy deficits in these cells and the subsequent build-up of free radicals. Haloperidol has the same effect. It can inhibit the complex I system selectively.

The magnitude of reduction of complex I activity in the platelets was found to be 42% of normal in persons taking neuroleptic medications and 46% in patients with Parkinson's disease, indicating that they inhibit this energy system to a similar degree. The concentrations of the neuroleptics medications necessary to depress complex I activity correlated directly with the dose needed to produce Parkinson's-like side-effects in patients. It is also known that the melanin in the neurons of the substantia nigra tends to concentrate these drugs, thereby exposing them to selective complex I inhibition, and sparing other areas of the brain. This would also make these energy-deprived neurons selectively hypersensitive to excitotoxin damage.

There is another bit of evidence that points to excitotoxins as a major contributor in the causation of Parkinsonism. A recent analysis of Parkinson's patients disclosed that the loss of neurons is a linerly progressive pathologic process.[241] This means that the number of neurons lost is the same every year. Such evidence is not compatable with a disease that suddenly accelerates or decelerates from year to year. Of all environmental exposures the one that would most exactly meet such criteria would be a food-borne toxin eaten every day. The excitotoxin food additives would certainly fulfill such a requirement. One would expect neuron loss under such exposure to be rather uniform.

AMYOTROPHIC LATERAL SCLEROSIS: LOU GEHRIG'S DISEASE

Amyotrophic lateral sclerosis, also known as Lou Gehrig's disease, is a neurodegenerative disease that primarily affects the anterior horn cells of

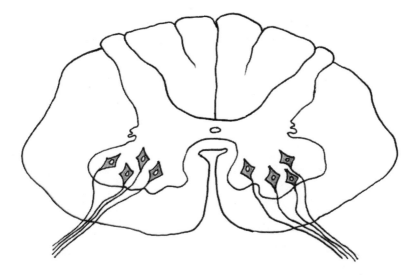

5-4 *Cross section of spinal cord demonstrating the anterior horn cell. These are the neurons destroyed in amyotrophic lateral sclerosis (ALS). These neurons are of the glutamate type.*

the spinal cord. (FIG 5-4) These are the primary neurons in the spinal cord that control muscle movements of the body. But these neurons do not operate by themselves, rather they are controlled from higher up in the brain by other neurons in the motor cortex which send fibers down the spinal cord, that in turn connect (synapse) with the anterior horn cells. This bundle of fibers from the cortex is called the corticospinal tract. In most cases of ALS these neurons are also affected.

Some have proposed that ALS is really many diseases.[242] This is because it can be present in many different forms. While most cases first appear after age forty, sometimes it strikes in the twenties or even teens. Most cases progress relentlessly for three to five years until the victim dies of respiratory failure or a related complication. But other cases seem to stabilize for decades. Dr. Stephen Hawkins, the astrophysicist, apparently has this form of the disease. Rarely, we see cases that progress very rapidly to death within a year.

The clinical presentation also varies. Some develop weakness first in the muscles of the face, while most begin with weakness in the muscles of the hands. This weakness slowly progresses up the arms. Still other cases affect primarily the legs and instead of the usual flaccid weakness, they experience spasticity and rigidity of the legs. Almost all cases spare sensation in the arms and legs and do not involve the mind. That the mind remains clear until the very end is one of the features that makes the disease particularly horrible.

Another unusual characteristic is that while most cases of ALS occur sporadically, some are definitely inherited. In one study of a Dutch family, researchers found the appearance of ALS in six generations.[243] In these cases the onset of the disease was earlier and the progression was more rapid than normal. Similar cases have been reported throughout the medical literature.

The excitotoxin hypothesis is able to explain many of these variables. As we have seen with Parkinson's disease, there are many factors at play in determining sensitivity to excitotoxins. For example, heredity plays a role in controlling enzymes that either generate energy for the neuron or protect it from dangerous accumulations of free radicals or excitotoxins. Other factors would include the integrity of the blood-spinal cord barrier (similar to the blood-brain barrier), the effects of aging on the neurons, and exposure to other toxins such as aluminum. All of these variables could account for differences in not only clinical patterns, but incidences of the disease.

As we have seen at the beginning of this chapter, a known plant toxin can produce a disease that is clinically indistinguishable from spontaneously occurring amyotrophic lateral sclerosis (ALS). The only pathological difference is the presence of numerous neurofibrillary tangles (microscopic fibrous bodies arranged as paired helical filaments seen in degenerating neurons) throughout the nervous system in the case of the Guam disease.[244] Spencer has pointed out that this may be the result of the type of toxin and not as a specific consequence of the disease itself.[245] This is further supported by the observation that even those who do not develop the clinical disease also have numerous neurofibrillary tangles throughout their nervous system.

In 1987 Dr. Andreas Plaitakis and James T. Caroscio reported that twenty-two patients they selected as having early signs of ALS responded differently to dietary glutamate than did normal controls and patients with other neurological diseases.[246] When they fed these patients MSG in a dose of 60 miligram per kilogram (after the patients had fasted overnight) they found that the ALS patients' blood glutamate levels were twice as high as compared to the control normal patients and persons having other neurological diseases. Not only were their blood glutamate levels grossly elevated, but so were their aspartate levels, while the blood levels of other amino acids were all normal.

But then they found something even more astounding. Even during the early stages of their disease, when fasting, these ALS patients have serum glutamate levels that are 100% higher than normal persons under the same conditions.[247] When these patients ate normal mixed meals containing protein, their glutamate levels also rose significantly higher than normal persons. It was obvious that these patients had a defect in their ability to metabolize glutamate. A related disorder, called atypical ALS, is known to have a defect in the enzyme glutamate dehydrogenase,[248] which causes glutamate from even a normal meal to accumulate in high levels in the blood and the nervous system. It is known that the corticospinal neurons and possibly the anterior horn cells are glutamate type neurons, thus making them sensitive to damage by high levels of glutamate and aspartate.[249]

Others have measured glutamate levels in ALS patients and have not found elevated levels.[250] But Dr. Plaitakis points out that glutamate is very difficult to measure in the serum and must be done under very exacting conditions. His review of the negative reports indicate that these precautions have not been used in these previous studies.

In a follow-up study, Dr. Plaitakis and his coworkers examined the glutamate and aspartate levels from the cerebellar cortex, frontal lobe, and two areas of the spinal cord in patients dying of ALS.[251] They found that glutamate levels were significantly decreased (21 to 40% lower than controls) in all areas tested. The cervical and lumbar cord, the areas containing the greatest number of motor neurons, showed the greatest deficit. Aspartate was significantly decreased in the spinal cord only (32 to 35%). This defect in the aspartate and glutamate pools in the brain and spinal cord of ALS patients could indicate that these specialized neurons are destroyed and as a result have lost their previously high concentrations of these excitatory amino acids.

One argument against this hypothesis is that the blood/spinal cord barrier should effectively exclude the glutamate and aspartate in the blood from entering the spinal cord. Again, as with the blood-brain barrier, this is hypothetically true. But, we know essentially nothing about the ongoing competence of this barrier from day to day and minute to minute. As with any barrier, it will tend to fail under certain conditions. For example, excessive physical stress, elevated body core temperature, infections, trauma, certain drugs and metals, and aging itself may all alter the competence of this barrier. Remember, blood glutamate levels are always elevated in persons subject to ALS, day and night, and even when they have not eaten meals containing high glutamate compounds. When they eat foods containing MSG their blood levels rise much higher than following normal meals.

But what is most important is that their highest blood levels occurs following ingestion of MSG. Apparently, persons destined to develop ALS have difficulty metabolizing ingested glutamate. If they eat any food containing glutamate or aspartate, their blood levels of this toxic amino acid become extremely elevated. Should they eat food manufactured in the United States, most likely it will contain a multitude of excitotoxins, most notably, aspartate and glutamate in various forms. I would estimate that the typical American diet contains anywhere from 10 to 20 grams of excitotoxins a day. (Some individuals will consume much higher amounts.) A study done in Korea found that the average per capita consumption of MSG was 4 grams a day, with some individuals consuming as much as 120 grams in a twenty-four hour period.[252] This is an enormous amount of neurotoxins even for those able to metabolize glutamate normally.

From Dr. Spencer's studies on L-BMAA we learned that ALS was most common in the experimental animals exposed to massive doses of this excitotoxin. Parkinson's disease occurred with lower doses spread over a longer period of exposure. This is most likely why people with the inherited enzyme defect (glutamate dehydrogense) develop ALS and not Parkinson's disease, because they are exposed to more massive doses of the excitotoxins.

A recent finding shed a new light on this terrible disease. Dr. Jeffery Rothstein, working at Johns Hopkins University in Baltimore found that ALS patients have a deficiency of glutamate transporter proteins.[253] These are special proteins that transport free glutamate from the fluid surrounding the neurons (extracellular space) into surrounding astrocytes. Remember, free glutamate in the extracellular space can kill the neurons. This removal process occurs very rapidly under normal conditions.

Loss of the glutamate transporter is a specific defect thus far seen only in ALS. Dr. Rothstein found that when he applied a drug known to block the glutamate transporter to a spinal cord slice in a culture, glutamate levels rose to high levels that persisted for weeks. During this time the neurons appeared normal. Then he began to see a process of slow death among the motor neurons (the neurons destroyed in ALS).

From this data it appears that ALS is a disease in which the glutamate transporter protein is lost (for some unknown reason) leading to a chronic rise in glutamate within the spinal cord. This high concentration of glutamate will eventually destroy the large motor neurons in the spinal cord. But as yet we do not know what causes the glutamate transporter to suddenly disappear.

There is a rare familial form of ALS in which there is a defect in the antioxidant enzyme—super oxide dismutase (SOD)—within the motor neurons of the spinal cord. When neurons have their SOD enzymes lowered experimentally to levels that are not very toxic and are then exposed to glutamate, one sees massive destruction of these motor cells. This again demonstrates the interplay between free radicals and glutamate toxicity.

It appears that ALS is a disease caused primarily by a rise in intrinsic glutamate rather than ingested glutamate. But, I would again caution those with the disease that it would be foolhardy to expose yourself to additional excitotoxins at such a critical time. We do not know what part food additive excitotoxins play in the progress of this disease, but extreme caution would be advised. It is entirely possible that food borne glutamate and aspartate may accelerate the disease process.

A second bit of the growing evidence that excitotoxins play a major role in ALS is based on studies of a related disorder called olivopontocerebellar atrophy or OPCA for short.

INHERITED GLUTAMATE SENSITIVITY

Olivopontocerebellar degeneration is a rare inherited condition that can appear anywhere from age 12 to 52, with 38 as the average age of onset. Most cases eventually develop a severe loss of balance (ataxia), spasticity of the legs, and Parkinson's-type symptoms. What makes this disease especially interesting is that it represents a neurodegenerative disease caused by an inborn defect in an important enzyme. This enzyme, known as glutamate dehydrogenase (GDH), plays a vital role in converting glutamate, the excitotoxin, into glutamine, the inactive storage form of glutamate.

Studies of patients with OPCA demonstrate that their white blood cells and fibroblasts (special cells in the skin), are deficient in glutamate dehydrogenase. This indicates that all of the cells in their body are deficient in this important enzyme and not just the neurons in the nervous system. In one study of OPCA patients, it was found that after an overnight fast, their blood glutamate levels were twice as high as that seen in normal people.[254] And after eating a normal meal containing one gram of protein, they had a marked elevation in both glutamate and aspartate. But even more importantly, when they were fed pure MSG in a dose of 60 miligram per kilogram of body weight, their glutamate levels rose three times higher than that of a normal person. At this blood level the glutamate concentration was equal to that used to produced neurological lesions in experimental animals.[255]

The brain normally contains glutamate concentrations 1000 times higher than that found in the serum. The GDH (glutamate dehydrogenase) enzyme keeps this level rather stable by shifting any excess glutamate into the astrocyte, where it is converted into glutamine. When GDH is deficient, glutamate can attain levels high enough to cause serious brain or spinal cord injury, which is, in fact, what produces the severe, but selective, destruction of the brain seen in OPCA. What this disease demonstrates is the enormous destructive power of excitotoxins when they are allowed to accumulate in the brain and spinal cord. There is little question that individuals with this disorder should be especially careful to avoid excito-toxins in their food. And with the new FDA rules that allow food manu-facturers to disguise the various forms of glutamate and other excitotoxins, this is becoming ever more difficult to do. Some doctors, unaware of this important connection, do not warn their patients to avoid these food additives.

It is also important to note that in OPCD, high blood levels of gluta-mate following a meal do indeed pass through the blood-brain barrier and, should that happen, it would produce severe brain damage in areas thought to be protected by this barrier.

One important point needs to be made at this juncture. Most of these terrible neurological diseases represent the full genetic expression of the dis-order. But often, especially in hereditary diseases, rather than the full blown disease, one may see incomplete genetic expressions of the disorder which would produce only minor weakness in the cells and their enzymes. As a result, these diseases may never present with obvious clinical symptoms. This is because, as in the case of OPCA, the enzyme defect is not total, so that enough enzyme exists to prevent severe glutamate accumulation, if only low doses of glutamate and aspartate are eaten. But, these individuals cannot tolerate the extremely high levels of glutamate or aspartate seen in many commercially prepared foods. The extra excitotoxin, as MSG, hydro-lyzed vegetable protein, or natural flavoring, taxes the enzyme system beyond its limits. There are quite possibly thousands of people walking around in a perfectly normal state of health, who have a weakness for one of these inherited neurodegenerative diseases. High levels of MSG, or one of the other excitotoxins, could tip the scales and precipitate the full blown disease—which is an excellent reason to avoid all excitotoxin food additives.

PREVENTION OF ALS

The ultimate aim of our research into the cause of ALS is to not only to treat existing cases but to prevent the disease altogether. This is not an unreasonable goal. More than likely we will eventually discover that the neurons affected by this disease are also deficient in energy production, thus making them infinitely more susceptible to excitotoxin damage. The anterior motor neurons in the spinal cord are the largest neurons in the nervous system and naturally would require large amounts of energy to sus-tain them. A combination of GDH deficiency (causing high blood and spinal cord glutamate concentrations), glutamate transporter loss, and energy deficiency of the neurons themselves would put such an individual at high risk for developing the disease.

It is also for this reason that persons with a strong family history of ALS should be very careful to exclude all food additive excitotoxins, such as MSG and hydrolyzed protein, from their food. This will require that you prepare most of your food fresh. You must also avoid all foods and drinks sweetened with aspartame (NutraSweet®), since it contains the powerful excitotoxin aspartate. In addition, all that we have learned about hypoglycemia and Parkinson's disease also applies to ALS patients. Low energy levels greatly magnify the toxic effect of MSG and aspartate on the spinal cord.

It should also be recalled that excitotoxins produce much of their damage by unleashing free radicals within the neurons. Out of all the therapies tried in ALS patients, the most successful have been those using antioxidants, such as vitamin E, and dietary supplements that increase cellular glutathione levels.

It has been shown that when individuals with ALS are given large doses of L-leucine (one of the branched chained amino acids) they significantly improve their neurological function and the progress of the disease is slowed. It is known that L-leucine is an important inducer of the glutamate inactivating enzyme GDH. In one study twenty-two patients with ALS were used in a clinical trial (double blind, randomized, placebo-controlled) in which they were given branched chained amino acids in large doses.[256] (These are given together to prevent interference in absorption.) The control ALS patients were fed unsupplemented meals and showed a progressive decline in their neurological function, whereas those treated with branched chained amino acids showed a significant slowing in their deterioration, especially toward the end of one year.

Finally, it is important that the diet contain foods that have significant amounts of magnesium, such as broccoli and spinach. I would go so far as to recommend magnesium supplements (as magnesium lactate or gluconate) to those at risk and with the early stages of the disease. It is also important to have an adequate supply of zinc containing foods in the diet. I would, however, be cautious about using high dose zinc supplements since there is evidence that although zinc totally blocks the NMDA type glutamate toxicity, it may enhance toxicity at the non-NMDA sites. Certainly one should not take more than 25 to 50 miligrams of zinc more often than three times a week.

These recommendations in no way imply that you can cure ALS or even totally prevent it from occuring merely by avoiding excitotoxin food additives or by taking supplements. But it is entirely possible that these measures may slow down the progress of the disease and may in some instances delay the onset of the disease in susceptable individuals. In the future, special drugs may be designed which can attain these lofty goals.

HUNTINGTON'S CHOREA

In 1872 Dr. George Huntington, a general practitioner from Pomery, Ohio, read a paper before the Academy of Medicine in which he reported several cases given to him by his father and grandfather from their practices. What he described was an unusual neurological disease that affected patients by suddenly appearing around middle-age. Before the onset of this disease the patients usually had led perfectly normal and healthy lives. Characteristically, the disease began with jerking movements of the face and then the arms, followed by a relentless deterioration of neurological function so that the patients were eventually bedridden as writhing, disoriented, and demented cripples.

Eventually, studies determined that this disorder originated from a single genetic mutation occurring in a family living in the tiny village of Bures in Suffolk, England. From this lone family, six descendents immigrated to North America in 1630, and account for all known cases of the disease today, as the story goes.[257]

The onset of the disorder usually begins subtly with changes in mental ability and personality. Early on, one may see irritability, eccentric and even psychotic behavior, and difficulty with memory. Eventually, the mental abilities begin to fail. For example, these individuals may be unable to identify the names of common objects or to remember the names of close friends. This may go on for years and even precede the more obvious motor symptoms.

The first motor signs to develop may be a twitching of the muscles of the face and shoulders. At first this may be put off as nervousness or fidgeting. Gradually, this evolves into obvious writhing and jerking movements of the face and limbs, until finally the entire body is contorted by uncontrollable waves of spasm-like writhing called choreaform movements. All attempts at normal movement are grossly exaggerated, especially the facial expression, which may resemble grotesque grimacing. I'm sure there are some readers who are now feeling a sudden twitch of the eye or jerk of the neck. Don't worry, this condition is inherited as an autosomal dominant trait, which means that you should know if one of your ancestors had the disorder. Besides, it is a very rare condition.

This disease has its onset in two age groups. One group has an onset from age 15 to 40 years, and the other from age 55 to 60 years. Those having an earlier onset usually end up more severely impaired. Most patients eventually die after 10 to 15 years of unrelenting progression. At the end, they are usually bedridden and mentally incapacitated. I recall that during my sophomore year in medical school one of my first patients was a thirty-three year old nurse who had developed the disease shortly after her marriage and at the beginning of her nursing career. I recall so well, standing by her bed looking down at this writhing mass of emaciated skin and bones, horrified at the thought that at one time this was a normal, vibrant, pretty young nurse with her whole life ahead of her. I was overwhelmed with a feeling of helplessness before nature.

When the brain of an individual dying with Huntington's disease is removed at autopsy and cut crosswise and examined, we see some very characteristic changes in its internal structure. Most noticeable is the fact that the paired nuclei lying adjacent to the frontal horn of the ventricles (called the caudate, putaman and globus pallidus) are badly shrunken from degeneration. (FIG 5-5) Collectively, these nuclei are called the basal ganglion or striatum. For the purpose of this discussion I will simply refer to these nuclei as the striatum. (FIG 5-6)

The striatum plays a vital role in stereotyped movements, such as swinging the arms, and certain complex patterns of arm and leg movements that are fairly automatic. These movements are already preprogrammed within the striatum so that you do not have to figure out how to perform them each time they are needed. If we examine the striatum of a typical Huntington's disease patient under the microscope, we will see that not all of the neurons in the striatum are destroyed. Rather, the most severe loss is to the small and intermediate sized neurons, with almost complete sparing of the larger neurons.[258] We will see some neuron loss in the frontal cortex as well. So, once again we see that the damage is very specific, wiping out some neurons and sparing others that are close by.

While scientists have been unable to produce an exact model of Huntington's disease they have come close. Thus far, only one class of chemicals can produce the type of selective damage that we see in human Huntington's disease. *These chemicals are excitotoxins.* In earlier research it was found that two excitotoxins could produce this characteristic pattern of neuron loss in the striatum—quinolinic acid, a by-product of tryptophan metabolism, and the experimental drug kainate. Both of these act on glutamate receptor type neurons, just as MSG does.

Kainate is what we call a glutamate agonist. That means it acts like glutamate. Yet kainate is a much more powerful excitotoxin than is glutamate.[259] We know that the striatum contains the highest number of kainate-

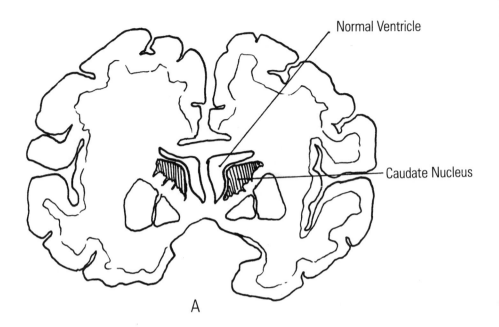

Normal Ventricle

Caudate Nucleus

A

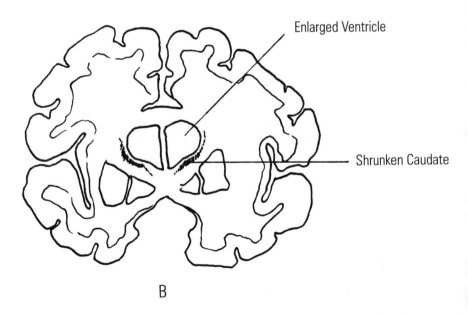

Enlarged Ventricle

Shrunken Caudate

B

5-5 *Drawing A demonstrates a cross-section of a normal brain. Drawing B shows the typical findings in a case of Huntington's Disease. Note the shrunken caudate nucleus and the adjacent enlarged ventricles.*

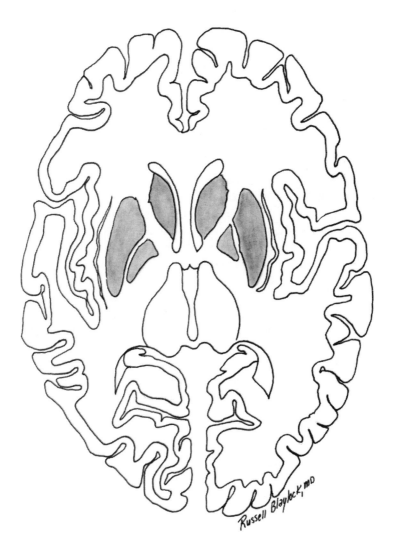

5-6 *Nuclei Affected by Huntington's Disease.*

type receptors of any part of the brain.[260] This is followed by the cerebral cortex and hippocampus of the temporal lobes. Injection of kainate into the striatum produces many similarities to the changes seen in human cases of the disease, such as sparing of the large neurons in the nucleus. Neuro-chemical studies in patients dying of Huntington's disease demonstrate a 50 to 70% reduction in kainate binding sites in the caudate and putamen.[261] The same thing is seen in experimental studies following kainate injection of the striatum in animals.[262] The problem with experimental studies is that rats do not develop the characteristic writhing movements seen in human cases of the disorder, called chorioathetosis. But they do develop some of the psychological changes seen in Huntington's disease. For example, rats will develop impaired learning of mazes, have altered daily activity, and exhibit abnormal feeding behavior, all of which indicate profound inter-ference with mental function.[263]

But there are problems with the kainate hypothesis. Mainly, kainate is not normally found in nature. Also, while many of the kainate receptors are lost in the striatum, they are not the main one's damaged. Recent studies have shown that 93% of the NMDA receptors in the striatum are in lost Huntington's disease.[264] A better candidate is quinolinic acid, the metabolite of the amino acid L-tryptophan. Injection of quinolinic acid into the striatum produces the same sparing of the large neurons but more closely resembles the other pathological and neurochemical changes seen in the disease.[265] It specifically kills glutamate neurons of the NMDA type.

Both of these excitotoxins drain the energy from neurons when injected into the brain. Experimental studies using mice demonstrate that when kainate is injected into the striatum, ATP and phosphocreatine energy molecules fall to drastically low levels.[266] Lactate levels, a measure of im-paired energy metabolism, doubled and glucose levels fell nearly fifty per-cent following kainate injection. This emphasizes the important role played by neuron energy requirements in this type of excitotoxin damage.

Similar changes can be seen in studies of living Huntington's disease patients utilizing the PET scanner.[267] This instrument allows scientists to study the metabolism of the living brain. In the past, studies of the brain's metabolism required either neurochemical analysis of brain tissue taken soon after death or the observation of isolated brain tissue in culture. Both of these methods were fraught with errors, the worst of which was the fact that one could not study how the brain metabolizes substances in every-day circumstances. The PET scanner allows us to observe the functioning of the brain by watching it metabolize special radioactive substances, such as radiolabeled glucose (2-(11C)-deoxy-D-glucose).

In one such study, scientists observed the metabolism of Huntington's disease patients in which the disease had developed from age 17 to 71. They found that the degree of hypometabolism (low brain metabolism) varied directly with the stage of the disease.[268] That is, patients having advanced deterioration showed the lowest levels of glucose metabolism in the striatum. They used the CT scanner, which gives a structural image of the brain's interior, to determine the degree of advancement of the disease.

We would expect advanced cases to have low metabolism in the striatum since the CT scanner showed this nucleus to be severely shrunken in such cases. But what surprised these scientists is that low metabolism could be detected even in cases showing no obvious shrinkage of the striatum. In fact, they demonstrated low metabolism in the striatum even in persons at risk for eventually developing the disease but who had none of the symptoms or signs of the disease.[269] In a follow-up study of fifteen of these high risk patients, they found that three out of four with the most advanced hypometabolism did eventually develop the full blown disease. Again, this emphasizes that these neurodegenerative diseases begin long before clinical symptoms develop and that impaired energy supplies to the neurons plays a vital role in this toxicity.

Doctors Olney and deGubareff have proposed that in Huntington's disease there is a defect in glutamate re-uptake, the normal elimination of glutamate by the brain.[270] If this were true, glutamate would accumulate in the striatum in concentrations that could kill striatal neurons. Others have proposed the idea that in Huntington's there is a defect in the membrane of the neurons within the striatum that makes them especially sensitive, and therefore vulnerable to excitotoxin damage. Whatever the mechanism, there is a high probability that excitotoxins play a vital role in the final expression of this enigmatic disease.

If this hypothesis is valid, then it may be possible that one can delay the onset, or even prevent the onset, of this disease by excluding excitotoxins from the diet. Most likely, it would also require the use of excitotoxin blocking substances and drugs to prevent the glutamate within the brain from causing damage. But it is obvious to even the casual reader that it is especially important for those at risk, or in the early stages of the disease, to avoid excitotoxins in their food, and to follow all of the other precautions outlined in my discussion of Parkinson's disease.

The reason I included this rare disease in the discussion of excitotoxins is that it, once again, demonstrates the importance of these toxins in producing known neurodegenerative disease. And it also points out a recurring pattern seen with excitotoxin accumulation: energy deficiency in the brain, impaired neural protective mechanisms, low magnesium, and high calcium accumulation in the neurons involved.[271]

· 6 ·

Alzheimer's Disease: A Classic Case of Excitotoxin Damage

There are more than twenty-five million persons over the age of sixty-five living in the United States. Of these, eleven percent, or approximately two million seven hundred thousand, suffer from mild to moderate dementia, and almost five percent are severely demented. But not all of these severely demented individuals have Alzheimer's disease. About fifty-five percent will have Alzheimer's disease and the rest will have dementia caused by multiple small strokes (called multi-infarct dementia) or a combination of Alzheimer's disease and strokes.

Chronic dementias account for almost 50% of nursing home admissions and cost six billion dollars annually. Demographic studies predict that by the year 2030 the population of people over age sixty-five will have doubled. This will mean that the annual cost of caring for the demented could reach thirty billion dollars by the year 2030. Enormous sums of money are spent not only caring for these unfortunate individuals, but also in an effort to find a cause and, hopefully, a cure for this devastating disease. This form of dementia not only destroys the lives of those afflicted by it, but it devastates their families as well. The following is the testimony of the wife of a victim of Alzheimer's disease before a Joint Congressional hearing on Alzheimer's disease:

"I can tell you that it is like a funeral that never ends. My husband was a handsome, vital, athletic man, a civic leader, a public speaker, a highly respected businessman. He was administrative vice-president of his company. He is now a statistic. He is permanently hospitalized, not knowing his family or speaking a word in the past 4 years. He requires total care as the physical deterioration takes its toll. I have a husband, but I speak of him in the past tense. I am not a divorcee; I am not a widow; but where do I fit?[272]

Unfortunately, the majority of attention concerning this disease has been directed at the various abnormal proteins found throughout the damaged parts of the brain. The most intriguing protein found thus far is called beta-amyloid, which accumulates within the dying cells of the brain. The accumulation of this unusual protein has been theorized to be caused by various mechanisms such as abnormal immune function, viruses, aluminum in the diet, or genetic disorders.

But, it may be that simpler mechanisms are operating and that this abnormal protein, rather than being a cause of the disease, is merely the result of the disease. That is, something else is injuring these neurons, causing them to accumulate amyloid protein.

THE EFFECT OF NORMAL AGING

To understand Alzheimer's disease we must first understand the process of normal aging of the brain, especially what changes take place in its structure and its chemistry. Even though we know a considerable amount about these changes, many mysteries remain. One thing that is agreed upon by pathologists is that the brain does shrink as we grow older. With the advent of computerized brain scanning, we can now see this shriveling of the brain in the aged while they are still alive. Part of this shrinkage is due to the death of brain cells, and some is secondary to a loss of the fatty insulation (myelin) surrounding fiber pathways within the white matter of the brain.

Studies of brain metabolism in the aged have yielded conflicting results. Some earlier studies indicated that there was a general decline in the metabolism of the brain as we get older.[273] But better conducted studies, in which healthy, active elderly were separated and studied as a group, indicated that there was no difference in the brain metabolism and that of younger persons. Much of the previously reported decline in brain metabolism had been the result of strokes or other diseases affecting the brain and not due to aging itself.

Metabolic studies in rats have disclosed very little change in the flow of blood and in the metabolism of oxygen and glucose by the brain with aging. Using the most modern techniques of studying metabolism of the living brain in humans, called positron emission tomography (also called PET scanning), it was found that the healthy, alert, and active elderly have normal metabolism in all areas of their brain.[274] This supports the idea that brain function does not necessarily have to decline with age.

Neurochemical studies of the brain indicate that there may be some decline of selected brain chemicals, such as acetylcholine, an important neurotransmitter.[275] But again, various reports are often conflicting and depend on the health and activity of the individual. What we must realize is that aging of the brain does not represent a progressive decline in neurological function until we eventually die. Often, the brain continues to function at a near normal manner until we die from other causes.

MICROSCOPIC CHANGES

If aged persons that are active and healthy are selected for study, we find that their brains contain the same total number of neurons, neuronal density (number of neurons per volume of brain), and percentage of cells in the cortex as younger persons.[276] But there are areas of the brain that do undergo significant cellular loss with aging. For example, as we age the nucleus, called the substantia nigra (which is related to Parkinson's disease) shows a progressive loss of the neurons that use dopamine as a transmitter. This decline usually begins at age thirty. In humans, this loss can be as great as 60% at the extremes of age, yet even with this degree of loss there may be a few clinical signs of medical problems.[277]

Certain zones of neurons within the hippocampus in the temporal lobes are also especially sensitive to the effects of aging. As you may remember from the chapter on how the brain works, the hippocampus is concerned primarily with learning and memory.

One microscopic change in the brain seen with aging which has not been disputed is the presence of and progressive accumulation of an "age pigment" called lipofuscin, a yellow-brown pigment known to collect in neurons of the elderly. Ironically, it has nothing to do with mental function, as brains with abundant lipofucsion exist in bright, active elderly persons.

Many years ago, neuropathologists discovered strange looking clumps of dark staining material scattered throughout the frontal and temporal lobes of individuals over the age of fifty. It soon became obvious that the presence of this unusual pigment was a normal consequence of aging, hence the name senile plaque.[278] As we grow older, more and more of these senile plaques develop. Today they are called neuritic plaques. (FIG 6-1)

It appears that these plaques represent failed attempts by neurons to sprout new dendritic processes (the receiving or input fibers of neurons). We often find that the brain attempts to repair itself and bypass the injured areas by sprouting these new dendritic spines, which is part of the brain's plasticity. Experimentally, this process has been shown to play an important part in learning. For example, animals exposed to various learning tasks (such as mazes) are found to develop extensive numbers of dendritic spines, while animals deprived of learning stimulation have considerably fewer spines. This sprouting process also appears to be a very important repair

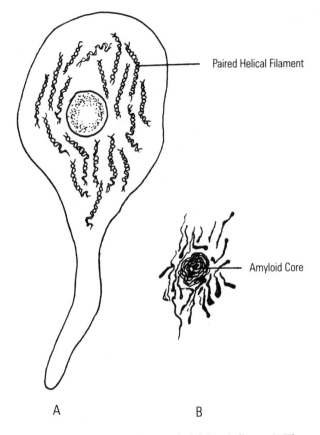

Paired Helical Filament

Amyloid Core

A   B

6-1 *Two microscopic bodies frequently seen in cases of Alzheimer's disease: A) The neurofibrillary tangles seen within dying neurons. Notice the paired helical filaments wrapped around each other. B) A typical neuritic plaque. Within its center is the amyloid core which contains high concentrations of glutamates.*

mechanism in aging.[279] Interestingly, the presence of neuritic plaques seems to play no part in any loss of brain function.

Another pathological feature of aging is the presence of twisted, dark-staining microscopic pigments called neurofibrillary tangles. These ''age tangles'' are seen commonly in the brains of active and healthy elderly persons, but only in small numbers. Extensive studies of these bodies indicate that they are twisted helical filaments of insoluble protein.[280] In the case of Alzheimer's disease, they became numerous throughout the brain, especially in the parietal and temporal lobes.

Recently it has been shown that there is an accumulation of calcium within the brain cells of aged rats.[281] Remember, it was calcium that was most associated with cell death in other neurodegenerative diseases such as Parkinson's disease and ALS.

CHANGES IN BRAIN FUNCTIONS WITH AGING

Many laymen believe that as we age we are doomed to become mentally slow and decrepit. While it is known that the elderly do not do as well as the young on timed test of mental ability, they will perform as well as when given more time to complete tests. And with training, they will show incredible improvements in mental function, including cognition and memory. This is even true of those elderly found to have impaired memory prior to the learning exercise.

One of the major causes of the decline in mental acuity and function seen with aging is a lack of involvement in academic and intellectual affairs, or using one's mind every day. The brilliant economist Ludwig von Mises continued to produce great economic works even into his nineties, and his student, F.A. Hayek, who just recently died in his nineties, produced one of his greatest works just before his death.

There is little question that a significant part of their ability to preserve their mental acuity was their unending involvement in intellectual pursuits. History is filled with stories of brilliant men and women who continue to produce intellectually well into their advanced years. Experimentally we know that growth of the dendritic processes (associated with learning) is stimulated by increased use of the brain and continues well into the extremes of age.[282] The brain, in this way, is much like a muscle; the more you exercise it the more powerful it becomes. Thinking is the exercise of the mind. Henry Ford once said that, "Thinking is the hardest form of work. That is why so few engage in it."

As we grow older, we often grow intellectually lazy. Rather than memorize a list of things to do, we write them down. With the rapid growth of using electronic tools that often obviate the necessity for concentrated thought, the lazier we become. Electronic calculators, computers, and other technologies keep us from fully using our brains.

There is also growing evidence that those with declining intellectual function, other than Alzheimer's disease, often have suffered from multiple insults to the brain. For example, many elderly have experienced several strokes by the time they reach their middle to late sixties. Often these strokes are silent.[283] The person may be totally unaware that anything has happened.

Strokes result when a brain artery is blocked, thereby depriving that part of the brain of its blood supply. If the blocked vessel is a major artery, such as the carotid artery in the neck, a serious stroke occurs with paralysis and numbness on the opposite side of the body. But should the blocked vessel be a small artery, not supplying blood to a critical part of the brain, the stroke may go unnoticed. Over a long period of time, usually over many years, several of these strokes may occur, until the accumulated damage finally kills off enough brain cells to result in serious malfunction of the brain. It is when this occurs that the elderly seem to deteriorate mentally more rapidly with age.

I remember one gentleman who came to my office complaining of difficulty with his memory. He ran a chicken farm and had for years been responsible for all of the details of the business, which included a lot of facts and figures. Of late he had been unable to recall the number of newly purchased feeders. This forgetfulness seemed to increase over the last several months to the point where it was interfering with his business.

I sent the gentleman for an MRI scan of his brain. I suspected that he had a dementia of early onset that was most likely caused by something other than Alzheimer's disease. Sure enough, his scan confirmed that he was suffering from multiple small strokes that over the years had taken their toll. These strokes appeared on his scan as multiple lucent (luminous) areas scattered throughout his brain. I knew that over time more of these strokes were likely to appear, further impairing his mental abilities.

There are a multitude of reasons for intellectual deterioration in the elderly. For example, low thyroid hormone production (hypothyroidism) can cause severe intellectual deterioration, often resembling Alzheimer's disease, as can severe depression. In fact, depression can clinically present exactly like Alzheimer's disease. This is one form of "dementia" that responds well to treatment.

Recently, it was discovered that low brain levels of the vitamin B_{12} can cause severe intellectual deterioration.[284] We know that B_{12} deficiency is more common in the elderly than many physicians realize. Unfortunately, some doctors are unaware that the blood levels of vitamin B_{12} can be within the normal range in the presence of dangerously low brain levels of the vitamin (even without anemia). This form of dementia can often be reversed by injections of vitamin B_{12}. But replacement of vitamin B_{12} works only if the treatment begins early in the course of the disorder.

In a recent study in which the levels of vitamin B_{12} were measured in the serum and the cerebrospinal fluid of persons with Alzheimer's disease, it was found that their median serum B_{12} levels were significantly lower than that of normal controls.[285] [286] Two patients were found that had high serum levels of B_{12} with low levels of the vitamin in the brain. This seems to indicate that these two patients had a defect in the mechanism that transports vitamin B_{12} across the blood-brain barrier into the brain.

There are a multitude of other causes of brain damage resulting in dementia. For instance, recurrent bouts of severe hypoglycemia can cause accumulated brain damage much like the mini-strokes we have talked about.[287] Some of the medications commonly used today to treat medical disorders can depress brain function, which is a special danger in the elderly who are often given a multitude of prescriptions from several different doctors. I see elderly patients frequently in my practice, often clutching a bag full of prescription bottles. Several of these drugs, such as blood pressure medications and tranquilizers, can have an adverse effect on mental function, especially when used in combination.

Now let us examine an abnormal aging disorder of the brain, Alzheimer's disease.

WHAT IS ALZHEIMER'S DISEASE?

Dementia has been recognized for thousands of years. Hippocrates described persons with mental dulling due to fevers, which he called phrenitis. But it was Celsus, in the first century A.D. who introduced the terms "delirium" and "dementia". Areataeus of Cappadocia classified dementia into acute and chronic types. The chronic type he associated with old age and with a "stupefaction of the gnostic and intellectual functions." Revolutionary hero and physician, Benjamin Rush, described dementias of the aged as "the brain becoming so torpid and insensible, as to be unable to transmit impressions made upon it to the mind." By 1830, senile dementia was recognized as a definite clinical disorder in the aged.

But of more importance were the sporadic reports of senility of the mind occurring before the age of sixty-five. In fact, cases were being reported as young as age forty. This condition was eventually referred to as pre-senile dementia, and was considered to be a different disorder than that seen in the elderly. In 1907 the neuropathologist Alois Alzheimer, using a newly discovered silver stain, described special microscopic bodies, or inclusions, in the brain tissue of a 51-year-old patient dying of pre-senile dementia. He called those bodies neurofibrillary tangles and senile plaques. Later, he discovered these same dark inclusions in the brains of persons dying with typical senile dementia of the aged.

It was not until 1977 that neurologists and neuropathologists agreed that the same disease process was occurring in both pre-senile and senile dementia. In other words, that senile dementia was not a normal aging process affecting the brain of the elderly. They agreed to call both forms of Alzheimer's disease, that is, the pre-senile and senile forms, the syndrome of dementia of the Alzheimer's type or SDAT for short.

Clinically, Alzheimer's disease is a very specific type of dementia. There are many causes of dementia, as we have seen, of which Alzheimer's disease is but one. Most people think of Alzheimer's disease as just a loss of memory. But, in fact, many of the higher functions of the brain are severely impaired as well. For instance, speech, cognition, orientation, visual perception, and even weakness can all develop with Alzheimer's disease. This deterioration of mental functions occurs either slowly over several years, or, on occasion, quite rapidly.

I remember one gentleman, a business executive, who appeared to be in his usual good state of mental health until one day when driving home from work he became completely disoriented and couldn't find his way home. After this initial episode he quickly deteriorated, losing all of his ability to recall recent events or develop new memories. His disorientation became crippling. Disorientation is a frequent presenting feature of Alzheimer's disease, and is a more specific finding than is memory loss.

Sudden onset of this type of dementia may also occur following blows to the head or even high fevers. I had one elderly gentleman as a patient who, according to the family, had been intellectually bright and active, but then suddenly began to deteriorate rapidly. I performed a brain scan which demonstrated a large collection of blood over one-half of his brain, a "chronic subdural hematoma". Normally, these are very favorable conditions, in which the patient usually returns to normal once the blood clot is removed. But in this case the man remained severely demented after his operation. It was later found that he suffered from Alzheimer's disease of an acute onset.

Most likely, such sudden onsets of Alzheimer's disease represent the final event of a long standing, but gradual and silent loss of brain cells over many years, even decades, rather than a sudden loss of massive numbers of neurons. As discussed before, the brain has an incredible ability to compensate when injured. Usually there are no clinical signs of the disorder until the majority of the involved brain cells have died. Therefore, the clinical presentation of the disease may not appear until the last 20% or so of these cells drop out. It is like the old adage of the straw that broke the camel's back.

As for memory loss, we know that one of the earliest types of memory loss is that affecting recent memory. This type of memory involves the laying down of new memories, for example, memorizing a list of numbers or words, or remembering what we ate for breakfast this morning. It is the hippocampus of the temporal lobes that appears to be most involved in recent memory. Pathologically, we know that the temporal lobes show extensive damage in Alzheimer's disease. Some researchers feel that it is the retrieval mechanism of memories that is faulty rather than actual storage of new memories.

Eventually, even long term memories begin to fade. The longer a memory has been stored in the brain the more resistant it is to loss through brain diseases or injury. So, one may forget events that happened several months ago, but remember other events clearly that happened in high school, or even childhood.

MICROSCOPIC CHANGES SEEN IN ALZHEIMER'S DISEASE

When Dr. Alzheimer peered through his microscope he found that two types of microscopic bodies were scattered throughout the shrunken parts of the brains of these demented patients. He called these dark staining bodies neuritic or senile plaques and neurofibrillary tangles. Since this observation, these two microscopic lesions (called inclusions) have been considered pathologic for Alzheimer's disease. But later he discovered that these same inclusions were also found in the brains of normal elderly persons. In fact, we see them in the brains of old monkeys, dogs, cats, and polar bears, but not rats.

This would tend to indicate that they are part of normal aging and the various pathological disorders that go with aging. There is growing evidence that these lesions are not the cause of Alzheimer's disease, but rather a consequence of it, or that they develop as a result of the death of neurons, but do not cause the neurons to actually die. We also see large numbers of these lesions in the brains of "punch drunk" boxers, as well as the brains of those having other chronic degenerative brain diseases.

But these lesions do correlate with the degree of dementia. There are many more neuritic plaques and neurofibrillary tangles in severe cases of dementia than in mild cases. Again, this may just represent the degree of damage to neurons and not a cause of their destruction. The distribution of these neurofibrillary tangles and plaques is characteristic of Alzheimer's disease, with large numbers being seen in the frontal and parietal cortex and in the hippocampus of the temporal lobes. Again, this is where most of the damage and neuron death occurs.

These two microscopic inclusions differ somewhat in importance ways. The neurofibrillary tangle is a microscopic mass consisting of a twisted collection of fibrils found within the dying neurons. (Under the electron microscope they appear as clusters of paired strands twisted on themselves, called paired helical filaments.) The number of neurofibrillary tangles correlates with the degree of dementia.

It is interesting to note that these neurofibrillary tangles are also primarily located in neurons having glutamate receptors. Analysis of the protein content of these tangles reveals that glutamate and aspartate are found in them in the highest concentration of any of the amino acid components.[288] Until recently, neuroscientists had little idea as to the origin of these unusual bodies. But in 1985 two scientists working with spinal cord cells in tissue culture discovered that prolonged exposure of these neurons to glutamate or aspartate (excitotoxins) resulted in the formation of paired helical filaments almost identical to those seen in Alzheimer's disease.[289]

The second of the inclusion bodies is the senile or neuritic plaque. This darkly staining body is located outside the neuron and in the same anatomical areas as the neurofibrillary tangle. What makes them unusual is that in the core of these plaques sits a very special protein called beta-amyloid. Until recently, most neuroscientists considered Alzheimer's disease to be a disorder resulting from the accumulation of this abnormal protein in brain cells. What could not be explained is why it only accumulated in certain neurons, especially those containing glutamate receptors, and not others.

Electron microscopic examination of these plaques reveals that they contain many distorted mitochondria and lysomes. Mitochondria, you will recall, are the energy generators of the cell. Lysomes can be thought of as suicide packets, since they contain a multitude of destructive enzymes that are released when a cell is severely injured. These enzymes break down the cell's components so that white blood cells and scavenger cells can carry the dead neuron fragments away.

Further examination of these plaques reveals that they have specific immunological staining characteristics. That is, they react only to very specific stains directed towards specific types of protein. (In fact, these immunological stains are used to diagnose Alzheimer's disease from brain biopsies.) Still, this does not change our general hypothesis that Alzheimer's disease is caused by an abnormal accumulation of excitotoxic amino acids in the brain. Rather, it strengthens the case since, as we shall see, these immunological markers can be produced by the very same metabolic derangement seen with Alzheimer's disease.

A more recent discovery that points to excitotoxins as a major player in the causation of Alzheimer's disease is the finding that beta-amyloid, when placed in a dish with normal neurons, causes them also to degenerate and die.[290] Further study revealed that this occurred because beta-amyloid made glutamate sensitive neurons even more sensitive to excitotoxin induced death. But why? Part of the explanation lies in the observation that beta-amyloid stimulates an abnormal flow of calcium into the interior of the neuron.[291] Remember, massive calcium entry into the neuron is what triggers the destructive reactions that ultimately kill the cell during high dose glutamate exposure. If earlier findings of high concentrations of glutamate and aspartate in neuritic plaques are true, then this would explain why these neurons are dying. They are being excited to death by high concentrations of excitatory amino acids.

EXCITOTOXINS AND ALZHEIMER-SPECIFIC PROTEINS

Examination of neuritic plaques and neurofibrillary tangles using immunological methods demonstrates that very specific types of proteins are found to exist in high concentrations (as far as we know) only in Alzheimer's disease.[292] The most specific immunologic staining test is called ALZ-50 which stains for a protein labeled A68. This protein is reported to occur in elevated concentrations only in the brains of people with Alzheimer's disease.[293] AlZ-50 immunoreactive staining is reported to be 56 times higher in Alzheimer's brains than in normal brains. Other Alzheimer specific immunoreactive proteins include 5E2 and ubiquitin.

Exposing cultures of normal hippocampal neurons to high concentrations of glutamate significantly increased the staining of these neurons to all three of these Alzheimer-specific immune stains.[294] Even more interesting was the finding that concentrations of glutamate below that which can kill neurons (subtoxic doses) also markedly increased the immunoreactive staining. This is an important observation since it strongly suggests that even lower concentrations of food borne excitotoxic taste enhancers and aspartame can result in the same specific immunoreactive stain changes seen in Alzheimer's disease.

To prove that it was the added glutamate that caused the accumulation of Alzheimer-specific proteins, these researchers next added specific glutamate blocking drugs to the culture medium and found that the effect was completely blocked. Removal of calcium (which is considered to be the mechanism by which glutamate kills neurons) from the medium also blocked the effect.

It has been shown that exposing normal neurons to extracts of Alzheimer's affected brains induced paired helical filaments very similar to those seen in the neurofibrillary tangles of Alzheimer's patients.[295] Likewise, exposing neurons to glutamate or aspartate (a major component of NutraSweet®) can induce paired helical filaments very similar to those seen in naturally occurring Alzheimer's disease.[296]

It has also been shown that exposing neurons to concentrations of beta-amyloid, the primary component of neuritic plaques, can markedly enhance the destruction of neurons by excitotoxins.[297] This enhancement of excitotoxicity was dose dependent, with higher concentrations causing greater enhancement. (Beta-amyloid acted through all three subtypes of glutamate receptors—NMDA, quisqualate, and kainate.)

So why is this important to know? Because these experiments show that: first, glutamate can induce the same Alzheimer-specific types of immunoreactive proteins and second, once the neurons begin to degenerate, they will form abnormal proteins in the form of beta-amyloid. This amyloid protein can further enhance the toxicity of glutamate and aspartate in a dose dependent manner, so that the more plaques that are formed (i.e., the higher the concentration of beta-amyloid) the more sensitive the surviving neurons become to excitotoxins. This would mean that further exposure to excess excitotoxins, both from food additives and from those normally within the brain itself, could accelerate the process causing the disease to progress more rapidly.

MEMORY LOSS IN ALZHEIMER'S DISEASE

Memory is one of the great mysteries of the universe. How is it that we can store all that we see, hear, feel, and envision in our minds and then later, even decades later, extract selected memories in vivid detail? There is evidence that we record every event entering our consciousness, the hissing of a radiator in the background, the singing of the birds outside our window, the color of another's eyes that we casually pass on the sidewalk— every minute detail of life. That is, we record events, impressions, and senses that enter our brain unconsciously.

But how can we store such an enormous amount of data? That it is actually stored was dramatically demonstrated by Dr. Wilder Penfield, Chief of Neurosurgery at the Montreal Neurological Institute, when he demonstrated this storage mechanism by stimulating various areas of the exposed temporal cortex in awake patients.[298] This is done by using small probes that emit microvoltage currents. The probes are gently placed upon the surface of the temporal lobes until a memory is elicited. One of his patients, during stimulation, commented, "I just heard one of my children speaking." She added, "It was Frank." Also she could hear "neighborhood noises" as well, which she described as "automobiles passing her house and other children."[299] Another patient heard an orchestra playing "White Christmas". She also could see "people walking". She added that they were strangers.[300]

What made all of these brain stimulation memories particularly interesting was that the memories were not vague recollections but rather it was as if the patient could actually see and hear all of the sights and sounds being replayed before them. Yet these patients were also aware that they were in the operating room. Somehow the brain is able to read through the billions of memory files stored in the temporal lobes until it finds the memory we wish to review. The brain is also able to suppress the background "clutter" that is unimportant.

One of the most commonly recognized features of Alzheimer's disease is the loss of memory. As I stated earlier, it is recent memory that is first lost. And there is considerable evidence that recent memory originates from a region of the brain called the hippocampus (Latin: meaning sea horse). This is a portion of the temporal lobes that looks like a scroll, tucked along the inside of the lobes. (The hippocampus is divided into various regions based upon its microscopic appearance. These are given names like CA1 and CA3.) (FIG 6-2)

In both experimental studies and in the pathological examinations of the brains of patients dying with Alzheimer's dementia, it is these microscopic areas in the hippocampus that have been most severely damaged by the disease. In humans, we know that injury to both hippocampi can result in a complete loss of all recent memory and the ability to form new memories. In one form of brain virus infection, herpes encephalitis, it is the hippocampi that are destroyed. When some of these patients recover from the infection, they are found to have a complete loss of recent memory, yet they can recall distant memories clearly.

One man, suffering from destruction of both temporal lobes, cried with joy every time his wife entered the room, as if it were the first time he had seen her in years. No matter how many times he read a book, on each occasion it was as if he were reading it for the first time. Yet his older memories were preserved. We are not certain where these older memories are stored. Some have proposed a hologram theory of memory, in which these older memories are stored all over the brain and reassembled on demand. Others have proposed that the problem in Alzheimer's patients is not the laying down of memories, but the retrieval mechanism. Thus far no one knows how we retrieve memories from the memory files of the brain.

It is known that hippocampal neurons appear to play an important part in laying down of new memories. We also know that the hippocampus contains high concentrations of NMDA-type glutamate receptor cells. Maragos and coworkers found neurofibrillary tangles to be localized in the same brain areas as glutamate receptor neurons—primarily in the hippocampus and the association cortex of the parietal lobe.[301]

Neuroscientists now know that glutamate plays a vital role in the

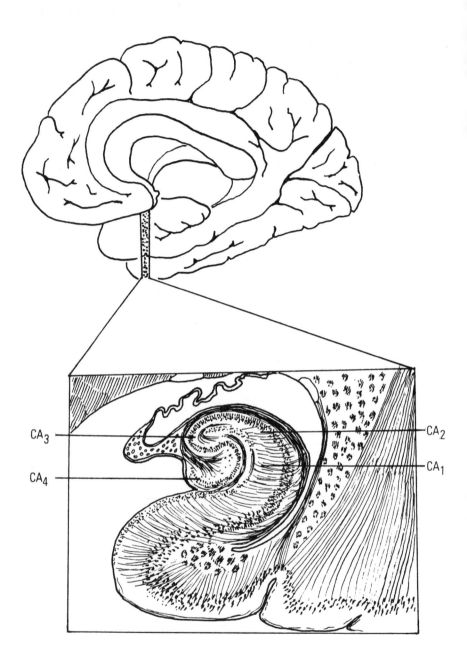

CA₃ — — —

CA₄ — — —

CA₂ — — —

CA₁ — — —

6-2 *Cross-section of temporal lobe with the various cellular layers. This is the area of the brain most sensitive to glutamate excess. It is thought to play a major role in memory. These neurons show extensive damage in Alzheimer's disease.*

memory storage process. Physiologically, memory is thought to involve a phenomenon called "long term potentiation", or LTP for short.[302] Basically, long term potentiation is a process that results in a network of neurons being fired for prolonged periods of time, sometimes lasting days or even weeks. Glutamate-type neurons play an important part in the initiation, but not the maintenance or continuation of LTP.[303] That glutamate plays a critical role in memory function has been demonstrated by giving experimental animals a drug that blocks NMDA type glutamate receptors. This drug causes these animals to exhibit difficulties not only in recent memory, but also in orientation, just as is seen in Alzheimer's patients.[304]

When experimental animals are given large doses of MSG, either by injection or in their diet, these same hippocampal cells degenerate.[305] While most of the damage done in Alzheimer's disease appears to be to the NMDA type of glutamate receptor, we also see damage to the other two types of glutamate receptors (quisqualate and the kainate).[306] [307] It is important to recall that all three of these receptors are damaged by MSG and aspartate.

WHAT CAUSES ALZHEIMER'S DISEASE?

This is the million dollar question. There are several hypotheses concerning this enigmatic disease—some quite clever. But until now none has met all the criteria that would explain the disorder fully. Critical problems existed in these explanations.

As you remember from chapter 5, one of the earliest clinical observations regarding this disease was that it appeared to develop over a relatively short period of time in otherwise normal individuals. This led to the burning question: What could make massive numbers of neurons, in specific anatomic locations of the brain, suddenly die? One of the most intriguing explanations concluded that these brain cells had defective genes that caused the neurons to age much faster than normal brain cells. As a result, parts of the brain became old and died before other parts.

As our scientific techniques became more sophisticated, we began to learn more about the various changes occurring in this intriguing disorder. Electron microscopists explored the neuritic plaques and neurofibrillary tangles, while biochemists probed the brain for changes in neurotransmitters and the energy pathways, and immunologists searched for evidence of wayward immune attacks upon the brain. Yet one of the most important advances in our understanding of the brain, especially when diseased, involved a new scanning technique we discussed previously, called the PET scanner (Positron Emission Tomography). With this instrument we could actually watch the living brain function and metabolize glucose for energy.[308]

All of this new information led us to realize that Alzheimer's disease does not represent a sudden loss of massive numbers of brain cells, but rather is a very slow degeneration of the brain over decades. Clinically, all we were seeing was the end stage of this gradual deterioration; that is, the point at which the brain could no longer compensate. (But it may be that as the disease progresses this deterioration accelerates toward the end.) It also became obvious that only very specific brain cells were dying.[309] In fact, other cells sitting right next to these dying cells appeared quite healthy. So, whatever was killing these neurons was a highly specific process or toxin. Somehow it could distinguish these particular cells from all the rest.

Scientists knew that some special viruses, called prions, could infect the brain and cause delayed killing of cells and even lead to dementia in humans. It initially sounded like a perfect answer to the puzzle. But there were problems with this theory. First, the virus tends to affect widespread areas of the brain rather than selected sites. Second, it caused symptoms not seen with Alzheimer's disease. And, third, the other pathological features did not match.

Several features of Alzheimer's dementia led scientists to believe that it was caused by an environmental toxin. For instance, it was known that while there is some genetic susceptibility to the disease, most cases were not purely genetically linked. While Alzheimer's diseases was more common in the offspring of Alzheimer's patients, more often they were spared the disease.

It was also known that some environmental neurotoxins could act on specific brain cells and spare others just as in Alzheimer's disease. But what really convinced scientists that a toxin was responsible was when it was recognized that a particular type of dementia occurred at a higher rate in persons undergoing dialysis treatment for kidney failure.

As discussed before, it was found that the dialysis bath used in the kidney machine contained high concentrations of aluminum. Experimentally, when aluminum is injected into animals it can produce some of the pathological features seen with human cases of Alzheimer's disease, such as neurofibrillary tangles. (But these tangles are different from those seen in Alzheimer's disease.) When aluminum was removed from the dialysis bath, the number of dialysis patients suffering from this dementia fell dramatically.

Neurochemical examinations of the brains of individuals dying with Alzheimer's disease indicated that there was a significant reduction in the neurotransmitter acetylcholine and the enzymes associated with its synthesis and destruction.[310] (Both choline acetyltransferase (CAT) and acetyl-cholinesterase are greatly reduced in the areas of the brain most severely damaged by the disease.) It had been known that the neurotransmitter acetylcholine played a vital role in the memory function of the brain.[311] Later it was discovered that much of the damage to these special fibers could be explained by destruction of one small pair of nuclei located at the base of the brain, called the basal nucleus of Meynert.[312]

Anatomical studies indicate that this nucleus sends a wide spray of fibers to the same areas of the cortex and hippocampus that are found to contain the most neurofibrillary tangles in Alzheimer's disease. (FIG 6-3) In most studies of Alzheimer's patient's brains, destruction of this tiny nucleus was seen. Further support of the cholinergic hypothesis came from the observation that drugs that block acetylcholine also blocked memory, and that choline, a food borne precursor of acetylcholine, could enhance memory in normal persons.[313]

Earlier experimental studies indicated that when the basal nucleus of Meynert was destroyed in animals it did not produce the characteristic neurofibrillary tangles and plaques seen with a typical Alzheimer's disease. But then in 1987, Dr. Gary Arendash and his coworkers found that destruction

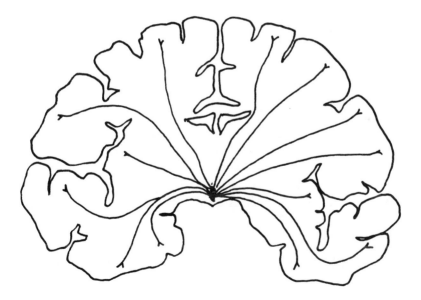

6-3 *The widespread connections of the basal nucleus of Meynert. These neurons use acetylcholine as their neurotransmitter even though the neurons within the nucleus itself use glutamate as a transmitter. It is damage to this tiny nucleus that is thought by some scientists to cause the memory loss in Alzheimer's disease.*

of these nuclei caused many of the chemical and pathological changes seen in Alzheimer's dementia.[314]

Critics previously charged that none of these experimental studies demonstrated the typical plaques or neurofibrillary tangles that were seen in virtually all cases of Alzheimer's disease. But the 1987 study demonstrated that if these same animals were allowed to survive longer than five months before they were sacrificed, neuritic plaque-like structures did indeed develop in the cortex and hippocampus, just like those seen in the Alzheimer's brain. Earlier experiments using this technique had sacrificed the animals well before this critical time. So once again we see that timing is important in the pathology of degenerative disease of the nervous system.

It appeared from these studies that a powerful case had been made that damage to the neurons that use acetylcholine for a transmitter is a key element in Alzheimer's type dementia. Based on this idea, studies were then conducted using drugs that would increase acetylcholine concentrations in the brains of patients suffering from Alzheimer's dementia. The results of these studies were disappointing, even though brain acetylcholine levels were measurably higher after the drugs were given. In some studies, memory did improve in a few of these patients but they continued to deteriorate as before.[315]

But there were problems with the theory as well. First of all, it didn't explain the selective death of glutamate neurons in the brain. In part, this could be explained by the finding that the neurons in the basal nucleus of Meynert (that controls the brain's acetylcholine system) can be destroyed by injecting powerful excitotoxins into the area. That is, these special nuclei contain glutamate-type neurons. This would explain why this nucleus is destroyed in the majority of cases of Alzheimer's disease.

There were other problems with this theory, however, that are not so easily explained. For example, it is known that in another neurological disease the nucleus of Meynert, thought to be the primary site of injury in Alzheimer's dementia, is also destroyed—yet these patients do not suffer from significant dementia.[316] Also, some Alzheimer's patients have normal levels of the enzyme CAT in their cortex.[317] Apparently the acetylcholine system plays only a part in this disease.

THE HIT MEN OF ALZHEIMER'S DISEASE

We now know that within the brain there exists a whole network of neurons that use glutamate (MSG is a sodium salt of glutamate) as their transmitter. All of these neurons were found to be excitatory. That is, they excite the brain to activity rather than calm it down. Biochemical examinations of the brains of individuals dying with Alzheimer's disease indicate that large numbers of glutamate-type neurons are specifically destroyed.[318][319] For example, in the cortex of Alzheimer's patients, over 35 to 40% of all glutamate receptor neurons are destroyed. But remember, there are three types of glutamate receptors (called NMDA, quisqualate, and kainate). Over 60% of the NMDA type glutamate receptor neurons are destroyed in Alzheimer's brains.[320]

Perhaps these specific neurons are reduced in number because most of the neurons die in the cortex as a result of this disease. But if we examine the other neuron cell types that use other transmitters besides glutamate and aspartate, we see that most remain unharmed even late in the disease. So, whatever is killing these brain cells in Alzheimer's disease, it is targeting, for the most part, very specific types of neurons—neurons that use glutamate and aspartate as a neurotransmitter.

When MSG is consumed in large doses or injected into the brain of experimental animals, we see that not all of the neurons are killed or damaged.[321] The toxic effect is very specific. The most frequently killed cells are pyramid shaped neurons (called pyramidal neurons, which are located in the deeper layers of the cortex), cells in the nucleus basalis, certain neurons of the hypothalamus, and pyramidal neurons in the hippocampus of the temporal lobes.[322] The distribution of cellular damage caused by large concentrations of MSG is very similar to that seen in human cases of Alzheimer's disease.[323]

But we also know that in Alzheimer's disease, other types of neurons are also damaged, that is, cells that use chemicals other than glutamate for their neurotransmitter. As we have seen, the cholinergic neuron (those using acetylcholine as a neurotransmitter) are also severely damaged. But these neurons make up only a small portion of the cells in the brain. Most neurons in the cortex and hippocampus affected in Alzheimer's disease use glutamate or aspartate as their neurotransmitter.[324][325]

Previously, I stated that the basal nucleus of Meynert was the nucleus of origin for most of the cholinergic neurons scattered throughout the brain. I also quoted an experiment in which this nucleus suffered destructive lesions. But what is interesting is that these experimental lesions were made using a powerful glutamate receptor toxin called ibotenic acid.[326] It is now known that this critical nucleus contains numerous glutamate receptor neurons. Other experiments have shown that when glutamate is applied to the cortex of the brain, neurons utilizing acetylcholine as a neurotransmitter within the basal nucleus of Meynert die.[327] As a result, all of the cholinergic damage seen with Alzheimer's disease could be explained by selective excitotoxin damage to this nucleus. Thus far most of the features of the disease seem to fit the excitotoxin hypothesis.

OTHER CONNECTIONS TO EXCITOTOXINS

When I discussed the other neurodegenerative diseases in the previous chapter, I stated that the final common effect of exposure to large doses of excitotoxic amino acids was the release of free radicals within the neurons triggered by the influx of calcium. A related phenomenon also triggered by calcium is the destructive outpouring of fatty acid compounds within the cells called prostaglandins. If excitotoxins are the primary cause of the neuron death seen in Alzheimer's disease, we would expect to see high levels of free radicals in these brain areas and evidence of prostaglandin activation as well.

In one study in which the brains of Alzheimer's patients were examined it was found that the areas most often affected by the disease demonstrated very high levels of these destructive enzymes and free radicals.[328] It has been demonstrated experimentally that glutamate in toxic doses can greatly increase the levels of destructive lipid products (prostaglandins) and free radicals within the cells.[329] In fact, in tissue culture experiments, vitamin E, a powerful antioxidant, can completely block the toxicity of glutamate. (This degree of protection has not been demonstrated in intact animals or humans.)

The finding of accumulation of very high levels of destructive lipid products (prostaglandin cascade) and free radical formations in the neurons exposed to high concentrations of glutamate may explain an interesting observation reported in the British medical journal, *Lancet*.[330] In this study a group of doctors examined the records of a large number of rheumatoid arthritis patients and a second population of clinically diagnosed Alzheimer's disease patients and found that the incidence of Alzheimer's disease in the rheumatoid arthritis patients was far below that expected for the age group examined. After studying a multitude of possible causes for this low incidence they concluded that the cause was a high and prolonged intake of anti-inflammatory drugs by the rheumatoid arthritis patients.

In the rare case of rheumatoid arthritis patients having Alzheimer's disease they found that almost all had discontinued taking their medications years before. We know that anti-inflammatory drugs not only reduce inflammation but do so by inhibiting the prostaglandin cascade, the same destructive reactions seen when neurons are exposed to excitotoxins. Another possible mechanism is that the anti-inflammatory drugs could help stabilize the blood-brain barrier so as to prevent toxic doses of glutamate and other excitotoxins from entering the brain.

Further evidence for the protective effect of anti-inflammatory medications comes from a recent study appearing in the journal *Neurology*.[331]

This study is even more impressive because elderly twins were used as the test subjects. What makes a study of twins so important is that it eliminates many variables that cannot be controlled for in other population studies. For example, in a twin study the subjects are the same age, they share the same early life environmental locations, the same basic nutrition, and the same exposure to toxins. But most important, they share the same genetic makeup.

In this study they found that those taking anti-inflammatory medications, either as steroids or non-steriod anti-inflammatory medication, had the lowest incidence of Alzheimer's disease. In fact, the best protective effect was seen when steroids were combined with non-steroidal anti-inflammatory medications. This doesn't mean that they took steroids regularly, but that they had taken them at one time before the onset of the disease in their twin.

The authors of the paper concluded that anti-inflammatory medications appear to delay the onset of Alzheimer's disease and may even prevent its development.

Earlier I stated that excitotoxins could stimulate the formation of free radicals within exposed neurons. It is also known that free radicals can, in turn, trigger the release of even higher levels of glutamate within the brain, resulting in even greater damage.[331] So we see that the process of destruction, once initiated, becomes self-generating.

One fact that we must keep in mind is that most studies demonstrating the toxic effect of glutamate have used it in very high doses. This is because researchers cannot wait ten or twenty years to observe the effect of prolonged exposure to lower doses. But we do know prolonged exposure of neurons to subtoxic doses (lower than needed to kill neurons) of glutamate can produce identical changes in the dendrites of neurons seen in cases of typical Alzheimer's disease.[333] Unlike most animals experiments using glutamate or asparate (which involve short exposures) with human cases of Alzheimer's disease the exposure to these excitotoxins would be expected to persist over decades—over a lifetime. This is especially true with the large number of foods now containing excitotoxin taste enhancers of various sorts and with the widespread use of aspartame. It is important to recall that excitotoxin damage is multiplied by the addition of several excitotoxins within one's diet. Glutamate plus aspartate is much more toxic than either one used alone. Many foods contain glutamate, aspartate and cysteine as hydrolyzed vegetable protein. Most diet colas contain aspartame, with a primary ingredient of aspartate.

Another piece of the evidence linking excitotoxins to Alzheimer's disease is the finding that the highest density of neurofibrillary tangles (the characteristic pathological finding in all Alzheimer's cases) is seen in the parts of the brain containing the highest concentration of glutamate-type neurons.[334] (FIG 6-4) Exposing human neurons in tissue culture to aspartate or glutamate can induce the formation of paired helical filaments similar to those seen in neurofibrillary tangles.[335] This is a very important finding because this particular structure is almost exclusively seen in neurodegenerative diseases.

The studies of Parkinson-ALS-dementia complex of Guam demonstrate that chronic exposure of humans and other primates to a plant excitotoxin (BMAA) can produce widespread damage to many parts of the nervous system.[336] Of equal interest was the finding that the final stage of the disease produced by the excitotoxin exposure depended on the concentration of the excitotoxin and the duration of exposure. For example, Spencer found that short exposures of high concentrations of the toxin most often produced ALS and Parkinson's disease, whereas more chronic exposures produced dementia.[337] This may explain why glutamate in our food (and asparate) can manifest as different diseases—ALS, Parkinson's disease or Alzheimer's dementia.

Another interesting discovery is that as our nervous system ages our

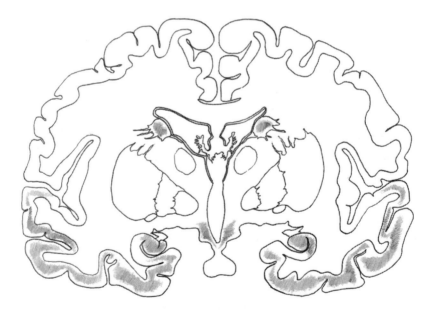

6-4 *A cross-section of the brain demonstrating those areas of the brain most sensitive to excitotoxin damage. These areas are also damaged in Alzheimer's disease.*

neurons (NMDA type glutamate neurons) have more difficulty controlling the influx of calcium into the cell.[338] This would mean that as we age our brain would become more vulnerable to excitotoxin damage. This is why the older we get the more cautious we should become about eating foods containing excitotoxins such as MSG and aspartate (NutraSweet®).

ENERGY: THE KEY TO BRAIN PROTECTION

In review, we now know that glutamate, if given in large doses, can kill neurons containing glutamate receptors. For this reason the brain must have some mechanism to protect itself from high concentrations of glutamate in the blood. It does this by the blood-brain barrier. Previously, it was thought that when this barrier system was working properly it could protect the brain from even massive concentrations of glutamate and aspartate in the blood. To some extent this is true.

The brain normally contains relatively low concentrations of glutamate and aspartate, which are used as metabolic fuels and as neurotransmitters. (Glutamate is the most common neurotransmitter in the brain.) But the concentration of these excitatory amino acids within the brain must be carefully regulated so as to prevent toxic amounts from building up around the neurons. To prevent this from happening, the brain possesses an elaborate system to prevent glutamate accumulation. It does this by using an energy dependent pump system that literally pumps excess glutamate found in the fluid circulating around the neuron into surrounding glia cells. Once in the glia cell the glutamate is deactivated by special enzymes. By carefully controlling the amount of glutamate near the neuron's glutamate receptor, the protective pumps prevent excess stimulation of the neuron. It works sort of like a thermostat in a tropical fish tank. If the water gets too cold or too hot, the fish will die. The thermostat keeps the amount of heat just right. But the thermostat in the fish tank requires electricity to operate. If the power fails, the thermostat also fails and the fish die. The energy driven pumps in the glia do the same thing, they keep the concentration of glutamate at just the right level, so that the neurons won't die.

If this protective system fails because of a lack of energy, glutamate will began to accumulate and stimulate the receptors on the surface of the cell membrane allowing calcium to pour into the cell. As a result the neuron will become overexcited. Also, excess calcium triggers a cascade of destructive reactions that can lead to cell death. Normally this protective mechanism is very efficient in keeping this from happening, but it requires large amounts of energy to operate efficiently. Fortunately, the neuron has a back-up or "fail safe" system should excess calcium enter the neuron. Once excess calcium is detected within the neuron, it will begin to pump this excess calcium back out of the cell. Normally this is a very efficient process, but it too requires large amounts of cellular energy for its operation.

So what can cause energy in the brain to fail? One of the most common causes is hypoglycemia—low blood sugar. The brain uses glucose, a simple sugar, as its primary fuel. In fact, the brain, which weighs only three pounds (2% of the body's weight), consumes over 25% of all of the glucose used in the body.[339] (FIG 6-5) Unfortunately, it cannot store energy, so when this supply of glucose is shut off, the brain quickly begins to fail. This is why some people have difficulty concentrating or they feel fuzzy-headed shortly after drinking a sweetened drink. The sudden rush of glucose causes their pancreas to secrete a burst of insulin, which in turn drives down their blood glucose. We call this rather common condition reactive hypoglycemia.

When hypoglycemia is severe and prolonged certain parts of the brain begin to die. These are the same areas of the brain destroyed when animals are fed large doses of MSG.[340] At first this seems illogical. Why should a lack

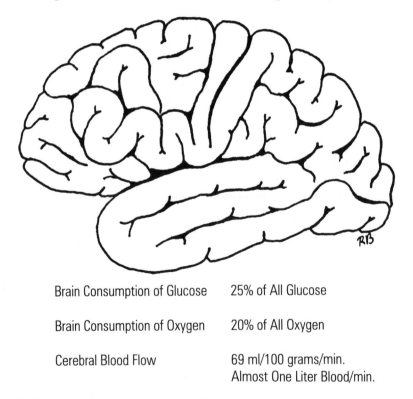

Brain Consumption of Glucose	25% of All Glucose
Brain Consumption of Oxygen	20% of All Oxygen
Cerebral Blood Flow	69 ml/100 grams/min. Almost One Liter Blood/min.

6-5 *The brain requires enormous amounts of energy to survive.*

of glucose in the brain cause the very same pattern of brain injury that is seen when large doses of a neurotoxin are given? But when you begin to appreciate the importance of energy, supplied by the glucose, in maintaining the protective systems that keep high concentrations of glutamate from accumulating around the neurons, it makes sense.

It appears that the brain damage caused by severe hypoglycemia is a result of the failure of these protective mechanisms and not from a lack of fuel to the brain cells themselves. The brain cells do not actually starve to death. If we remove brain energy using another method, such as by preventing blood from reaching the brain, or by cutting off the brain's oxygen supply, the same excitotoxin pattern of destruction is seen.[341] So it doesn't matter what the cause of the energy failure is because the result is identical—glutamate accumulates in the brain in high levels and destroys glutamate-sensitive neurons.

This hypothesis can be further tested by seeing if glucose can protect the brain from the effects of excessive glutamate. And, as expected, it works; at least partly. When rats were fed glucose plus large amounts of MSG, the amount of brain damage seen was considerably less than when glucose was denied.[342] This has also been shown in cell cultures.[343] While glucose can markedly reduce the amount of neuron damage caused by high doses of glutamate, the protection is not complete. The cells are still damaged but much less so than when glucose is absent. What this means is that chronic exposure to high levels of glutamate or aspartate will cause less brain injury when one's diet contains adequate levels of carbohydrates, but the cumulative damage over many years can still be substantial.

This energy protection also seems to exist in humans. The defenders of MSG safety frequently cite a study in which human volunteers were fed large doses of MSG combined with a mixed meal of protein and carbohydrates.[344] Only 10% developed a headache. Most were unaffected. But when the study was repeated using 14 human volunteers, this time keeping the subjects without food overnight, all developed headaches, tightness in the chest, and other symptoms of neurological toxicity related to MSG.[345] So merely going without food overnight can greatly increase the toxicity of MSG. In another study involving 1529 persons, it was found that 25% developed adverse symptoms after eating foods containing MSG.[346] Children have been reported to develop "shudder attacks," shivers, and migraine-like syndromes which stopped when MSG was eliminated from the diet.[347]

While the brain may be able to use some fatty acids for fuel to obtain its energy, the primary fuel for the brain is glucose, a type of simple sugar. The nervous system's appetite for this sugar is voracious. Under normal conditions the brain absorbs twice as much glucose as it uses.[348] This offers a large measure of protection under conditions where the brain's energy needs are greatly increased, such as with seizures and during the early stages of brain injury. But, unlike other tissues in the body, the brain is unable to store energy. When its glucose supply runs out the brain dies, or at least specific parts will. As we have seen the loss of cells under conditions of extreme hypoglycemia resembles brain damage caused by MSG.

It is known that not all areas of the brain transport and consume glucose at the same rate.[349] For example, the hippocampus has a much narrower margin between its supply and its needs than does the cerebellum. This means that when glucose supplies are low it is the hippocampus that is injured first and most severely. In fact, the cerebellum is quite resistant to hypoglycemia. We often see this demonstrated in cases of uncontrolled seizures where the brain is consuming enormous amounts of energy, frequently exceeding its glucose supply, thereby resulting in brain damage. The brain of a person dying with uncontrollable seizures consistently shows severe damage in the hippocampus but sparing of the cerebellum. So we see that the brain's supply of glucose is very critical.

It appears that the death of these cells is the result not of starvation, but rather a hypersensitivity to excitotoxins. Under such conditions of insufficient energy supply, even low doses of glutamate and aspartate can kill neurons.[350] This is because the cell's protective mechanisms require large amounts of energy to work. When energy supplies are low, excitotoxins open the calcium channels for much longer periods of time and as a result destructive reactions are triggered that will eventually kill the neurons.

It has been shown that patients with Alzheimer's disease consistently demonstrate low metabolism in certain parts of their brain, particularly in the parietal lobes and temporal lobes.[351] This has been most dramatically demonstrated with the PET scanner, which displays metabolism of the brain in living subjects.[352] It gives us an ongoing picture of the brain's metabolism during thinking, anger, sleeping, and other everyday conditions.

It may have occurred to you that the decreased metabolism is to be expected since these areas of the brain are dying. Dead and injured brain, after all, doesn't require much energy. But at least one study has shown that even before any pathological changes or clinical impairment has taken place there is substantial slowing of the brain's metabolism of glucose in these areas.[353] We also know that the brain's metabolism, as measured by PET scanning, does not decline with normal aging.[354]

Is Alzheimer's disease caused by energy failure of the brain? There is growing evidence that it plays at least a major part in the story. For the brain to receive an adequate amount of glucose on a constant basis three conditions are necessary. First, glucose must be absorbed from the intestines and enter the blood. Second, the glucose in the blood must be transported across the blood-brain barrier into the brain. And finally, the brain cells must be able to convert the glucose into usable energy, primarily ATP.

GETTING GLUCOSE TO THE BRAIN

In 1983, Dr. Gosta Bucht and coworkers, working at the Department of Geriatric Medicine at the University of Umea in Sweden made a most remarkable observation.[355] They found that out of 839 demented patients studied only sixty-three were diabetic, and none of these had Alzheimer's disease. (They all had dementia of other causes.) Statistically, you would expect at least one Alzheimer's patient to have diabetes in this age group. They then studied the Alzheimer's patients to see how they responded when given a high concentration of glucose, with a glucose tolerance test. The patient is given 100 grams of glucose as a drink, after which blood glucose and insulin levels are determined on an hourly basis for six hours. These Alzheimer's patients' responses were then compared to patients having vascular dementia (due to multiple strokes), vascular disease without dementia, and normal healthy elderly persons.

They found that Alzheimer's patients had lower fasting glucose blood levels than did the control patients, but the same insulin levels. But, following the glucose challenge the Alzheimer's patients had significantly lower glucose levels and higher insulin levels than did the control patients. The study seemed to suggest that diabetes and Alzheimer's disease never co-exist in the same patient and that Alzheimer's patients demonstrated reactive hypoglycemia.

A similar study was repeated in 1991 by Dr. Yoshikatsu Fujisawa and his associates in Japan.[356] While they did not find lower blood glucose levels in the Alzheimer's patients while fasting they did see significantly lower glucose levels and higher insulin levels after the glucose drink. And, as in the previous study, they did not see these changes in other types of dementia or in normal control patients. In this study, Dr. Fujisawa also measured the level of insulin in the cerebrospinal fluid of these individuals and found that Alzheimer's patients have significantly higher levels of insulin than was seen in dementia of other causes. These high cerebrospinal fluid insulin levels were seen even before the glucose drink was given.

So what do these findings mean? It could indicate that persons destined to develop Alzheimer's disease have an abnormal response to simple sugars in their diet, that is, they have reactive hypoglycemia. Since insulin has to pass through the blood-brain barrier it could also mean that in Alzheimer's disease this barrier is impaired. This would not only allow insulin to enter the brain but it would also allow glutamate and aspartate from the diet to enter as well.

As we have seen, when brain cells are starved for glucose they become extremely vulnerable to destruction by excitotoxins such as MSG. In fact, even normal levels of glutamate can damage energy deficient neurons. And as we have learned, a typical diet of processed foods contains enormously high levels of MSG and similar excitotoxins. Frequently, the elderly are left to prepare their own food. In today's world of prepared dinners and packaged meals it is much easier for the elderly to eat these foods than to prepare their meals from scratch. This puts them at high risk of being exposed to large amounts of food additive excitotoxins. It is important to remember that following a meal containing MSG the blood level of glutamate remains high for at least three hours. This would mean that after three spaced out meals a person's blood glutamate level would remain high all day long and well into the night. Under such conditions, this glutamate could continuously leak through the impaired blood-brain barrier, flooding the energy impaired and hypersensitive brain with extra glutamate.

THE GLUCOSE TRANSPORTER SYSTEM OF THE BRAIN

Because of the brain's voracious appetite for glucose a mechanism is needed that will continuously supply this simple sugar to the neurons. Glucose cannot simply diffuse across the blood-brain barrier, rather it has to be escorted across. The blood-brain barrier, remember, is primarily formed by tightly fitting vascular cells (endothelial cells) that excludes certain substances within the blood from easily entering the brain's interior space. Within these endothelial cells there exists a system to transport glucose to the other side of the vessel wall allowing it to enter the fluid space around the cells of the brain. This escort system, called the glucose transporter, does not require energy to operate and is very specific for glucose.[357] (FIG 6-6)

This transporter system is very efficient when you consider that the microvessels feeding the brain make up only 1% of the brain's weight yet supply glucose for the entire brain.[358] Equally impressive is the fact that the glucose transporter can deliver ten times its weight in glucose every minute. The survival of the brain is entirely dependent on this transporter system. Should it malfunction, the brain can become deficient in energy supply and ultimately die as a result.

Does this glucose transporter system malfunction in Alzheimer's disease? The answer appears to be, yes. When the microvessels from the brains of persons dying with Alzheimer's disease were examined it was found that

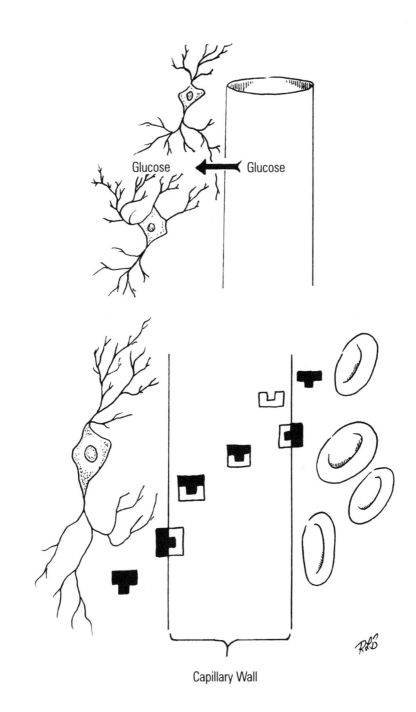

Glucose ← Glucose

Capillary Wall

6-6 *The Glucose Transport System*

they contained significantly less glucose transporter than did the micro-vessels from normal brains in persons of the same age.[359] Other studies have confirmed these findings.[360] It appears that damage to the brain's glucose transporting system is specifically related to Alzheimer's disease.

Clinical studies have shown that the degree of dementia is closely cor-related to the degree of metabolic malfunctioning of the brain's cortex.[361] That is, when glucose metabolism and energy production are impaired in specific brain regions one sees all of the typical finding of Alzheimer's dis-ease, memory loss, disorientation, etc. Once a person begins to develop severe dementia each additional decline in glucose metabolism greatly mag-nifies the degree of mental impairment.[362]

Not only is the function of the glucose transporter impaired with Alzheimer's disease but there is ample evidence that it is physically damaged as well. Doctors Arnold Scheibel, Taihung Duong and Roland Jacob studied the microvessels from Alzheimer's patients with scanning electron microscopy (this allows the researcher to examine the vessels in 3-D) and found that the capillary walls were irregularly swollen and distorted throughout their course in the brain.[363] In a large number of Alzheimer's cases they found that the capillaries looked like "swiss cheese". They con-cluded, "It is difficult to conceive that in a wall structure as physically dis-torted as this, the blood-brain barrier function could continue intact."

In another study of microvessels taken from the brains of Alzheimer's patients it was found that the capillaries were filled with a protein substance causing the vessels to be congested and distorted.[364] Yet, when the micro-vessels from normal elderly persons were examined they were found to be normal. Other studies have confirmed these findings.[365]

There is yet another bit of evidence for the failure of the blood-brain barrier in this disease, though less direct. It has been known for some time that Alzheimer's patients have a particular protein (called amyloid) within their brain tissue. This substance is not normally found within the brain and is not manufactured by it.[366] Amyloid is a large protein and under normal conditions is blocked from entry from the blood by way of the blood-brain barrier. Therefore the only way it can enter the brain is by pass-ing through the barrier, which would indicate that the barrier malfunctions in Alzheimer's disease.

There is also evidence that glutamate itself can impair the entry of glu-cose into the brain. When mice were fed high doses of glutamate and then given radioactively labeled glucose (so that it could be traced into the brain) researchers found that the glutamate lowered the amount of glucose allowed to enter the brain by 35 percent.[367] This effect appears to be dose related, that is, the larger the dose of glutamate the greater the lowering of brain glucose. At very high concentrations of glutamate brain glucose fell by as much as 64 percent.

It would not be unreasonable to conclude that in a person with Alzheimer's disease who already has impaired glucose transport, adding glutamate to their diet will only magnify the problem by further interfering with glucose transport into the brain. And, as we have seen, with Alzheimer's disease the brain is already trying to operate with severely limited energy supplies. Also, with an impaired blood-brain barrier glutamate could enter the brain freely from the diet, thereby further endangering glutamate-type neurons that have already been made hypersensitive by energy depletion. Remember, energy depleted neurons can be killed by even low doses of glutamate.

There appears to be adequate evidence that because of damaged capillary walls and depleted glucose transporter in Alzheimer's disease, the brain, in essence, becomes hypoglycemic, and it can be hypoglycemic even when the blood sugar is normal. This is important to remember because most of us would assume that if we were hypoglycemic we would have all of the symptoms that go with it, such as weakness, trembling, severe hunger, and light headedness. But if only the brain is hypoglycemic many of these symptoms, such as trembling and hunger, would be absent.

If you have ever had a severe attack of hypoglycemia you know well the feeling of confusion and disorientation that can occur. These are the same symptoms that occur with Alzheimer's disease. The difference is that with hypoglycemia (unless severe and prolonged) the symptoms are reversible once glucose is supplied to the brain.

With malfunctioning of the glucose transporter the brain would, in essence, remain hypoglycemic for extended periods of time. And with a defective blood-brain barrier, high levels of glutamate could enter the brain and damage glutamate sensitive neurons. Also, in the face of low brain energy supplies these neurons would be even more sensitive to excitotoxin damage and eventual death.(FIG 6-7) With the normal three meals a day and frequent MSG-tainted snacks and aspartate sweetened drinks and desserts, blood glutamate levels can remain dangerously high. The importance of prolonged elevations of blood excitotoxin levels was demonstrated in the experiments of Eugene Toth and Abel Lajtha, who studied the effects of chronic administration of several amino acids on brain levels of these supposedly "excluded" substances.[368] They found that by keeping blood levels of glutamate and aspartate elevated in rats, brain levels of these excitotoxins could be increased as much as 30 to 60 percent. This is a significant increase, especially under conditions where neurons are made energy-deficient. They concluded from their study that while the brain is able to exclude certain

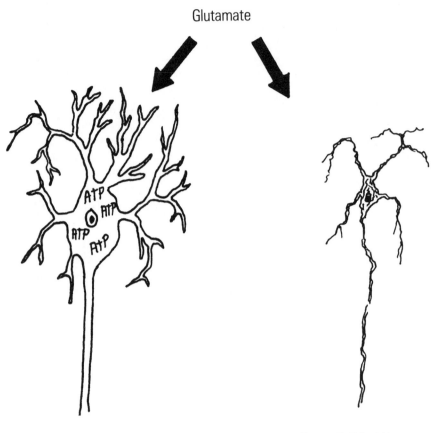

Glutamate

Abundant ATP   Energy Deficient Neuron

6-7 *When neurons have abundant energy supplies, they are very resistant to glutamate toxicity. But when energy deficiencies exist the neurons become vulnerable even at low doses.*

amino acids when elevated for short periods of time, it cannot when these amino acids are elevated for long periods of time, as would be the case when excitotoxin taste enhancers are added to foods and drinks. It is important to note that this study was done in animals having a normal intact blood-brain barrier.

DEFECTIVE ENERGY PRODUCTION IN ALZHEIMER'S NEURONS

Thus far we have seen that there are conditions associated with Alzheimer's disease that impair the delivery of energy-giving glucose to the brain. We have also seen that in the case of Parkinson's disease metabolic energy defects have been identified within the specific neurons responsible for this disease.[369] Similar findings have been demonstrated in the case of Alzheimer's disease. For example, there is evidence that one important energy enzyme within the mitochondria (called cytochrome oxidase) is deficient in the brain tissue of most Alzheimer's patients studied.[370] The enzyme deficient in Parkinson's disease is called Complex I and the deficiency in Alzheimer's disease is of complex IV. Both enzymes are part of the electron transport system which generates most of the ATP energy molecules in the cell.

In 1985, Doctor Kwan-Fu Rex Sheu and his coworkers demonstrated that there is another important energy producing enzyme deficient in Alzheimer's disease.[371] This vital energy enzyme (called pyruvate dehydrogenase) was not only deficient in badly damaged areas of the brain but was extremely deficient in areas of the brain that appeared normal as well. It appears that this deficiency is an enzyme defect seen in all brain cells. But why would the equally energy starved neurons within other areas of the brain be spared?

The difference appears to lie in the fact that they contain very few glutamate-sensitive neurons whereas the hippocampus, which is severely damaged in Alzheimer's disease, contains one of the highest densities of glutamate receptors in the entire brain.[372] It is glutamate overstimulation that causes the energy deficient neurons to be damaged in the first place.

Some critics have charged that one would naturally expect enzymes to be deficient in areas of severely damaged brain based purely on the fact that the cells have been damaged. But beside the fact that normal nonglutamate sensitive brain neurons also have very low concentrations of the enzyme, even the severely damaged cells still have normal levels of the other mitochondrial enzymes.[373] Therefore it is not a general effect of neuron damage, but rather a specific and, possibly, primary cause of the energy failure of the neurons.

There is also evidence that the defective energy producing enzymes are not only found in brain cells but are seen in other body tissues as well.[374] In fact, over forty studies have reported such defects in Alzheimer's patients.[375] A recent study has disclosed another interesting deficiency in cellular energy production in Alzheimer's patients. In this study it was found that neurons from the brains of patients dying with Alzheimer's disease were deficient in three particular types of energy-producing enzymes that are dependent on thiamine (vitamin B1) for their normal operation.[376] (These enzymes are called pyruvate dehydrogenase complex, transketolase, and ketoglutarate dehydrogenase complex. Vitamin B1 is attached to these enzymes and acts as a co-enzyme or helper.)

These researchers studied several regions of the diseased brains and found that all three of these enzymes were dramatically reduced in all areas of the brain but were so low as to be almost undetectable in the temporal lobe, the area of the brain most affected by Alzheimer's disease. Again, these enzymes were also extremely low in areas of the brain unaffected by Alzheimer's cellular injury, ruling out the possibility that the enzymes were low because of the injury itself.

A loss of these three vital energy-producing enzymes correlates well with the observed decrease in the brain's oxidation of glucose seen with studies done on individuals with the disease.[377] This is not to say that vitamin B1 can reverse the effects of this energy loss, because evidence so far indicates that feeding large doses of this vitamin to patients with Alzheimer's disease is of little benefit. Apparently the injury to these enzymes is more serious than that seen with vitamin deficiencies alone.

There is one other interesting finding regarding these three enzymes. It has been shown that when they are deficient the normal metabolism of glutamate and its precursor, glutamine, is also deficient.[378] This could possibly lead to an accumulation of dangerous levels of glutamate in the brain.

It is known that patients with Alzheimer's disease in its early stages have a high rate of brain glucose metabolism in certain regions of the cortex. This would further confirm the finding of enzyme deficiencies within the energy production system of neurons, since such defects would cause more glucose to race through the impaired energy cycle in a effort to produce more energy. Similar hypermetabolism has been shown to occur in patients with Parkinson's disease.

We have seen that in the face of low neuron energy levels (while the neuron is exposed to glutamate), the cell's protective systems will fail causing a rapid and sustained flow of calcium into the inside of the neuron. This calcium influx then triggers a cascade of destructive reactions (involving free radicals and prostaglandin products) that will eventually kill the neuron. Studies of neurons damaged in the brains of Alzheimer's patients consistently demonstrate high levels of calcium within the damaged neurons and within the plaques and neurofibrillary tangles.[379]

Remember also that experimentally we can produce the very same neurofibrillary tangles merely by poisoning the energy-producing reactions in the mitochondria. (These specific poisons block the electron transport chain stopping the production of ATP by the cell. This process is called uncoupling.) These experimentally produced "tangles" are antigenically the exact same material found in human cases of Alzheimer's disease. Further evidence of an energy deficit as the primary cause of this disease comes from the microscopic finding of distorted mitochondria within the typical plaques of Alzheimer's disease.[380]

Doctor Richard C. Henneberry and his coworkers found that when glutamate type neurons are placed in cell culture and exposed to fairly high concentrations of glutamate in the presence of both glucose and magnesium the cells remained normal.[381] But when magnesium was removed and the glucose remained the glutamate became a fairly potent toxin. When conditions were reversed, that is glucose was removed and magnesium remained, the same dose of glutamate became an extremely potent toxin. It became obvious to these investigators that when the neuron was deficient in energy production even normal to low doses of glutamate could become extremely toxic.

Thus far we have seen that there are several steps involved with energy production within the brain that are malfunctioning in Alzheimer's disease—delivery of glucose to the blood-brain barrier, transport of glucose into the brain itself, and the actual production of ATP within the neuron. I have also demonstrated that under such energy-starved conditions even low doses of glutamate can cause neuron injury and ultimately, if unrelieved, death. The same mechanism that injures the glucose transporter system also damages the blood-brain barrier itself. This could allow high levels of glutamate and aspartate to leak into the brain and spinal cord and cause widespread damage to the nervous system, ultimately resulting in one of the neurodegenerative diseases. While this scenario has not been proven, its component parts have been demonstrated experimentally and several investigators have proposed this mechanism as a major contributing cause, if not the cause, of Alzheimer's disease.[382] [383] [384] [385] [386]

At this point I want to emphasize that I am not making the claim that food borne excitotoxins are the primary and only cause of Alzheimer's disease or that by avoiding food borne excitotoxins one can totally prevent or arrest the disease. So far, the bulk of the evidence points to excitotoxins manufactured within the brain itself, in conjunction with neuron energy failure, as the primary culprit in this disease. But, high levels of dietary excitotoxins, such as MSG and asparate, could greatly aggravate the condition and cause it to progress more rapidly. And it may be that some cases of the disease are precipitated by glutamate and other excitotoxins in the diet. For example, elderly persons having had strokes and hypertension would be at great risk of developing brain damage from food additive excitotoxins. This remains to be proved.

We do know, for example, that glutamate can damage the mitochondria of neurons and that it can produce the very same plaques and neurofibrillary tangles seen with Alzheimer's disease. Also, as I have shown, glutamate circulating in the blood has been demonstrated to impair the passage of glucose into the brain. This would make the brain hypoglycemic (energy starved) even when the blood sugar was normal. So eating foods high in excitotoxin additives throughout the day could produce a condition that would make the brain vulnerable to even low doses of glutamate.

FAILURE OF THE GATEKEEPER: THE BLOOD-BRAIN BARRIER

One of the primary arguments that the defenders of the excitotoxic food additive industry make is that the brain is protected from glutamate and aspartate by the blood-brain barrier, and therefore they pose no danger to the brain. But, as I have cited above, it has been shown that this protection appears to exist only with short-term exposures to high blood concentrations of glutamate and aspartate. Experimentally, it has been shown that with prolonged exposure to high blood levels of glutamate and aspartate these excitotoxins do seep past the blood-brain barrier and enter the brain.[387]

Under normal conditions most people are exposed to multiple foods and drinks containing MSG, hydrolyzed vegetable protein, and aspartate due to the widespread use of these taste enhancers by the food industry. In addition, we consume these foods and drinks all day long (as snacks as well as meals) and with each dose of glutamate the blood level of these excitotoxins rises for many hours afterwards. This constant barrage of the brain's gatekeeper by excitotoxins means that a significant amount could enter the brain and spinal cord.

We must also raise the possibility that a certain number of individuals will be unable to metabolize glutamate normally, as we saw in the case of ALS. These individuals would develop enormous blood levels of glutamate following a meal containing MSG or aspartate. And these high glutamate levels would persist for many hours, so that their nervous systems would be assaulted by glutamate levels much higher than is normally seen.

Alzheimer's patients, most of who are elderly, will frequently have areas of small strokes (silent strokes) that may not be noticed by the individual or their family. These tiny strokes may act as ''holes'' in the barrier which can allow excitotoxins from the blood to seep past the gatekeeper and diffuse widely throughout the brain. Again, large amounts of excitotoxins in the diet would be expected to significantly raise the concentrations of glutamate and aspartate in the blood and increase the risk that they would enter the brain. If this mechanism exists, as has been shown in a several experiments, then adding MSG, hydrolyzed vegetable protein, and other excitotoxins to the food would be fool hardy and irresponsible.

I asked a prominent neuroscientist doing research with excitotoxins the following questions: What if it could be shown that the blood-brain barrier was defective in Alzheimer's patients? Would that significantly strengthen the case for dietary excitotoxins as a contributing cause for the neurodegenerative diseases? His unequivocal answer was, "Yes."

On this basis, I began to search the medical literature for answers to this vital question. Initially, I expected to find very little on this subject, but to my surprise I found enough to at least partially answer these questions. There is, as yet, no firm consensus on this proposition.

Dr. William M. Pardridge concluded, after a study of the effects of aging on the blood-brain barrier, that indeed there are changes in the neurons, astrocytes, and blood vessels that may adversely effect the brain's gatekeeper.[388] In a separate study, Dr. I. Elovaara and coworkers, found that Alzheimer's patients had consistently higher spinal fluid concentrations of IgG, transferrin, and albumin.[389] These are all large proteins usually not seen in the spinal fluid in high concentrations, which would indicate that the gatekeeper had failed to keep them out.

Drs. Arnold B. Scheibel and Taihung Duong found, in their study of Alzheimer's patients, that 90% demonstrated structural changes in their brain capillaries consistent with an altered blood-brain barrier.[390] Interestingly, these changes were not seen throughout the brain but only in those areas that were known to be effected by Alzheimer's type damage. Under the scanning electron microscope they observed large numbers of holes and craters in the basement membrane, which forms an integral part of the blood-brain barrier. (FIG 6-8)

Not all investigators agree with these conclusions. Dr. K. Blennow and coworkers also studied the gatekeeper in Alzheimer's patients, but they divided the study into those with some evidence of vascular disease and those without.[391] They found that alteration in the blood-brain barrier correlated best with age-related vascular disease and not a general decline in barrier function with aging or Alzheimer's disease. The problem with this investigation was that it was based on a study of a rather large molecule, albumin, and did not test passage of smaller molecules, such as glutamate and aspartate.

Drs. William Banks and Abba J. Kastin did study smaller molecules and, indeed, found that with aging there was an alteration in the barrier that allowed their passage.[392] It has been demonstrated that as we age we develop many diseases and conditions that alter blood-brain barrier function. Hardening of the arteries, diabetes, hypertension, poor blood oxygenation, various infections, head injuries, and tumors all can alter the functioning of the gatekeeper.

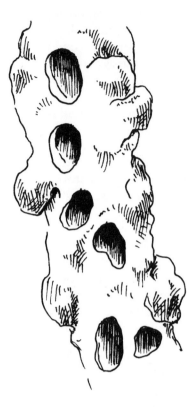

6-8 *Drawing made from scanning electron micrograph of a typical capillary from a 79-year-old woman with Alzheimer's disease. Notice the lumpy, nodular appearance and the multitude of "holes" in the wall of the vessel, giving it a "swiss-cheese" effect.*

One of the more definitive studies was conducted by Alafuzoff and colleagues who used a sophisticated immunocytochemical method to study the blood-brain barrier in both Alzheimer's patients and the aged. They found that not only was the barrier disrupted in Alzheimer's disease but it was also malfunctioning in the non-demented elderly. From this study they concluded that the blood-brain barrier is labile and can be damaged by drugs, seizures, strokes, hypertension and other factors common to many of the middle-aged and elderly.

One of the more important implications of this study is that with the blood-brain barrier being damaged in the aged, many toxins normally excluded by the barrier, including glutamate and aspartate, can now enter the brain's environment. This would mean the elderly would be at a high risk when exposed to food borne excitotoxin taste enhancers.

But if most elderly eventually develop an incompetent barrier system why don't they all develop Alzheimer's disease or one of the other neurodegenerative diseases? A good question. There are several explanations. Remember, neurons are relatively resistent to excitotoxins as long as their cellular energy-producing systems are efficient. It may be that individuals with impaired energy production are the ones more likely to develop this disease earlier. The older we get the more likely we are to develop Alzheimer's disease. After age 85 years more than 40% will develop the disease. Advancing age may be associated with impaired brain energy production, low brain magnesium levels, exposure to other toxins, strokes, and nutritional deficiencies, all of which can increase vulnerability to excitotoxins.

Experimentally there are many ways to disrupt the blood-brain barrier, either totally or partially. Electroshock, blunt head trauma, heating the brain, extreme physical stress, brain infections, exposure to radiation, alkalosis, and ischemia/hypoxia, can all disrupt the barrier system.

But what about in humans? Are the results of these environmental stresses the same? In fact, it is known that throughout our lives we are exposed to many conditions that can alter the competence of the brain's gatekeeper. For example, fever or heat stroke can both increase the core temperature of the brain to such a degree that the barrier system may be temporally weakened. Infections, such as encephalitis and meningitis can alter the barrier, sometimes for prolonged periods of time. Little is known about the long term consequences of such severe infections on the gatekeeper. It is possible that it is permanently altered to certain smaller molecules, such as the excitotoxins.

Exposure to radiation can adversely effect the blood-brain barrier. This would include children receiving whole brain radiation for the treatment of leukemias. Today, with cure rates for some leukemias being over 50%, this could mean a significant number of children would grow up with impaired barrier mechanisms. Another problem seen in children is exposure to excess lead from the environment, such as old lead paint. We know that lead exposure can easily disrupt the blood-brain barrier. In fact, it is a method commonly used in laboratory experiments.

The strength of the blood-brain barrier also varies with age. It is known that at birth the barrier system is very poorly developed and that it takes many years before it reaches adult maturity. One stark example of this slow development is a condition known as "flash edema". Normally, when an adult receives a blow to the head the brain may react with a slowly developing swelling of the brain. This occurs because fluid gradually leaks across the blood-brain barrier. But in children, even up to age 16 or 17, the barrier may suddenly become unhinged so that this fluid pours across the barrier causing the brain to swell so fast as to result in rapid death. From this it obvious that the blood-brain barrier doesn't reach its full state of maturity until quite late in life. Children, therefore, may be very susceptible to the effects of these excitotoxins, especially during times when the brain's gatekeeper is impaired.

Recently, neurosurgeons have devised a method to purposely disrupt the blood-brain barrier.[393] Why would they want to do such a terrible thing? One of the basic problems with treating some brain tumors is that it is very difficult to get chemotherapy drugs across the blood-brain barrier to the tumor. It was then found that you could disrupt, temporally, the barrier by infusing hypertonic solutions into the artery feeding that part of the brain. The chemotherapy agent then could reach the tumor in high concentrations.

The problem with this method is that it leaves the brain vulnerable to all sorts of other toxins circulating in the blood, including excitotoxins. But from this we have also learned that there are probably other drugs and conditions that can also disrupt the brain's gatekeeper.

One common cause of an impaired barrier mechanism, as we have seen, is a stroke. Basically a stroke occurs when a brain-feeding artery is blocked off. As a result the part of the brain fed by this artery fails to receive oxygen and glucose. If this blockage is not relieved quickly, this brain tissue dies. But things, as so often occurs in nature, are not so simple. Surrounding this area of dead brain is a zone of injured brain, that has the potential of recovering.

But something strange happens. The pattern of brain cell death resembles that seen with the injection of large doses of excitotoxins. How can this be explained? Simple—we know that the mechanism that prevents glutamate accumulation in the brain requires large amounts of energy, and hence, oxygen. When the blood supply is marginal, these protective systems cannot work and glutamate begins to accumulate locally in very high concentrations. This causes a delayed death of these sensitive cells.

Recently, scientists have shown that the effect of strokes in experimental animals can be markedly reduced by giving the animal a substance that blocks the toxic effect of glutamate. One such substance is a drug called Nimodipine, which blocks the calcium channels in the neurons.[394] Now, if we take an animal and totally shut off the blood supply to its brain, we see a pattern of brain cell death that closely resembles the effect of feeding massive doses of MSG to an animal. Nimodipine can block this toxic effect.

Should a person survive a stroke, not only will intrinsic or internal glutamate levels rise, but glutamate from the diet will also have access to the brain, since the gatekeeper has been damaged. It makes sense that persons having had a stroke should avoid MSG and other food borne excitotoxins. Some scientists will undoubtedly counter that the damage to the blood-brain barrier is short lived and would have no long term impact on oral excitotoxins. But we really have no idea what the total long termed effect of this injury will be on the barrier system, especially as regards such small molecules as glutamate and aspartate. It has been known for many years that recovery of the blood-brain barrier following various types of injuries varies with the type of injury and the size of the molecules in the blood vessels of the brain. In brain trauma even large molecules, such as albumin, may seep through such a leaky barrier for as long as three months.[395] Smaller molecules, such as glutamate and aspartate, may continue to leak into the brain's environment for much longer; perhaps for a lifetime.

Experiments in animals have shown that small zones of blood-brain barrier failure can allow excitotoxins to seep in and damage much larger areas of the brain. Millions of elderly people who have had mini-strokes are at particular danger because of the holes created in the blood-brain barrier system, which can then allow noxious substances to seep into the brain, such as glutamate and aspartate.

It is obvious that as we age our brain is assaulted by many diseases, injuries, and disruptions that leave us more vulnerable to excitotoxin damage. It appears that the very young and the elderly are at greatest risk. But, it is possible that decades of assault by these food additive toxins throughout our lives, such as MSG, results in much of the damage that is eventually seen, such as dementia.

Recently, scientists have isolated a group of excitotoxins, primarily cysteine, that can penetrate a perfectly healthy blood-brain barrier. Cysteine is now being added to some bread dough.

More evidence for the passage of so-called restricted substances past the blood-brain barrier exist. For example, it is accepted that most metals are restricted from entering the brain by the gatekeeper. But calcium in elevated concentrations will eventually get past this barrier as well.[396] So there appears to be substantial evidence that the blood-brain barrier does indeed fail in the case of Alzheimer's disease. While there still exists controversy about the gradual failure of the blood-brain barrier with normal aging, there is some compelling evidence there as well.[397]

If this turns out to be true, then the elderly and the very young, will be at extreme risk of brain injury from excitotoxin additives in the food. Remember, the brain (because of the damaged barrier system) will be assaulted by high concentrations of glutamate and aspartate in the blood for many years, even decades. The damage that occurs will be slow and accumulative. This would be consistent with what we see in the case of all neurodegenerative diseases.

DOMOIC ACID: MUSSEL MADNESS

Occasionally nature provides us with opportunities to observe phenomenon otherwise seen only under experimental conditions. Such an opportunity occurred in late November of 1987 when the Canadian Health Agencies of New Brunswick and Quebec received reports of three persons who had developed a strange neurological illness.[398] In each of the three cases the victims developed disorientation, confusion, and memory loss within twenty-four hours of eating mussels.

Soon more cases were reported and before the event ended in December of 1987, some 107 cases had been reported.[399] In most instances the symptoms were limited to gastrointestinal complaints such as nausea and vomiting, abdominal cramping, and diarrhea. In many of these cases the symptoms were severe enough to require hospitalization. But a third of the cases developed serious neurological symptoms within one to forty-eight hours of eating the mussels.[400]

The neurological symptoms included mutism, seizures, purposeless chewing and grimacing of the face and emotional lability such as uncontrollable crying and aggressiveness. Seven of the victims lapsed into a coma. A study of those less affected by the poisoning found that most suffered from a loss of recent memory.[401] But surprisingly, these individuals retained normal cognitive functions. They could perform mathematical computations, use logic, and think. The more severely affected individuals had great difficulty learning verbal and visuospatial test material and had extremely poor delayed recall on memory tests.

While many of these symptoms were related to toxic reactions in the brain, there were also signs that it was affecting the spinal cord as well. All of the victims were found to be very weak and had difficulty with their balance.[402] Most of the weakness was in the lower parts of the legs. In many ways it resembled the clinical presentation of ALS.

Further studies using the PET scanner to evaluate the brain's metabolism of glucose, indicated that those with memory deficits had low metabolism within the hippocampus.[403] In addition, they found impaired metabolism in the amygdaloid nucleus, which would explain the aggressiveness and emotional lability in these patients. Severe memory loss correlated well with the degree of impaired brain metabolism within the hippocampal lobes. Interestingly, no structural damage caused by the toxin was seen on the CT scans of these same patients. This would indicate that the damage was on a cellular level.

Four of these patients died, which gave investigators an opportunity to study the pathological changes caused by the poison. Microscopic examination revealed a severe loss of glutamate-sensitive neurons in the hippocampus and amygdaloid nucleus.[404] It was obvious to other researchers that the pattern of neuron loss was identical to that seen when kainic acid is given to experimental animals.[405] (Remember, kainic acid, a power excitotoxin, reacts with non-NMDA type of glutamate receptors.)

The unanswered question was what was the toxin that made these people so sick and destroyed their memories. At first researchers assumed the causative agent was a shell fish toxin. But further investigation clearly indicated that some entirely different toxin was at fault. When the involved mussels were examined it was found that their digestive systems were clogged with a particular type of diatom (algae), called *Nitzschia pungens forma multiseries*.[406] Analysis indicated that this particular algae contained large amounts of a known excitotoxin called domoic acid.

But why weren't more people affected? After all, tons of Canadian mussels were being consumed in Canada and the United States every year. As chance would have it, there happened to be an extensive bloom of this one particular diatom from November to December of 1987, and it occurred only along a 450 meter strip of the Cardigan river estuary off of Prince Edward Island.[407] These cultured blue mussels fed primarily on these diatoms.

Domoic acid is of particular interest because its chemical structure is very similar to that of glutamic acid.[408] But, unlike glutamic acid, it reacts only with the kainate type of glutamate receptor. (Kainate is isolated from a family of algae known as *Digina simplex*.) Domoic acid is very resistant to heat so it is not inactivated by cooking. While it kills the same types of neurons, domoic acid is two to three times more powerful than kainate and thirty to one hundred times more powerful than glutamate as an excitotoxin.[409]

Domoic acid has other properties it shares with glutamate. They are both better absorbed from the gastrointestinal tract of rats than primates such as monkeys.[410] But, when domoic acid enters the blood stream it is just as toxic in monkeys as rats. Based on the structure of domoic acid (being chemically similar to glutamate) one would predict that it should not pass through the blood-brain barrier. But it does!

Some have hypothesized that, like glutamate, it enters the protected brain by way of the periventricular areas that are known to have a poorly developed barrier system. If this were true then it would mean that gluta-mate would also seep into the so-called "protected" brain and do harm. Being a weaker toxin, the damage from glutamate would be subtler and more prolonged than that seen with acute domoic acid poisoning.

Others have suggested that the damage to these "deep structures" was due to seizures caused by the domoic acid.[411] There are two problems with this idea. First, if true it would mean that domoic acid (and perhaps glutamate as well) penetrates the cortex of the brain and causes the neurons to be stimulated, resulting in a seizure. The defenders of glutamate safety could never allow this. Second, it is interesting to note that out of the fourteen sickest victims, only five developed seizures.[412]

So this theory would not explain the damage in the remaining nine patients. The most likely explanation is that domoic acid does indeed penetrate the blood-brain barrier, which would mean that glutamate and aspartate may as well.

Research with domoic acid has turned up another interesting property. It was found that subtoxic doses of domoic acid when combined with subtoxic doses of aspartate and glutamate can produce severe damage to neurons.[413] We also know this to be true with other excitotoxins. Their toxic effect is magnified greatly when they are combined.

There is one final interesting observation from these cases. It is interesting that in general older individuals seemed to be more severely affected than younger people. Several explanations are possible. The author of the study suggested that one common denominator was impaired renal function in those most affected by the toxin, causing the toxin to appear in higher plasma concentrations.[414] While this is certainly a possibility, I would offer a different explanation. The most severely affected people were in their late seventies and eighties, an age in which you would expect silent strokes to occur. This was confirmed on some of the CT scans. Also, we know that with aging the blood-brain barrier loses its competence (becomes leaky) as a barrier, especially to smaller molecules. This would allow the domoic acid access to the brain's interior in these older individuals, and not in the younger victims. Remember, two-thirds of those who were sick did not have neurological symptoms; most were in the younger age groups.

What these cases demonstrate is that glutamate-like molecules can enter the brain and cause severe damage to glutamate neurons; that the worst damage occurs in individuals in the older age group, suggesting that the blood-brain barrier loses competence with age; and that an excitotoxin can damage the hippocampal lobes in humans causing a loss of recent memory.

MAGNESIUM AND ALZHEIMER'S DISEASE

Important to the discussion of Alzheimer's disease is a consideration of nervous system magnesium levels. We know from chapter two that magnesium plays a central role in the NMDA-type of glutamate receptor. It is also known that magnesium plays a critical role in the functioning of over three hundred enzymes, many of which play an important part in energy production. There are many facets to the story of magnesium and the protection of neurons.

FREE RADICALS AND MAGNESIUM DEFICIENCY

There are many serious problems caused by magnesium deficiency. It has been recently demonstrated that low magnesium levels can not only magnify free radical damage, but can also precipitate the production of free radicals as well.

In one study utilizing cell cultures of epithelial cells, it was found that low magnesium levels in the culture medium increased the levels of free radicals in these cells by two fold.[415] When these cells were examined microscopically, it was found that 95% of the low magnesium cells had died, whereas only 55% of the cells grown in normal amounts of magnesium died.

In a second part of the experiment, cells were tested for intracellular damage when free radicals were added to the culture. It was shown that cells grown in low magnesium media were twice as susceptible to free radical damage as were cells grown in normal amounts of magnesium. That is, magnesium deficiency greatly magnifies the effects of free radical damage, increasing the amount of free radicals being formed within cells and then doubles their damaging effect when they do develop.

Glutathione peroxidase is a vital free radical neutralizing enzyme found within all cells, including neurons. While this experiment measured only the effect of low magnesium on epithelial cells, it can be safely assumed that the same effect would occur with neurons. When these cells were tested for glutathione content it was found that cells grown in low magnesium conditions had slightly low glutathione levels. But of more interest was the finding that when free radicals were added to the low magnesium cell culture the glutathione levels fell much more rapidly, making the cells infinitely more susceptible to free radical damage.[416] Remember, a fall in the glutathione levels of the cells within the substantia nigra appears to be one of the earliest findings in Parkinson's disease.

A similar study was conducted using the red blood cells from hamsters fed low magnesium diets.[417] In this study it was shown that the RBCs were much more susceptible to free radical damage when the serum magnesium levels were low. Vitamin E was found to add significant protection against this damage in the magnesium deficient animals. One interesting observation was that low magnesium appeared to alter the fluidity of the cell membrane, thus making it more susceptible to destruction and changing its permeability. This effect was caused by a significant reduction in the content of a vital membrane lipid (sphingomyelin) apparently caused by the magnesium deficiency.

It has been shown by several investigators that rats deprived of magnesium may develop an acute metabolic encephalopathy; in other words, they can have widespread injury to their brains.[418] This occurs when the spinal fluid magnesium and brain magnesium levels are very low. Chutkow has shown that replacing this lost magnesium is a slow process. In rats it takes thirty minutes for injected magnesium to correct spinal fluid magnesium levels and even longer for brain levels to correct. For example, it took one to two hours for the cortical and cerebellar levels to return to normal, and four to six hours for the deep brain structures and brain stem magnesium levels to return to normal.

It should be remembered that correction of magnesium deficiency in other body tissues by taking magnesium supplements can take as long as six months to be completed.[419] So dietary correction of magnesium deficiency can be a very slow process.

But what about humans? How do they react to low magnesium levels? There is evidence that similar neurological problems do occur in humans. For example, one journal article reported the case of an elderly lady who had taken diuretics for hypertension.[420] As a result her serum magnesium levels became very low. She was admitted to the hospital with severe weakness and quickly developed an overt psychosis with paranoid delusions. She completely recovered within twenty-four hours following injections of large doses of magnesium. No other abnormalities were found to explain her condition.

THE MYSTERIOUS CASE OF THE SICK FOOTBALL PLAYERS

It was purely by accident that I came upon the next, most interesting, case report in the medical literature. But it plays an important part in this story. The incident involved eleven young football players and was investigated by the FDA.[421] According to the article the boys' coach became concerned because of their frequent complaints of leg cramps, so he gave them a supplement containing calcium. It was a hot south Florida day and the boys were playing very hard. Soon after half-time eleven of the boys became disoriented and had difficulty walking. The coach noticed that their speech was slurred, they complained of muscle spasms, and were breathing very deeply. Within an hour, eight of the players fell to the ground and had a full blown seizure. Two of the boys had repeated seizures.

It was noted that those having the worst symptoms were the players that had been practicing the hardest. Thirteen other players reported headaches, blurred vision, muscle twitching, nausea, and weakness. Eventually all of the boys recovered.

An analysis of this most interesting incident indicated several important features common to all of those affected. They all had dietary evidence of a low calcium and low magnesium diet; fast-foods consisting mainly of carbohydrates and fats, and sodas containing phosphoric acid. It was hypothesized that the low calcium stimulated the release of excess parathyroid hormone. This hormone drives calcium as well as magnesium into the bone. When the boys took the calcium supplement, the excess calcium, along with magnesium from their blood, was driven into the bone. Since they were already magnesium deficient, the additional magnesium lost into the bone was enough to precipitate the "crisis".

But how does the magnesium produce the neurologic symptoms? One possible mechanism is the hyperactivation of the glutamate system in the face of low magnesium. We know that low magnesium levels can allow even normal levels of glutamate and aspartate to be toxic. There is a good chance that the fast food the boys had eaten contained significant amounts of glutamate and aspartate or even other excitotoxins. Under the conditions of heat exhaustion that would occur after playing a vigorous game of football in the south Florida heat, we can surmise that the boys' blood-brain barriers were at least temporarily and partially disrupted. This would allow the excess dietary excitotoxins to enter their brains.

What makes these cases especially interesting is that the neurologic syndrome produced closely resembles domoic acid poisoning described earlier.

Grass Tetany: The Case of the Drunk Livestock

The condition seen in the young football players closely resembles a disorder seen in veterinary medicine. It has been known for some time that when some farm animals are first allowed to begin their spring feeding on grasses and clover, they will shortly afterward began to wander around as if they were drunk.[422] Closer examination shows that their muscles go into spasm, they salivate, and breath very rapidly, especially when they are handled or exposed to noises.

It has been found that all of these animals suffer from a common problem, low serum, and especially, spinal fluid magnesium levels.[423] If the magnesium deficit is not corrected the animals will continue to seizure and eventually lapse into a coma and die. Magnesium supplements fed to the animals throughout the winter months will prevent the illness.

The mechanism of the disorder in the animals appears to be identical to that seen in the football players. During the winter months these animals are fed diets that are low in magnesium. In the spring they are allowed to feed on grasses and clovers that are low in magnesium and high in calcium. The calcium precipitates a further dip in the animal's tissue magnesium triggering the toxic reaction.

Consistently, researchers have found that areas with a high incidence of grass tetany have soils that are high in calcium and low in magnesium.[424] For example, Michigan has an especially high incidence of grass tetany where as its neighbor, Wisconsin, has a very low incidence. The soil, and hence the grass and clover, in Michigan is high in calcium and low in magnesium, whereas the soil in Wisconsin is high in magnesium. Magnesium appears to be the key element involved in both human disease and the animal disease.

It is interesting that chemical studies of the brain's of people dying from Alzheimer's disease consistently shows they have very low levels of magnesium within the effected neurons as compared with normal brains.[425] It has also been shown that Alzheimer's patients have especially low magnesium levels within their hippocampal tissue, an area consistently damaged in this disease.[426] What is especially important is that the total brain magnesium may be normal while localized areas damaged by the disease show magnesium depletion. Similar low levels of magnesium within the affected neurons have been seen in ALS as well.

ALUMINUM AND MAGNESIUM ABSORPTION IN THE BRAIN

It is known that affected brain neurons in Alzheimer's disease have significantly higher levels of aluminum than normal neurons.[427] It is also known that these same neurons have very low concentrations of magnesium.[428] It has been proposed that these lower magnesium levels may result from poor dietary intake, impaired absorption of magnesium from the gut, or the use of drugs that deplete the body's magnesium. These are all conditions that are commonly seen in the elderly. It is also known that aluminum directly impairs the function of magnesium requiring enzyme reactions, many of which catalyze energy production in the cell.[429] Aluminum is also known to inhibit the enzymes involved in producing the neurotransmitter acetylcholine, which is important in memory functions of the brain.[430]

Recently it has been proposed that the dementias result from magnesium depletion rather than the direct toxic effect of aluminum. It is known that severe neurological syndromes (encephalopathies) can result when other conditions cause extremely low levels of brain magnesium. It can be seen with chronic use of diuretics, something millions of people do to control high blood pressure. These neurologic conditions can present as seizures, delirium, coma, mutism, or psychosis. They are quickly reversed by administering large doses of intravenous magnesium.[431]

Magnesium brain levels can also be extremely low even when plasma magnesium levels are normal. This occurs when the brain is exposed to toxic metals.[432] It appears that the metals compete for magnesium entry into the brain cells. This is why measuring the blood magnesium level is not always an accurate way to determine brain magnesium levels.

Experimental studies indicate that magnesium deficiency can significantly interfere with complicated maze learning in the aged rat.[433] Treatment of these deficient rats with magnesium restores normal maze learning. We also know that magnesium is depleted within the hippocampus of patients with Alzheimer's disease.[434] It is the hippocampus that controls memory.

But why would brain levels of magnesium be low when the rest of the body and plasma have normal amounts of magnesium? Dr. J. Leslie Glick has recently proposed a very clever answer to this intriguing question.[435] He has proposed the idea that there are two types of albumin. One that has great difficulty getting through the blood-brain barrier, and another that can pass relatively easily. Normally, the altered form of albumin is in short supply, but in Alzheimer's disease it increases to much higher levels. This altered form easily and preferentially combines with aluminum.

Normally magnesium is bound to this altered form of albumin, but in Alzheimer's disease aluminum displaces the magnesium and changes the conformation of the albumin molecule so as to make entry into the brain easier. As a result aluminum prevents magnesium from entering the neuron. This produces a condition in which the brain suffers from magnesium depletion while the rest of the body has normal magnesium levels. (Selective brain deficiency of magnesium.)

While thus far this is purely theory there is growing evidence that it may indeed be true. If it is, then a case can be made for recommending dietary supplementation with magnesium and rigorous control of aluminum intake. There are several conditions in which magnesium deficiency is common. These include alcoholism, chronic diarrhea, renal disease, chronic use of diuretics, diabetes, and it is commonly seen in a high percentage of patients undergoing cardiac surgery.[436]

There is another interesting piece of this puzzle that bears mentioning. It has been found that not only is aluminum bound to albumin but that it can form a complex with glutamate that can easily pass through the blood brain barrier.[437] If aluminum passes through the blood-brain barrier as a glutamate complex one of the first places it will go, according to Deloncle and Guillard, is the regions using glutamate as a transmitter, the cortical association areas, the amygdala and the hippocampus—areas known to be sites of primary damage in Alzheimer's disease.

The authors of the study propose a different mechanism of neuron death than excitotoxicity, but their study demonstrates another way for dietary glutamate to pass through even an intact blood-brain barrier. From what we know so far it is reasonable to conclude that many systems can be altered by aluminum binding and magnesium insufficiency in the brain. Aluminum can cause energy deficits in neurons thereby making them much more sensitive to excitotoxin attack. Magnesium deficiency can increase free radical formation which will stimulate further glutamate release from surrounding glia cells. This excess glutamate can generate even more free radicals which eventually will destroy the neurons. Also low magnesium magnifies the toxic effect of glutamate on the NMDA type receptor.

So we see that low magnesium can have a devastating effect on neuron function and if uncorrected can lead to cell death.

CONCLUSION

Magnesium appears to play a vital role in the neurodegenerative diseases. From experimental studies we know that it is critical at many levels of the cell's physiology. It is intimately involved in over three hundred enzyme reactions, from energy production to protein synthesis. As we have seen, in some cells low magnesium can increase free radical formation and increase the cells vulnerability to free radical attack. Free radicals appear to play a major role in the neurodegenerative diseases. It is also known that the excitotoxins can stimulate the release of free radicals and that likewise free radicals can stimulate the release of glutamate, precipitating a vicious cycle. All of these reactions damage cells, including neurons, and can eventually produce cell death.

CYSTEINE: ANOTHER CANDIDATE FOR NEURODEGENERATIVE DISEASES

In 1967 doctors described an infant who rapidly developed severe mental retardation, blindness, spastic paralysis of all four limbs, and shrinkage (atrophy) of the cerebral hemispheres of the brain. At age two and one-half years the child died. It was found that all of the child's tissues were deficient in a critical enzyme, cysteine oxidase, used in metabolizing L-cysteine. As a result, an abnormal metabolite of L-cysteine called cysteine-S-sulfate, accumulated in the child's nervous system. When cysteine was injected into infant rats it was found to cause the same pattern of neuron destruction seen with high doses of glutamate or MSG.

Cysteine is one of the sulfur containing amino acids and can be manufactured in the body from two other amino acids, serine and methionine. Dr. John Olney and others found that when L-cysteine is given orally to mice in large doses it produces a pattern of brain damage identical to that of glutamate.[438] This damage is limited to the circumventricular organs having no protection from the blood-brain barrier. Based on this observation, L-cysteine was felt to be an excitotoxin.

But then they discovered something very unusual about this particular excitotoxin. When it was given in lower doses it produced a devastating neurotoxic syndrome in which there was widespread damage to the cerebral cortex, hippocampus, caudate, and thalamus.[439] Unlike the high dose, this lower concentration produced its damage at a much slower rate (4 to 6 hours). This same dose of L-cysteine was found to cause damage to the brains of developing lab animal babies when given, either orally or by injection under the skin, or to pregnant mice late in their gestation. Unlike the high dose, the lower dose easily passed through the blood-brain barrier.

The next question researchers asked was, "Will glutamate antagonist block the effect of L-cysteine, since L-cysteine appears to act on glutamate receptors?" Using such a blocking drug, called MK-801, they found that it afforded complete protection from the toxic effects of L-cysteine.[440] (MK-801 works only on the NMDA-type of glutamate receptor.) Next they tried another powerful NMDA receptor blocker, zinc. Sure enough, zinc completely blocked the excitotoxic effect of L-cysteine. Interestingly, they found that at lower concentrations L-cysteine acts via the NMDA receptor and at higher concentrations it also operates through the quisqualate type glutamate receptor, which may explain why the effects of the two doses (high or low) are so different.

L-cysteine is interesting in that its toxicity depends of the presence of the bicarbonate ion.[441] Bicarbonate is a natural buffer used by the blood to neutralize acids. The neurotoxin from the cycad seed, BMAA, is also activated by bicarbonate.[442] L-cysteine is a more potent neurotoxin than BMAA. Remember, BMAA can produce disorders identical to all three of the neurodegenerative diseases—ALS, Parkinson's disease, and Alzheimer's disease.

L-cysteine is found normally in the brain. Exactly how its concentration is controlled is unknown. But we do know that it can pass freely through the blood-brain barrier, which makes it an especially dangerous environmental toxin. **Some bread manufacturers are adding L-cysteine to their dough.**

Recently, Dr. M. Thomas Heafield and coworkers made a remarkable and vital discovery.[443] They examined a carefully selected group of patients having either Parkinson's disease, ALS, or Alzheimer's disease, for the presence of abnormal metabolism of L-cysteine. They discovered that while all had the same amino acid patterns as normal controls, they had a statistically significant elevation of their cysteine to sulfate ratios.

Cysteine is a normal intracellular amino acid in the brain that functions as a donor of sulphate groups. As discussed, cysteine is quite toxic in high doses and is therefore carefully regulated by the brain. There is evidence that when it accumulates in the brain cells it can cause abnormalities in protein synthesis and the conformation (shape) of the proteins that are produced. This, Heafield says, could explain the abnormal microscopic protein bodies seen in all three of these diseases—Lewly bodies in Parkinson's disease, Bunina bodies in ALS, and amyloid proteins in Alzheimer's disease.

There is also evidence that certain chemical reactions involving intracellular metals and cysteine could generate free radicals. One of these metals is aluminum, which is known to accumulate in degenerating neurons in Alzheimer's disease and ALS.

Heafield suggests that in all three diseases there exist an inborn defect in metabolism of L-cysteine, which causes an accumulation of abnormal metabolic products. While he rejects the idea that cysteine is acting as a direct neurotoxin, it seems obvious that Dr. Olney's demonstration of the powerful excitotoxic properties of L-cysteine makes a good case for such toxicity.

WHAT DO ANIMAL STUDIES
TELL US ABOUT HUMANS?

Most of what we know about the damaging effects of excitotoxins comes from experiments on animals other than man. Many people, especially laymen, want to know what "rat experiments" have to do with human disease. This is an important question. Sometimes, because of the radical differences in human and the physiology of lower mammals, the two can not be equated.

But Dr. John Olney has shown that MSG and the other excitotoxins produce the same damage to neurons in all animals species tested—dogs, rats, mice, chickens, and even primates. And in each case, it is the same types of cells that are affected, those with glutamate receptors. There is one major difference, however, between man and animal. Humans accumulate higher amounts of MSG in their blood following a similar oral dose of MSG than does any known animal. And, it appears that human brain cells are just as sensitive to the damaging effects of excitotoxins as laboratory animals, and in some cases, even more sensitive.

It is also important to compare how the test dose of MSG was given. Was it injected directly into the brain? If so, was it a microinjection into a specific area of the brain? Remember, injection bypasses the blood-brain barrier. Such studies do tell us that should glutamate or aspartate accumulate in this particular brain region it will produce a specific injury. It is important to know the effect of oral doses of excitotoxins versus injections into the abdominal cavity. We know that MSG given orally is about 75% as effective as injected forms. But it produces the same type of neuron damage. (Animals will consume enough glutamate as MSG orally to produce the same brain lesions seen with injected MSG.[444])

It is also important to know the differences in species sensitivity and even differences between animals of the same species. For example, we know that some animals of the same species require higher doses of the toxin to produce the same toxic effect as a similar animal of the same weight and age. Apparently there are some differences in the ability of certain animals to resist the toxic effects of these compounds. The same is undoubtedly true in humans.

Sometimes these compounds are tested in tissue culture, where specific living cells are isolated in a media dish. While this is a far cry from how the cells will react in the intact brain, it does give us some important clues as to the mechanism of action of these poisons. A new method utilizes whole brain slices, so as to more closely resemble the intact brain. With this technique, a thin slice of, say, the temporal lobe, is placed in a special nutrient medium and tested with various excitotoxins. The importance of this method can be appreciated in a recent experiment in which it was shown that neurons alone in tissue culture are one hundred times more sensitive to MSG as when astrocytes are also present. As we have seen previously, the astrocytes, by their ability to absorb excess glutamate, are important in the protection of neurons from the toxicity of glutamate. In the whole brain, the neurons are surrounded by millions of astrocytes. This must be considered when interpreting research data.

We should also appreciate that most of these studies are short term studies. For example, a mouse tested with MSG may receive a massive dose in one single injection, or over a series of injections. While this tells us a lot about the acute effects of exposure it tells us nothing about chronic exposure seen in most humans. Even so-called long term studies rarely extend beyond a few months. What about years or even decades of exposure? There are no similar studies to date. (It can be argued that in comparative terms the length of exposure in the mouse and rat equals prolonged exposure in humans. But there still can be differences.)

That the time of exposure is important is seen in the studies in which destructive lesions were made in the nucleus basalis, considered to be central to the cholinergic theory of Alzheimer's disease. Multiple studies of this kind were considered to be a failure because none demonstrated the typical neurofibrillary tangle lesions characteristic of Alzheimer's disease. Yet, all of these animal studies used animals killed within a few weeks of the time the experimental injury was made. But when the animals were allowed to live past six weeks, all developed these characteristic "Alzheimer's" lesions. The same may be true in studies with MSG and other excitotoxins. More chronic studies are needed.

It is obvious that animal studies can never tell us everything we need to know about how certain diseases develop, but they can give us important clues. There are so many variables introduced into the lives of ordinary people that the same conditions can never be reproduced in a laboratory situation. The real value in animal studies is that we can learn how these toxins work, and possibly how to avoid their harmful effects.

One final word. Critics often attack those who seek to warn the public of the danger of excitotoxins in processed foods by quoting older studies which failed to demonstrate histologic damage in animal studies using MSG. At first I was greatly concerned by these negative experiments. But then I came across a study which pointed out that histological changes, that is changes that can be seen with a microscope, only occur with severe injury and as a late stage in the injury process. A more sensitive method would involve measuring the physiological damage to the living cell caused by low dose excitotoxins, and may not be detectable by examining the cells under the microscope. (We know that some of the negative studies were fraught with poor laboratory techniques and by workers who were looking in the wrong areas of the brain. It is now well accepted by neuroscientists that excitotoxins cause these brain lesions.)

When these same negative studies are repeated using physiological and biochemical measurements to test how these cells were actually functioning following MSG exposure, consistent severe abnormalities were seen. This is also seen in the studies on human subjects with Huntington's disease and other of the neurodegenerative diseases. For example, utilizing the PET scanner to measure the living brain's metabolism of glucose and other substrates, it has been shown that metabolic changes occur long before pathologic changes can be seen. The same is true for Alzheimer's disease.

As a result, because of the short term studies done in experiments and their reliance on crude histologic changes, these older studies fall far short of adequate methods to demonstrate the toxicity of the excitotoxins in question. It has been shown that when using lower doses of excitotoxins many of these cells are severely damaged without actually dying. But, as a result of this damage, they operate at a much reduced level of efficiency. Certainly, we want our brains to operate at peak efficiency. Also, repeated injury to these damaged neurons will eventually kill them. Unfortunately, the only experiments to demonstrate these long termed effects in humans are being conducted on you, and me, and our families by the food industry and the producers of aspartame and MSG.

WHAT SHOULD THOSE WITH ALZHEIMER'S DISEASE DO?

First of all, you must recognize that nothing doctors have tried so far has been shown to cure Alzheimer's disease or even to significantly slow its natural course. But dietary changes, especially avoiding excitotoxin food additives, has not been tried. In truth, the most sensible thing to try would be to use all that we have learned through our research and apply it to a large group of patients with early Alzheimer's disease.

One of the problems faced by those who early on advocated using chemotherapy for cancer was that all human experiments were carried out in patients with advanced cancers especially those already near death. You would not expect to see much improvement under such dire circumstances. But once chemotherapy began to be used in patients during the early stages of cancer, a definite benefit was seen. The same would be true of Alzheimer's disease. The best chance for stopping, or at least slowing down the progression of the disease, would be to use treatment soon after the diagnosis is made. Even more important would be to improve our diagnostic methods so that we can detect those individuals destined to develop Alzheimer's disease. In this way we could attack the disease long before the brain cells were irreversibly injured.

The following is a list of observations made concerning this disease that could possibly be applied to its treatment and/or prevention.

1. High levels of excitotoxins within the brain appear to play a major role in Alzheimer's disease. It is essential that individuals with a strong family history of Alzheimer's disease and those having had a stroke or high blood pressure avoid excitotoxin food additives. The simplest way to do this is to restrict foods from your diet that contain excitotoxin taste enhancers such as MSG, hydrolyzed vegetable protein, and aspartame (NutraSweet®).

2. Free radicals appear to play a major role in the ultimate damage seen with this disease. The most efficient free radical scavengers (neu-

tralizers) are found naturally in the form of certain vitamins and minerals. Among the most important of these are vitamin C, E, and beta-carotene. The minerals selenium, zinc, and magnesium also play a part in reducing free radical damage. New, more powerful, free radical scavengers are being developed by the pharmaceutical companies. They may have a more powerful effect and be better localized in the neurons that need them than naturally occurring compounds.

3. There is a suggestion that persons who take regular doses of aspirin or other anti-inflammatory drugs get Alzheimer's disease far less than those who do not. At least theoretically, there is evidence that the destructive changes triggered by excitotoxins involves the prostaglandin system, which is responsible for inflammation reactions, within the cells. Aspirin and the other anti-inflammatory drugs act by inhibiting this system.

While taking one or two aspirins a day is probably safe for those not having a history of ulcer disease, doses high enough to prevent these changes are associated with a high incidence of bleeding from the stomach. But there is an alternative. A special oil (called omega-3-fatty acids) found in the skin and flesh of fish (especially cold water fish) can have the same action as the anti-inflammatory drugs.

One way to increase the level of these oils within your brain is to eat fish at least three times a week. But it would be difficult to eat enough fish to significantly raise the brain levels of this compound. Fortunately, this same oil can be obtained from most health food stores in capsules. As far as I am aware no one has tried these types of oils as a treatment or as a preventative.

4. The blood-brain barrier is usually disrupted or "leaky" in cases of Alzheimer's disease. Since we do not know what causes the barrier to be injured it is difficult to say what needs to be done to restore its function. There is some evidence that the anti-inflammatory drugs such as aspirin, other anti-inflammatory drugs, and the omega-3-fatty acids can restore some of its function in certain conditions.

5. The brain is starved for energy for many different reasons. Glutamate in the blood can impair the entry of glucose into the brain. This is another good reason to restrict excitotoxins from the diet.

It is important that the brain receive adequate glucose from the diet. This would require that you eat plenty of complex carbohydrates and some sugars as a mixed meal. Reactive hypoglycemia usually results when simple sugars are eaten alone and especially when consumed in the liquid form, such as with soft drinks. This disorder must be treated early and vigorously. Regular exercise (not aerobics) is also important in maintaining a stable blood sugar and avoiding hypoglycemia.

The future treatment of errors in cellular metabolism appears to lie in utilizing various compounds known to bypass these damaged systems. There is some evidence, for instance, that L-carnitine, co-enzyme Q and vitamin C can bypass such energy deficits and thereby prevent damage by certain types of excitotoxins.[445]

6. Previously, I described the protective actions of magnesium on the NMDA-type of glutamate receptors. Magnesium appears to prevent excess activation of this glutamate receptor, thereby protecting the neuron from the devastating effects of sudden influxes of calcium.

Dr. J. Leslie Glick has proposed that Alzheimer's patients have a defect in magnesium transport into the brain.[446] It is known that Alzheimer's patients do have lower brain magnesium levels than do normal persons. Recent nutritional studies have shown that up to seventy-five percent of adults in the United States have a significant magnesium deficiency. This deficiency increases with age and would add to the brain's vulnerability to glutamate and aspartate, since the normal magnesium protective blockade would be impaired. Phosphate, as found in most colas, is known to deplete the body's magnesium. Children and teenagers consume enormous amounts of colas in this country and eat diets poor in magnesium.

Based on this knowledge, it would be reasonable to supplement the adults, and especially the elderly, with magnesium so as to maintain normal brain levels of this vital mineral. Several studies have indicated that the elderly frequently do not eat the vegetables or other foods that are known to be high in magnesium, such as broccoli and spinach. Experimentally, we know that neurons are many times more sensitive to the lethal effects of excitotoxins when magnesium is absent or low. Likewise, adding magnesium can greatly reduce the toxicity of these excitotoxic compounds on the brain and spinal cord. But it is also important to note that magnesium, while very effective against excessive activation of the NMDA receptor, is ineffective against activation of the quisqualate and kainate types of glutamate receptor. Also, magnesium protection is lost once the neuron is activated, such as might be the case during hypoglycemia.

Magnesium is important in preventing free radical damage and activation. It is also important in the operation of enzyme systems necessary for cellular energy production.

Zinc blockade of the NMDA receptor is not interfered with by activation of the neuron as is seen with magnesium blockade. But there is some evidence that zinc can mildly stimulate the quisqualate and kainate receptors. Zinc supplementation may represent a two-edged sword, since Alzheimer's disease involves all three types of receptors. Zinc also plays a vital role in many of the enzymes utilized by the brain for its normal function. Normally, high concentration of zinc is found in the hippocampus. I would just caution the reader to avoid excess doses in the forms of supplements. (No more than 25 milligrams twice a week.)

7. While there is as yet no proof, it makes sense that general stimulation of the nervous system should be avoided by individuals at the greatest risk of developing one of the neurodegenerative diseases, such as Alzheimer's disease, ALS, and Parkinson's disease. Caffeine is a mild brain stimulant. Seizures are known to occurs when large doses of caffeine are ingested. When caffeine stimulates the brain cells it increases their metabolism and hence demand for energy. As I have pointed out, several of the neurodegenerative diseases have been shown to demonstrate an impaired ability of the neurons to produce energy. By stressing the neurons, you could tip the scales causing the neurons to die sooner.

World wide consumption of caffeine from various sources now approaches 80,000 metric tons a year. In the United States this is primarily through coffee consumption (75%) while in Canada 60% is from coffee drinking. Teenagers the world over consume substantial amounts of caffeine from drinking colas. The average nine ounce cola contains about 30 milligrams of caffeine, which is higher than a cup of coffee. Most teenagers drink at least three or four colas a day.

Interestingly, a cup of hot chocolate contains up to 40 milligrams of caffeine and a chocolate bar about 20 milligrams. But there are a lot of sources of caffeine of which most people are not aware. For example, many headaches preparations, cold medicines, appetite suppressants, and "wake-up" pills contain varying amounts of caffeine. One brand of the latter, called "Zoom", advertises it as a "legal upper with the smooth-riding qualities of a snort of cocaine."

All nervous system stimulants, in my opinion, should be avoided by persons at high risk for developing one of the neurodegenerative diseases. The best indication of risk is the presence of at least one direct relative (especially a parent) with one of these diseases. In a society that is saturated with a multitude of brain stimulants as recreational drugs, such as cocaine, amphetamines, and designer drugs, a large segment of our population is at risk for developing these horrible diseases.

The most commonly used nervous system stimulant still remains the excitotoxin taste enhancers that have been added to our food and drink. But by adding these other stimulants you are greatly compounding the risk.

· 7 ·

Other Neurological Disorders Related to Excitotoxins

This chapter will review briefly some of the other neurological conditions associated with, and made worse by, excitotoxins. This list grows almost daily. Rather than provide an exhaustive review of the medical literature on the subject, I have touched on the major areas of research. For some of these disorders the connection to excitotoxins, especially those that are added to our food, is controversial. I shall provide the reader with citations from the medical literature from both sides of the controversy. But it is also important to keep in mind that the food industry not only paid for some of these studies, but has also hired scientists for the specific purpose of demonstrating the safety of these additives.

The fact that a study is funded by a food manufacturer is not *prima facie* evidence of guilt of wrong doing. But these studies must be viewed critically, at least to the extent that all other medical studies are, or should be, viewed critically. In some instances it can be shown that the experiment was either designed to show the desired result or did so through poor design and shoddy experimental work.

SEIZURES

Those who oppose excitotoxins used as food additives frequently cite that they can either precipitate seizures in persons known to have a history of seizures, or they can actually cause seizures. This became especially prevalent with the introduction of the artificial sweetener aspartame or, as it is better known, NutraSweet®.

Early studies demonstrated that glutamate, when injected directly into the brain, could cause seizures in animals. With the development of powerful analogs of glutamate, such as kainate, it was found that these analogs could also cause seizures whether given by injection, ingested orally, or injected directly into the brain.[447] In fact, kainate was found to induce a type of seizure, called status epilepticus, that persisted long after the drug had disappeared from the blood stream.

What was even more incredible was the finding that this excitotoxin-induced seizure could damage the brain at a distance far removed from the site of the original injury, and that this remote lesion could be prevented by cutting the fibers leading to this distant site. We know that a similar mechanism occurs in cases of human epilepsy, especially in temporal lobe epilepsy. Prolonged seizures arising in one temporal lobe will eventually produce a zone of damage in the opposite temporal lobe. This is referred to as a mirror focus.

WHAT IS A SEIZURE?

As we have learned so far, the brain is made of cells that either stimulate or suppress activity. The balance between these two systems is very carefully controlled. The inhibitory cells and their neurotransmitters prevent the excitatory cells from overreacting. As discussed, this also involves various minerals such as calcium, magnesium, and zinc. Sometimes these balancing forces are so altered that the excitatory cells are released from their inhibitory control, or even stimulated to fire excessively.

When this happens impulses are fired repetitively down the nerve fibers that are connected to these cells. This results in a seizure. The final effect of this abnormal firing of neurons depends on the function of the particular group of cells involved and on whether or not this focus of abnormal firing will spread to other areas of the brain. In many instances the seizure begins in a well defined focus of cells. In this case the seizure is defined by what anatomical and functional portion of the brain is involved. For example, seizures occurring in the temporal lobe (called temporal lobe epilepsy) can result in hypersexuality, sudden attacks of *deja vu*, or outbursts of violent behavior. Those occurring in the motor strip can cause sudden jerking of one or more of the limbs. There are a large variety of focal seizures.

Sometimes the entire brain seems to go berserk, causing its hapless owner to fall to the floor, jerking uncontrollably. These are called grand mal seizures. Actually, most grand mal seizures begin as silent seizures originating in a single focus and rapidly spread to the entire brain.

A seizure, or convulsion, as they are sometimes called, is really a symptom and not a disease in itself. It just indicates that something has gone awry within the brain. Sometimes the seizure is triggered by a small scar caused by an injury, a brain tumor, or an abnormal collection of blood vessels (called an arteriovenous malformation). Sometimes seizures are caused by metabolic derangements, such as with uremia of kidney failure, chronic alcoholism, certain vitamin deficiencies, and liver failure. Hypoglycemia, when severe, can also cause seizures. Certain of the illicit drugs can precipitate seizures, such as cocaine and amphetamines.

Whatever the cause, ultimately a focus of brain cells is produced that is very sensitive to any stimulus that can cause these neurons to fire. Epileptics may have their seizures precipitated by fever, drinking excessive water, hyperventilation, low blood sodium levels, low blood sugar, and a multitude of other homeostatic derangements.

When a seizure occurs, the brain undergoes some drastic biochemical changes. As would be expected, the brain's metabolic rate increases enormously, and with this, glucose and oxygen consumption increases to supply needed energy. Unfortunately, the oxygen delivery system is unable to keep up with the enormous demands being made by the seizuring brain. This means that the brain becomes oxygen starved and must shift its metabolism to a much less efficient energy producing system called glycolysis. As a result, lactic acid builds up in the brain and, if the seizure is not stopped, the neurons begin to die.

As we have seen before, when the brain's energy supply is deficient, it becomes much more vulnerable to the toxic effects of glutamate and aspartate. There is some evidence that glutamate plays a vital role in the neuronal damage caused by seizures.[448]

Do Excitotoxin Food Additives Cause Seizures?

This is a hotly debated subject and one that will not be settled quickly. Soon after aspartame had been approved for use as an artificial sweetener, clinical reports began to surface implicating its use in seizures, both in adults and children. But most of these reports were anecdotal. For example, in 1985 Dr. Richard J. Wurtman reported three such cases in the journal *Lancet*.[449] One case involved a forty-two-year-old secretary who developed a seizure following a practice of drinking seven liters of NutraSweet® containing beverages per day. She had no previous history of seizures. The second case was a twenty-seven-year-old computer programmer who had a single grand mal seizure after drinking 4 to 5 glasses of "Crystal Light" containing NutraSweet®. It is interesting that this patient also experienced "twitching, trembling, jerking, and hyperventilation." What makes this interesting is that it resembles the "wet dog shakes" seen when dogs are given large doses of the excitotoxin kainate. The last case was a thirty-six-year-old professor who drank one liter of ice tea sweetened with Nutra-Sweet® every day. After several days of this practice he developed a grand mal seizure.

Critics of anecdotal cases such as these counter that other mechanisms could explain the seizures. For example, water overload is also known to precipitate seizures. And this is true. But generally it requires much larger volumes of water consumption over a shorter period of time to precipitate a seizure than is seen in these cases, except perhaps the lady who swilled down seven liters a day.

Another criticism is that several of the cases attributed to NutraSweet® were in people known to have conditions that could predispose them to seizures. For example, in the last case, the professor was found to have a venous angioma in his brain. But this still does not preclude the idea that aspartic acid and other excitotoxins could precipitate seizures in these individuals. We know that these silent lesions produce a focus of hyperexcitable cells. The excitotoxins act by stimulating brain cells.

It is known that seizures may be precipitated by a number of factors and that these may act in conjunction. For example, we know that water overloading, low magnesium, low sodium, fever, and low blood sugar can all precipitate seizure, especially in those harboring silent brain lesions. When more than one of these factors are present, the chance of a seizure is greatly magnified. When excitotoxins are added in addition to these factors, one would expect the likelihood of a seizure to be even greater.

Another anecdotal case is of particular interest.[450] This case involved a fifty-four-year-old woman with no known medical problems, other than a twenty year history of depression. She had been maintained on one of the psychotropic medications for approximately five years. Without any warning, she experienced a grand mal seizure, which was followed by a profound behavioral change. Her psychiatrist categorized her symptoms as manic, that is, a state of hyperactivity of the brain. She also experienced insomnia, irritability, and agitation.

During their work-up her doctors discovered that she, for many years, drank large amounts of tea, even up to one gallon per day during the summer months. But, interestingly, she had always sweetened her tea with sugar, that is, up until two weeks before her seizure, at which time she began to use NutraSweet®. She had also gone on a weight loss diet. Her doctors stopped all of her medication and eliminated NutraSweet® from her beverages. Within four days all evidence of her manic activity stopped. When seen one year later the patient had been completely free of seizures and behavioral problems. She continued to drink large volumes of ice tea, but she used sugar rather than NutraSweet®.

This case is important, since the only variables that could explain her sudden seizure were: the recent use of NutraSweet®, the large volumes of fluid she ingested daily, and her medications. But she had been on the medication for five years without difficulty, and she continued to drink large volumes of fluid without precipitating a seizure. So the only real change in her dietary behavior was the addition of the NutraSweet®. And when it was eliminated, the seizures, as well as the behavioral problems, disappeared. It is important to note that the patient decided to use Nutra-Sweet® because of her concerns with weight gain. So, once again, we have a case of low caloric intake aggravating the toxic effect of a known excito-toxin by lowering brain energy levels.

One comment about anecdotal evidence: the scientific purists frequently discount such "evidence" as unscientific. This is so even when such cases are being reported world-wide and by different observers. And, indeed, one should approach such cases with a critical, but not, skeptical eye. Many of our medical and scientific discoveries began as anecdotal observations. What distinguished the innovators and the great men of science from their less well known peers was the ability and willingness of the former to accept anecdotal observations as valid, or at least as a starting point. Today, the scientific elitists are too quick to dismiss such accounts out-of-hand without so much as a moment's consideration. This is poor science.

In fact, it is human nature for them to react negatively when someone outside of their circle dares to suggest that they as well could make a contribution to the field. This reactionary stance is frequently seen. For example, when Linus Pauling first suggested that vitamin C had significant anti-viral activity in large dose, and later suggested that it may even retard the growth of some cancers, the scientific community reacted with shock and even anger. He was attacked and vilified in many of the most prestigious medical journals. And what is shocking is that these eminent scientists never once examined his data or attempted to test his hypothesis, at least not until much later.

The anti-viral actions of vitamin C are now well accepted after years of heated battle and denials by the scientific elitists. Also accepted, although reluctantly, is that vitamin C plays a significant role in preventing some cancers. Examples of this arrogance on the part of the scientific world abound. Now let us look at some experimental studies.

EXCITOTOXINS AND EXPERIMENTAL SEIZURES

In the early 1950's it was reported that when sodium glutamate (MSG) was injected into the cortex of dogs all developed seizures.[451] Since this early observation others have confirmed that excitotoxins can precipitate seizures in many animal species. Aspartame is known to make the EEG discharges worse in children with certain types of epilepsy.[452] The powerful glutamate analog, kainate, can, in fact, precipitate seizures when given orally. Yet, seizures are not usually seen with MSG, even in high doses, when fed to experimental animals. Likewise, aspartate, a major component in Nutra-Sweet®, has not been shown to precipitate seizures in normal experimental animals. But can the excitotoxins precipitate seizures in animals prone to develop seizures?

To test this, scientists used chemicals that are known to precipitate seizures in animals, such as pentylenetetrazol and flurothyl. Pinto and Maher found that aspartame, when given orally in doses of 1000 to 2000 milligram per kilogram, did potentiate the convulsant action of these two chemicals.[453] They also found that aspartame decreases the time of onset of seizures and increases the number of animals showing tonic-clonic convulsions when exposed to pentylenetetrazol. This was confirmed by Guiso and Garcia working in an independent lab.[454]

In another study Dailey and coworkers found that aspartame did not increase the seizure incidence in animals exposed to these convulsant chemicals.[455] It should be noted that this study was supported by a grant from the NutraSweet® Company. This is not to say that their studies are not valid. But when there is a serious difference of opinion involving several laboratory studies, one must be intellectually critical of studies funded by the company manufacturing the excitotoxin in question.

It may be that the design of the negative studies has more to do with their negative results than bias. For example, it is known that rats require twice the dose and mice seven times the dose of aspartame as humans require to produce the same increase in plasma phenylalanine. It is the rise in brain phenylalanine that is thought by some to cause the seizures. More likely is the direct excitatory effect of the aspartate itself. Phenylalanine may act to potentiate this irritability. In one study the blood phenylalanine levels rose thirty fold following a one gram dose of aspartame.

As with other excitotoxin studies, chronic exposure may play an important role in the causation of the destructive pathology known to occur with human seizures. Most of the experimental seizure studies used short-term exposure to the excitotoxin. We know that excitotoxins have a cumulative effect when given chronically, as the toxic damage accumulates with each successive dose given. One must also consider other concomitant factors, such as diet, water intoxication, and other metabolic derangements. As we have seen, some people have difficulty metabolizing certain amino acids, thereby resulting in an accumulation of toxic substances.

Roger Coulombe and Raghubir Sharma demonstrated that the rise in brain phenylalanine following aspartame ingestion was not evenly distributed throughout the brain.[456] And, they point out, that other experimental studies reporting little brain accumulation of phenylalanine were due to the method of using whole brain homogenates rather than testing individual brain regions. They found, for instance, that even with low doses of aspartame, levels of phenylalanine rose significantly in the hypothalamus, medulla oblongata, and corpus striatum, even though the whole brain phenylalanine levels were not elevated significantly.

Elevations of dopamine and phenylalanine in the brain have been associated with several known behavioral disorders including schizophrenia and seizures. This would explain the symptoms seen in the lady consuming large amounts of tea sweetened with NutraSweet®. Of equal concern is the effect on endocrine control by the hypothalamus. As discussed previously, excitotoxins play a major role in the circuits of the hypothalamus. It is also known that norepinephrine and dopamine, both produced by the metabolism of phenylalanine in the brain, play an important role in controlling the release of several pituitary hormones (vasopressin, prolactin, oxytocin, luteinizing hormone, growth hormone, and thyroid stimulating hormone).

From what we do know, it is conceivable that NutraSweet® can, in commonly consumed doses, cause abnormalities of this delicate endocrine control system, especially in the developing infant and child. As more and more foods containing NutraSweet® are added to our diets, the greater the danger to ourselves and our children grows. According to the FDA, in 1985 America consumed 3,500 tons of aspartate as NutraSweet®. Even more foods contain this excitotoxin sweetener today, and it continues to be promoted by a series of powerful advertising campaigns. With over a 100 million persons in the United States alone consuming NutraSweet® on a regular basis, these questions demand answers. And until these answers are forthcoming NutraSweet® should be banned from foods.

Magnesium and Seizures

Another piece of indirect evidence linking excitotoxins and seizures comes from the observation that magnesium raises the threshold for seizures, reducing the chances of a seizure developing.[457] Likewise, experimental studies have shown that low magnesium significantly lowers the threshold for seizure, i.e. makes them more likely to occur.

It has also been observed that the temporal lobes normally contain rather high levels of zinc. Both zinc and magnesium, you will recall, act to block the effect of excitotoxins on the special NMDA type glutamate receptors.

HEADACHES

This is the number one complaint by consumers using products containing NutraSweet®. As with seizures, the connection is hotly debated. Again, the NutraSweet® manufactures have marshalled scientific studies which disclaim a connection to headaches. And, as with seizures, much of the human connection is anecdotal. In a letter to the *New England Journal of Medicine*, Dr. Donald R. Johns reported what appeared to be a connection between a case of migraines and the consumption of large amounts of NutraSweet®-containing beverage.[458] It involved a thirty-one-year-old woman with a known history of well controlled migraine headaches, that is, well controlled until she began to drink six to eight 12 ounce cans of diet cola sweetened with NutraSweet®, 15 tablets of aspartame and other foods containing aspartame (approximately 1000 to 1500 mg) daily. Approximately two hours after ingesting the drinks she noticed stomach upset and a throbbing headache.

When she was taken off of dietary aspartame she noticed a significant improvement in her headaches, which eventually disappeared altogether. To make sure that it was the aspartame that was precipitating her migraine headaches, her doctor challenged her with a solution containing 500 mg of pure aspartame, after which her headache reappeared within one and one-half hours.

In 1987 Dr. Susan S. Schiffman and coworkers conducted a study at Duke University to see if aspartame could indeed precipitate headache. They used 40 subjects who had on several occasions reported headaches following aspartame ingestion.[459] She found that the incidence of headaches in those taking the aspartame was essentially no different from the subjects taking placebos. This would appear to lay the argument to rest. It should be noted that this study was funded in part by a grant from the Nutra-Sweet® Company.

But in the May 1988 issue of the *New England Journal of Medicine* three letters appeared which threw Dr. Schiffman's study into serious question.[460] In the first of the letters, Dr. Richard B. Lipton and coworkers at the Montefiore Headache Unit reported that in their studies using 171 patients, they found 8.2% of the patients who had headaches were sensitive to aspartame. While they acknowledged the negative study of Dr. Shiffman, they also noted that the connection of migraines with exposure to dietary chocolate also failed to pass the double blind study, yet it is widely accepted as a trigger for migraines.

They further noted that stress and tension are also triggers for migraines and other headaches and that the test itself is often stressful enough to precipitate a headache. They concluded that double blind testing is not a good method for testing substances that can precipitate headaches. It is interesting that Dr. Schiffman found that 35% of their patients developed headaches following aspartame exposure, which is considerably higher than

Dr. Lipton's figure of 8.2%. The difference could be secondary to the stress factor.

The second letter was written by Dr. Robert Steinmetzer and Dr. Robert Kunkel of the Cleveland Clinic and pointed out other equally important shortcomings in the Schiffman study. They note that the challenges using placebo or aspartame were separated by only 48 hours, yet it is known that migraine can occur as late as 72 hours following exposure to a known triggering substance. They also criticized the study for using only a single challenge. They concluded that it was a little premature to "exonerate" aspartame as a triggering substance for migraine, and that persons with migraine and other vascular headaches should be warned to avoid NutraSweet®.

The third letter was from Dr. Louis Elsas of Emory University, who found that the Schiffmann study did not measure the blood levels of phenylalanine. He also criticized the failure to perform a chronic study, which would resemble a person drinking diet drinks over a long period of time. Dr. Elsas also noted that encapsulated aspartame, as was used in the Schiffmann study, is poorly absorbed (50%). The doctor concludes, "Perhaps a more through, unbiased peer review of the clinical research protocols would have produced a better designed experiment. The NutraSweet® Company, which supported this experimental design, may have an interest in protocols that would find that their product had no untoward effects."

I have discovered another flaw in the study which may also help explain their negative results. They designed the study so that the subjects received normal meals for three to five days, and then after a "washout" period, which I assume was a period of fasting lasting 24 hours, they were given the aspartame pills. It has been estimated that anywhere from 10 to 15% of persons become hypoglycemic after a 24 hour fast. Hypoglycemia is not only a trigger for migraine, but it also triggers its own headache. And indeed Dr. Schiffmann reported that those patients in the treatment group did have lower blood glucose than those in the placebo group. Unfortunately, the figures for the blood glucose were not given in the paper and since clinically symptomatic hypoglycemia can occur within the lower range of so-called "normal" blood sugar, this information would be important.

It is not necessary for the glucose level to be drastically low to precipitate headache. Some laboratories report the lower limit of normal at 60mg%. Many people, including myself, will develop an excruciating headache at this level. And as we have seen throughout this book, hypoglycemia aggravates or magnifies the adverse effects of all excitotoxins, including aspartate. Going back to Dr. Steinmetzer's comment about the 72 hour delayed effect of known triggers, the 24 hour washout period would allow food triggers to appear in this study as well. So, in essence, the Schiffmann study settles nothing.

I recently received a most interesting letter from a gentleman and his wife who have been studying the question of MSG safety for many years, Mr. Jack L. Samuels and Adrienne Samuels, Ph.D. In this letter Mr. Samuels makes the statement that the glutamate industry has been engaged in "scientific fraud" as regards the safety of their product. This is a bold statement to make.

But he and his wife have some compelling evidence to back up their accusations. It appears that one of the prime organizations supporting the use of MSG, the International Glutamate Technical Committee, has known all along that placebos used in testing the safety of MSG contained a powerful excitotoxin themselves.

The Samuels sent me a copy of correspondence sent to Sue Ann Anderson, R.D., Ph.D., a senior staff scientist at the Life Sciences Research Office in Bethesda, Maryland, from the Chairman of the International Glutamate Technical Committee, Dr. Andrew G. Ebert, in which Dr. Ebert states that aspartame (NutraSweet®) has been used as a masking sweetener in both the MSG samples and the placebos in tests conducted on the safety of MSG.

A placebo is used in such a test as a control so that the test subject cannot tell which sample they are taking: the active drug or the control substance. To prevent them from tasting the MSG researchers had been using sucrose in both samples. But since 1978 the sweetener was changed to aspartame. This was done because sucrose was thought to alter the absorption of the MSG.

Placebos are supposed to be completely inert substances. Otherwise they would produce a physiological effect all of their own and ruin the experiment. In the case of MSG toxicology studies, the placebo used to test the excitotoxin glutamate is NutraSweet®, which contains the excitotoxin aspartate. It has been clearly shown in a multitude of studies that aspartate produces the identical destructive reactions on the nervous system as MSG. It would seem obvious even to the layman that you would not use a control substance to compare to a known toxin if the control contained the same class of chemical toxin. But that is exactly what is being done.

Are the representatives of the glutamate industry aware of this basic scientific fact? It is hard to believe otherwise, especially in the face of the fact that one of their own representatives presented evidence before a public hearing at a meeting of the Federation of American Societies for Experimental Biology in which tables were presented showing that aspartame produces the same types and incidences of reactions as MSG.

Did these scientists disclose in their scientific papers the fact that the placebos also contained a known excitotoxin? The answer is an emphatic "no," and I have reviewed dozens of these studies. In fact, I was not aware of this deception until I received the proof from Dr. Samuels. In many cases the powder used to mix the placebos was supplied by the International Glutamate Technical Committee (IGTC). It is interesting to note that the Ajinomoto company, the chief manufacurer of MSG and the raw materials of aspartame, is an active member of the IGTC.

This company funds extensive research programs and provides funds to major universities for research on the safety of MSG. In my personal opinion, I have to believe that both the company representatives, and certainly the scientists doing the research, must know that such studies are questionable at the very least.

So far I have been talking only about NutraSweet®. But what about other food additive excitotoxins? Dr. Alfred Scopp, co-director of the Northern California Headache Clinic, in a recent paper for the journal, *Headache*, notes that while MSG is a known trigger of migraine headache, foods frequently contain from 3 to 5 grams of MSG per meal. The headache produced by MSG ingestion is not always immediate, and can sometimes be delayed for several hours, especially when eaten with food. He has found that by eliminating MSG and other "hidden" forms of the excitotoxin from the diet, migraine suffers have far fewer and milder attacks.

I have found this to be true in my own practice. Once patients eliminate all forms of excitotoxic food additives from their diet, most find they have a dramatic reduction in the number and the severity of the attacks. I also instruct them to take 500 milligrams of magnesium lactate or gluconate daily for one week and then to switch to a maintenance dose of 250 milligrams a day thereafter. I have found that this regimen works for the majority of migraine suffers.

Take the case of Mary G., a twenty-eight-year-old lady who has suffered from recurring migraine attacks for the last five years. She had visited several neurologists before coming to me. Like most migraine sufferers, she had gone through the entire gamut of anti-migrainous medications, from Cafergot to long-acting beta-blockers. Most worked temporarily, but either caused incapacitating weakness and sleepiness, as with the beta-blockers, or eventually failed to control the headache. As regular as clockwork, the poor lady spent at least two or more nights a month in the emergency room. Their solution was injections of narcotics.

When I saw her in my office she was desperate. After taking her dietary history, I discovered that she consumed an enormous number of foods heavily laden with excitotoxin food additives (especially MSG and hydrolyzed vegetable protein). I outlined a diet for her and the importance of avoiding particular foods and beverages. I also prescribed the above mentioned magnesium regimen.

When she returned, she happily informed me that she had experienced only one attack since her last visit and that the pain was minor. After following her case for one year, she reported that for the first time in five years, she had been virtually headache free.

I have found that the women who have migraines triggered by their menstrual period have the most difficulty in controlling their headaches. In these instances I add fish oil capsules (omega-3-fatty acids), one capsule three times a day. There is clinical evidence that the omega-3-fatty acids can reduce the number and severity of migraine attacks. This conforms with the excitability hypothesis for the etiology of migraine. We know that excitotoxins precipitate the destructive, inflammatory reactions within the cell, triggered by the entry of calcium into the cell interior. Omega-3-fatty acids have been shown to block the inflammatory step in this reaction.

Some patients find the fishy taste of the capsules intolerable. I have found that this can often be overcome simply by keeping the capsules in the refrigerator. I would also caution the reader to take 400 IU of vitamin E twice a day to prevent the fish oil from becoming rancid. Recently, it has been shown that a class of anti-inflammatory drugs known as NSAID (non-steroidal anti-inflammatory drugs), when taken on a daily basis greatly reduces the incidence and severity of migraine headaches. This group of drugs includes such medications as Motrin, Naprosyn, and Lodine. Unfortunately, when taken on a daily basis many people develop potentially severe gastrointestinal complications, such as burning of the stomach, diarrhea, and abdominal cramping. The fish oil capsules work the same as the anti-inflammatory drugs but without the gastrointestinal side effects.

There is some evidence that tension headaches are related to migraine type headaches. In fact, we frequently see the two occurring together. It has been my experience, as well as that of others, that the combined headache is the most difficult to cure. This may be because this type of headache has an element of muscle inflammation involved in it as well.

One additional bit of data that seems to strengthen the relationship between migraine and excitotoxins, is migraine relationship to hypoglycemia. I have observed in many of my patients, and in my own case as well, that often both tension headaches as well migraine headaches, are precipitated by bouts of hypoglycemia. On several occasions I have had classical migraine attacks occur following a vigorous workout in the gym.

In one instance, I had just returned to the office following a workout when I noticed a collection of glowing spots in the right half of my visual field. Slowly, like a spreading pool of spilled milk, the vision began to disappear in half of my visual field. Even though I knew what was happening, it was terribly frightening. I quickly took a NSAID pill (this was before I knew about magnesium and fish oils). Within twenty minutes I was back to normal.

Since that time I started my daily regimen of fish oil capsules and magnesium supplements. The only time I have even a glowing spot in my vision is when I forget to take one of my supplements. It is important to prevent migraine attacks since sometimes permanent strokes can result. Before I had discovered these preventive measures I saw a man in my office who had developed the identical symptoms I had suffered, but his blindness persisted. His migrainous attack was so intense that he had a stroke in the visual part of his brain that left him blind in one half of his visual field.

EXCITOTOXINS AND BRAIN INJURY

For many years it was assumed that when the brain was injured, for example from an auto accident or from a blow to the head, all of the injury to the brain that was to be ultimately seen occurred at the time of the impact. But now it is known that most of the injury occurs many hours following the initial impact. This is because the brain slowly swells, releasing toxic chemicals into the injured areas of the brain.

Recently, it has been shown that such injuries to the brain also cause the brain to accumulate high concentrations of glutamate.[461] In one study it was shown that brain injury was associated with an eight to thirteen fold increase in extracellular glutamate and a six to seventeen fold increased concentration in the cortex.[462] There is also some experimental evidence that treatment of spinal cord and brain injured animals with antagonist (excitotoxin blocking drugs) of glutamate can reduce the severity of the injury.[463]

One early consequence of brain and spinal cord injuries is the development of edema (swelling) within the area surrounding the injury. A recent study found that following experimental brain injury, glutamate accumulates in concentrations 10 to 20 fold higher than normal.[464] There is also some evidence that glutamate itself can cause the brain to swell. Interestingly, it has been shown that glutamate, when initially secreted in the brain, can stimulate the release of additional amounts of glutamate, thereby greatly compounding the damage. And glutamate can promote the production of dangerous free radicals within neurons, making the problem even worse.

There is evidence that a similar process develops following head injury in humans. In a recent study of twelve severely brain injured patients it was found that their cerebrospinal fluid glutamate levels remained elevated longer than three days.[465] In one case in which levels were measured for a week, glutamate remained in high concentrations the entire time. The levels attained were high enough to cause destruction of neurons. Glutamate began to accumulate by twenty-four hours and peaked at forty-eight to seventy-two hours. This means that the severely injured brain is exposed to high concentrations of glutamate and aspartate for a great period of time. It is interesting to note that many of the tube feeding formulas used to feed patients during this critical time contain glutamate and aspartate.

In another interesting study using rats it was found that a blood clot placed over the surface of the brain (simulating a subdural hematoma in humans) caused a state of increased metabolism in both temporal lobes.[466] Analysis of the temporal lobe tissue demonstrated a three fold rise in glutamate and aspartate. It was proposed that the elevated metabolism was caused by accumulation of the excitotoxins within the temporal lobes. The hippocampal lobes contain the highest density of glutamate receptors in the brain. Scientists also know that one of the most common areas of damage seen following fatal brain injuries is to the temporal lobes. The pathological damage resembles the type of damage seen following exposure to high concentration of glutamate.

It is well known that brain injury can disrupt the blood-brain barrier. This can, in turn, allow glutamate and other excitotoxins from the blood to enter the brain, again further damaging an already injured brain. No one knows for sure how long these barrier defects persist. There is some clinical evidence that they may persist for a lifetime. I have seen patients who have recovered from brain injury suddenly get worse following a bout of high fever. That they did indeed have recurrent brain edema (caused by blood-brain barrier defects) was confirmed by MRI scanning.

The point is that persons who have had a brain or spinal cord injury should be especially diligent in avoiding excitotoxin food additives such as MSG, hydrolyzed vegetable protein or NutraSweet®. This is because these defects in the blood-brain barrier can act as points of entry for otherwise excluded toxic molecules to enter the brain and spinal cord. The manufacturers of tube feeding and hyperalimentation formulas must become aware of the real danger imposed by high glutamate and aspartate additions to these formulas.

STROKES: ISCHEMIA-ANOXIA

The pathological findings seen with strokes closely resemble the selective neuron damage observed with exitotoxins.[467] Once again, the neurons having glutamate receptors are destroyed and those without them are spared.

There are several medical conditions during which either blood supply or oxygen supply is interfered with (ischemia and hypoxia, respectively). For example, strokes, cardiac arrest, problems with oxygen supply during birth, and head and spinal cord injuries all result in either ischemia or hypoxia, usually both.

In the case of strokes, we know that there is a wedge-shaped zone of brain death in the territory supplied by the blocked artery. This dead brain tissue is said to be infarcted. But surrounding this "dead zone" is another zone where the cells are operating under reduced blood supply, but are just barely able to function. Scientists refer to this marginal area of survival as the penumbra, named after the hazy shadow surrounding the absolute darkness of an eclipse. It is these injured but surviving neurons in the penumbra that determine the clinical severity of a stroke, for they can potentially be saved.

In earlier experimental studies scientists completely shut off all blood supply to the brain (called global ischemia) for a variable period of time, after which they would re-establish blood flow. These studies demonstrated a set pattern of changes:

1. The neurons in the zone of infarction began to increase their rate of firing before they died.
2. They observed increased glucose metabolism in these dying and hyperexcited neurons.
3. **They observed significant elevation of excitatory amino acids, especially aspartate and glutamate, in the region of the infarction.**
4. Finally, they found that excitotoxin-blocking drugs greatly reduced the degree of neuron death seen.

In one such study it was found that cats made globally ischemic exhibited a ten-fold increase in aspartate and a thirty-fold increase in glutamate soon after the blood vessels were occluded.[468] But after thirty minutes of complete cessation of blood flow to the cat's brain, glutamate levels in the brain increased one-hundred-fold. Similar findings have been reported in other animal species.[469]

One of the real puzzles facing scientists studying strokes is the cause of the dramatic hyperactivity of neurons soon after the blood supply is shut down. A clue to this puzzle appeared almost fifty years ago when the biochemist H.A. Krebs demonstrated that glutamate could significantly increase the metabolism of both the brain and the retina.[470] This is because glutamate acts as an excitatory stimulant to certain neurons.

Roger Simon has demonstrated in his laboratory that the area destined to die always demonstrates a very high rate of glucose metabolism before death occurs.[471] This means that the injured brain is rapidly exhausting its supply of energy. Remember, these neurons still have the possibility of surviving the stroke if conditions improve. It has been shown that this state of hypermetabolism can last up to two hours after the blood supply is shut off. It is important to remember that energy starved neurons are infinitely more vulnerable to excitotoxin damage.

What makes this important is that this may represent a window of opportunity for saving this zone of injured brain cells. This, of course, could mean the difference between a small, recoverable stroke and a devastating one that could result in paralysis of one side of the body, a loss of speech, or even death. (FIG 7-1)

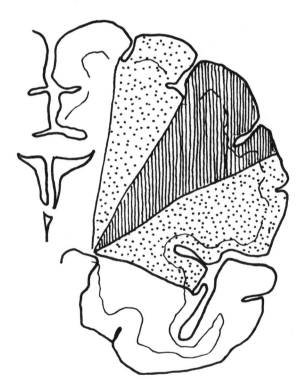

7-1 *A stroke that is affecting one hemisphere of the brain. The hatched zone represents dead brain while the stippled area (the penumbra) represents brain cells that are injured but not killed. High concentrations of glutamate are seen in this zone. Drugs that block glutamate toxicity can prevent those cells from dying.*

To better pinpoint the cause for this hypermetabolism Dr. Simon used a special method to analyze the content of the brain substance within this penumbra of damage. He found that during the first 90 minutes after occlusion of one of the major arteries to the brain (middle cerebral artery) there was a significant rise in glutamate, aspartate, and GABA levels. He also found that the levels of glutamate remained high for at least eighty minutes after occlusion of the artery.

To confirm that it was the accumulation of excitotoxic amino acids that was causing the damage, Dr. Simon next tested animals that were treated with a chemical known to block the harmful effects of excitotoxins. He found that the size of the area infarcted was markedly reduced.

Others have confirmed the protective role of glutamate blocking drugs. Hadley and coworkers, using twelve male baboons, found that Nimodipine, a drug that blocks calcium entry into the neuron, resulted in a smaller area of infarction following occlusion of the middle cerebral artery of the brain than did controls.[472] But, the size of the infarcts were not statistically significant.

Germano and coworkers did find a difference in treated and untreated animals that was statistically significant.[473] They found that the treated animals had smaller infarcts and better neurological outcomes. There is also evidence that other drugs known to block various stages of the glutamate reaction can reduce the size of the infarction and improve the clinical outcome after a stroke. More recently, Dr. Guoyang Yang and coworkers demonstrated that by giving animals a glutamate-blocking drug (MK-801) the damaged amount of the brain, the amount of brain swelling surrounding the stroke, and the neurological outcome of the animals could be greatly improved.[474] This study also demonstrated that MK-801 prevented a breakdown of the blood-brain barrier that usually caused it to become "leaky". We know that in cases of strokes in humans, high levels of glutamate accumulate in the brain. It remains to be demonstrated if high plasma levels of glutamate from the diet can also disrupt the blood-brain barrier, but the possibility exists. It may be even more likely in situations where there is already a weakened barrier due to aging, infection, high fever, or any one of a number of causes.

I have referred to the protective ability of magnesium on several occasions, especially when dealing with NMDA type receptor excitotoxins. Dr. S. Rothman found that high doses of magnesium could protect neurons from prolonged periods of anoxia (a lack of oxygen).[475] We have learned previously that neurons deficient in magnesium were much more sensitive to the damaging effects of excitotoxins. This becomes important when you realize that most Americans eat diets that are deficient in magnesium. In fact, dietary studies and metabolic balance studies indicate that the amount of magnesium in the American diet has been declining during most of this century.[476] According to a survey of 37,000 people conducted by the U.S. Department of Agriculture, only 25% of people had a dietary magnesium intake equal to or above the RDA for magnesium. In fact, 39% had magnesium intakes less than 70% of RDA.[477]

We know that stress greatly increases magnesium excretion, as does many diseases and even medications. This is especially true of chronic debilitating diseases, such as heart failure, chronic lung diseases, multiple sclerosis, and the other neurodegenerative diseases. In such cases, not only is there an increased excretion of magnesium but often the diet is poor secondary to a loss of appetite. Diuretics are also known to cause an abnormally large loss of magnesium by excretion. Alcohol and phosphates have been shown to significantly lower body magnesium levels. Carbonated beverages such as colas are high in phosphates. The ingestion of such beverages is epidemic in our society as well as the world.

I have seen far too many seriously ill patients lying in the hospital beds for weeks, or even months, without any effort by their doctors to replace magnesium losses. This is especially true with stroke patients. Even specialists are notorious for ignoring the metabolic and nutritional needs of their patients. Remember, experimental studies indicate that the stroke penumbra, that area of the brain containing struggling neurons, remains hypermetabolic for long periods of time after the stroke has occurred. This means that these cells need oxygen and glucose to survive. Also, when these vital nutrients are deficient, these neurons become especially vulnerable to the damaging effects of excitotoxins. When you add low magnesium levels on top of this, the neurons are even less likely to survive.

Thus far, I have tried to demonstrate that excitotoxins, especially glutamate and aspartate, play a major role in strokes and conditions in which oxygen is in short supply. This excitotoxin accumulation is secondary to release within the brain itself and not due to that taken in the diet. But, knowing that the blood-brain barrier is damaged by strokes and during hypoxia, one logically must assume that high levels of dietary excitotoxins can pose a significant threat to the survival of these floundering neurons in the penumbra zone. In addition, we know that some people are unable to metabolize glutamate from their diet, resulting in abnormal, toxic accumulations in the blood, and hence, within the injured brain. At present we have no inexpensive way to determine who these unfortunate people are.

We have seen that our normal diet contains enormous amounts of excitotoxins in various forms. Those in liquid form, such as NutraSweet®

sweetened beverages and MSG containing soups, are more rapidly and completely absorbed and therefore pose the greatest risk. Some hospitals add these excitotoxin food additives to the patient's food. In fact, several nutritionists are recommending that glutamine (the precursor of glutamate) be added to the diet of seriously ill patients to improve intestinal function. And cardiologists in some medical centers have concocted a cocktail containing high concentrations of MSG, with the idea that the glutamate will improve cardiac function. Patients on the heart pump frequently have multiple micro-strokes, which would make them very susceptible to occult brain damage. In my opinion, this practice should be stopped.

HYPOGLYCEMIA

We have seen that the supply of energy to the brain and spinal cord cells plays a vital role in protecting these cells from the damaging effects of excitotoxins. For example, a total loss of energy has been shown to increase neuron sensitivity to damage one hundred fold. We also know that hypoglycemia causes an outpouring of glutamate from within the brain and that the microscopic damage is indistinguishable from that seen when large doses of excitotoxins are given to experimental animals.[478]

When hypoglycemia is severe, the brain's supply of ATP is rapidly depleted.[479] This in turn knocks out the mechanism the brain uses to protect itself from abnormal accumulations of glutamate and aspartate. As with strokes, much of the brain damage produced by hypoglycemia can be reduced by using drugs known to block the harmful effects of glutamate.

It is evident from the medical and research literature that hypoglycemia appears to play a key role in glutamate excitotoxicity, and that this hypoglycemia is not always clinically evident. That hypoglycemia, as a separate syndrome, even exists as a widespread clinical problem is hotly debated among doctors and nutritionists. The conventional wisdom is that it is a rare clinical finding and more often the symptoms ascribed to hypoglycemia are psychological.

When the supporters of hypoglycemia as a common disorder demonstrated that a large segment of the population had a hypoglycemic response using the standard glucose tolerance test, the critics simply attacked this time honored test. They claimed that it didn't reflect the true conditions in everyday life. They insisted that a mixed meal be used. Unfortunately, most hypoglycemics do not become hypoglycemic with a mixed meal, especially if it contains complex carbohydrates. Rather, they develop very low blood sugars after ingesting foods containing primarily simple sugars, especially beverages.

I have seen quite a few patients suffering from hypoglycemia in my practice. All improve dramatically when placed on diets high in complex carbohydrates and low in simple sugars. The old standby of a high protein-low carbohydrate diet only makes the symptoms worse. Plus, the high protein usually contains a high proportion of glutamate or aspartate or both. The hypoglycemic state makes the brain even more vulnerable to the effects of the excitotoxins and for that reason should be avoided.

AIDS DEMENTIA AND EXCITOTOXINS

One of the tragic consequences of the advanced stages of AIDS is the development of profound disorders of the mind. This can vary from paranoid behavior and overt psychosis to severe dementia resembling Alzheimer's disease.

At first doctors assumed that this dementia was a result of the brain being infected by the virus. But later studies indicated that the neurons and glia cells within the brain were virtually free of the virus. The only sign of infection within the brain itself was within the white blood cells surrounding the blood vessels. Doctors knew that patients with full blown AIDS often had severe infections within their intestines. They proposed that the dementia and other nervous system disorders were caused by poor nutrition resulting in a deficiency of vitamin B_{12} or folate.

But recently researchers have found a more likely cause. It appears that the critical link is the activation of brain excitotoxins. Doctor Stuart A. Lipton and his coworkers discovered that the protein coat of the HIV virus could activate the NMDA receptor of neurons causing calcium to pour into the cells, triggering their death.[480]

Dr. Melvyn P. Heyes and his co-workers measured the levels of a powerful excitotoxin called quinolinic acid in the cerebrospinal fluid of patients having AIDS.[481] They found that during the early stages of the disease the levels of this excitotoxin were twice as high as that found in normal persons. But when the patients became severely demented or developed obvious neurological complications, their level of quinolinic acid rose twenty times higher than normal.

Interestingly, a recent study indicates that MSG exposure during the suckling period of mice produces a severe defect in cell-mediated immunity when they reach adulthood.[482] Cell-mediated immunity is important in fighting viruses, bacteria and cancer. It was suggested that this defect in immunity was caused by damage to the hypothalamus induced by neonatal exposure to MSG. It is known that the hypothalamus plays a vital role in immunity.[483] If this effect also occurs in humans exposed to MSG at an early stage of development, it could mean that they would suffer similar immune deficiencies as adults, which would mean more infections and a higher incidence of cancer, since the immune system would not be as efficient in fighting these diseases.

At present, the source of this excitotoxin is unknown. It may be produced within the brain or enter from the blood. It is obvious that with the brain already under excitotoxin attack, patients with HIV infections should avoid excitotoxin taste enhancers in their food.

ASPARTAME, BRAIN TUMORS AND THE FDA

It is interesting to note that the first experiments done to test the safety of aspartame before its final approval in 1981 disclosed a high incidence of brain tumors in the animals fed NutraSweet®.[484] In fact, this study was done by the manufacturer of NutraSweet®, G.D. Searle. In this study 320 rats were fed aspartame and 120 rats were fed a normal diet and used as controls. The study lasted two years. At the end of the study twelve of the aspartame fed rats had developed brain tumors (astrocytomas), while none of the control rats had. This represented a 3.75% incidence of brain tumors in the rats fed aspartame, which was twenty-five times higher than the incidence of spontaneous brain tumors developing in rats (0.15%).[485]

The study divided the rats into those exposed to low doses of aspartame and those exposed to a high dose. In the low dose group five of the rats developed brain tumors for and incidence of 3.13%. In the high dose group, seven developed brain tumors (4.38%). This indicates a dose related incidence of brain tumors. The higher the dose of aspartame, the more brain tumors were induced.

When Dr. John Olney pointed out these findings to the FDA "Aspartame Board of Inquiry" he was told that the high incidence of tumors was the result of spontaneous development of brain tumors in rats. That is, that some rats develop brain tumors naturally, just as humans do. Dr. Olney is a trained neuropathologist as well as a neuroscientist. He reviewed the incidence of spontaneously occurring brain tumors in rats and found that out of seven studies using a total of 59,000 rats, only 0.08% developed brain tumors—the aspartame fed rats had a forty-seven fold higher incidence. But to be fair, he even accepted G.D. Searle's references for spontaneously developing brain tumors in rats and arrives at a figure of 0.15%. This was still a twenty-five fold higher incidence in the aspartame fed rats than in the controls.

It was then observed that when brain tumors develop spontaneously in rats, the rate at which they appear begins to accelerate after two years of age, exactly when the Searle's study ended. Importantly, brain tumors are extremely rare before age one and one-half in the rat. So in truth the incidence of spontaneously occurring brain tumors would be even less than cited above. Yet, the aspartame fed rats developed two tumors by sixty weeks of age and five tumors by seventy weeks.

In a collective study of 41,000 rats no tumors were seen to occur before sixty weeks and only one by seventy weeks. The fact that 320 aspartame fed rats developed six brain tumors by seventy-six weeks indicates an "incredible and unprecedented" occurrence. Within the final twenty-eight weeks of the study six more brain tumors occurred in the aspartame fed group. Dr. Olney notes that "one must assume that many more (brain tumors) would have occurred after 104 weeks."

It became obvious that the G.D. Searle company was trying desperately to protect their potential billion dollar plus money maker. They claimed that more brain tumors were found because they searched the pathological slides so diligently. But, they searched just as diligently in the control rats and found none. Besides, neuropathologists examining the slides later stated that the tumors were large enough to be seen with the naked eye.

Because of the criticism submitted by Dr. Olney, the G.D. Searle company conducted a second study which was designed to be more comprehensive. Instead of a two-year study, this would span the entire lifetime of the rats, from intrauterine life to death. The results of this study can only be characterized as bizarre. This time they reported five brain tumors in 120 control rats (an incidence of 3.13%) and four brain tumors in 120 control rats (an incidence of 3.33%). While this was designed to show that aspartame was not the cause of the brain tumors, if accepted, the study would indicate that both groups had a brain tumor incidence thirty times higher than the known rate of spontaneous brain tumor occurrence in rats.

But the story gets even more interesting. Dr. Olney hypothesized that one possible cause of the tumor induction was a by-product of aspartame metabolism called diketopiperazine (DKP). When nitrosated by the gut it produces a compound closely resembling a powerful brain tumor causing chemical—N-nitrosourea.

The G.D. Searle company conducted a separate study to test the carcinogenicity of diketopiperazine (DKP). The results of this study were not submitted to the FDA until after aspartame had already been approved for general use by the American population. This study was not a lifetime study but rather a 115 week study which consisted of feeding rats their normal feed mixed with DKP. There were 114 control animals and 216 that supposedly ate the DKP. (Not all of the animals were even examined for tumors.) There were two brain tumors in the controls (1.62% incidence) and three (1.52%) in the DKP groups. But strangely enough, the incidence of brain tumors found in both groups were sixteen times higher than would be expected from spontaneous occurring tumors. That did not make sense.

So how can we explain these strange findings? It is instructive at this point to know that in 1975 the drug enforcement division of the Bureau of Foods investigated the G.D. Searle company as part of an investigation of "apparent irregularities in data collection and reporting practices." The director of the FDA at that time stated that they found "sloppy" laboratory techniques and "clerical errors, mixed-up animals, animals not getting the drugs they were supposed to get, pathological specimens lost because of improper handling, and a variety of other errors, [which] even if innocent, all conspire to obscure positive findings and produce falsely negative results."

The drug enforcement division carried out a study under the care of agent Jerome Bressler concerning Searle's laboratory practices and data manipulation (known as the Bressler Report). He found that the feed used to test DKP had been improperly mixed so that the animals would receive only small doses of the chemical to be tested. (I have seen a photograph of the feed mix and can attest to the "sloppy" method used.) The commissioner also charged G.D. Searle company with "failure to maintain control and experimental animals on separate racks and failure to mark animals to ensure against mix-ups between experimentals (animals fed aspartame and DKP) and controls." This vital and telling report was buried in a file cabinet, never to be acted on by the FDA.

Such poor techniques would explain why both control animals and those eating aspartame had exceptionally high brain tumor rates, since they, most likely, were both eating the aspartame feed. What is ironic is that the FDA would accept studies from a company with an obvious heavy financial interest in having aspartame approved. But even more amazing is that they would depend on this same company to provide studies that they, FDA, knew beforehand were highly questionable and possibly fraudulent upon which they would make such an important public safety decision.

Thus far, no independent studies have been done to examine this vital issue. As a neurosurgeon I see the devastating effects a brain tumor has, not only on its victim, but on the victim's family as well. To think that there is even a reasonable doubt that aspartame can induce brain tumors in the American population is frightening. And to think that the FDA has lulled them into a false sense of security is a monumental crime.

While it does not prove that aspartame causes brain tumors in humans, it is interesting to note that from 1973 to 1990 brain tumors in people over the age of sixty-five have increased sixty-seven percent.[486] During this same period, brain tumors in all age groups jumped by greater than ten percent.[487] The greatest increase in brain tumors has occurred during the years 1985, 1986 and 1987. Dr. H.J. Roberts, who has written an excellent book on the dangers of aspartame, has collected some evidence that one particular type of brain tumor may be associated with NutraSweet®.[488] This tumor is known as a primary lymphoma of the brain. It is a particularly nasty tumor with a high mortality rate.

Some primary brain lymphomas are associated with immune depression seen with AIDS. One would expect these to increase. But there is also a dramatic increase in these previously rare tumors in individuals without AIDS.[489] Some have suggested that the recent increase in brain tumors merely reflects better diagnostic methods. But a recent study found this not to be true; the increase is real.[490] Dr. Roberts feels that an association with the tremendous rise in the use of aspartame products in the last decade may hold the answer.

The use of aspartame has grown astronomically in this country: by 1985 eight hundred million pounds of aspartame were consumed in the United States alone. Worldwide consumption has increased dramatically over the last several years. It is estimated that over 100 million people drink aspartame-sweetened drinks, including a large percentage of children. In my opinion, aspartame should be banned from foods and drinks until this issue has been properly studied by independent researchers in the neuro-oncology field.

CONCLUSION

As we have seen, there are a growing number of conditions affecting the nervous system that are related to toxic accumulations of excitotoxins. Recently, it has been suggested that even the encephalopathy and dementia seen in the terminal stages of AIDS may be due to glutamate accumulation in the brain and not as a result of the virus itself.

Glutamate accumulation in the brain appears to be a common denominator in several devastating conditions and the list of neurological conditions either caused by or related to excitotoxin damage continues to grow.[491] Therapeutic treatments directed at methods to reduce excitotoxin damage have shown significant success in both experimental trials and some clinical trials.

Conclusion

In the introduction I stated that the purpose of this book was to point out to the reader some of the dangers of excitotoxins, especially those added to our food and drink as taste enhancers and sweeteners. We have seen that excitotoxins can have a devastating effect on the nervous system throughout all of its stages of development, from embryo to adult. But of primary concern is the effect of these powerful brain cell stimulants have on the developing brain of the infant and child and the later development in the adult of neurodegenerative diseases such as Parkinson's disease, Alzheimer's dementia, Huntington's disease, and ALS. The brain not only utilizes the excitatory amino acids as normal neurotransmitters, but there exists a delicate balance of excitatory and inhibitory chemicals in the brain. When this balance is upset, serious disorders of the nervous system can result.

When MSG was first being added to foods as a taste-enhancing substance, glutamate receptors had not been discovered, and no one knew that excess glutamate could cause brain cell death. The food industry invested millions of dollars in developing the use of MSG and hydrolyzed protein. It was only after tons of these "taste enhancers" were being added to our foods and beverages that scientists had their first hint that excitotoxins carried a serious side effect.

Unfortunately, this discovery remained buried in the medical research literature for over a decade before someone recognized this danger. And, as we have seen, this toxic compound was being added in large doses to foods given to newborns and small infants, despite the fact that it had been demonstrated that it was the developing brain that was most vulnerable to the toxic effects of excitatory amino acids. They were so toxic, in fact, that researchers renamed them excitotoxins. Abundant research had demonstrated that these excitotoxins not only damaged the cells of the retina of the eye, but also that they were extremely toxic to the nerve cells in the

215

hypothalamus and other vital areas of the brain.

It is important to appreciate that many of the toxic effect of excitotoxins occur at a time when no outward symptoms develop. The child does not become sick or throw up, or have any behavior that would alarm the parents that something was wrong. When toxic doses of MSG are give to baby animals they continue to act in an entirely normal way. But when their brains are examined microscopically, vital groups of neurons are found to be permanently destroyed in the hypothalamus. This has been referred to as a "silent brain lesion." Such silent lesions are frequently seen in neurology and neurosurgery practices.

It is also important to remember that following MSG ingestion, humans concentrate glutamate **twenty times higher** in their blood than do monkeys and **five times higher** than mice. Humans may be **five times more vulnerable to MSG toxicity than mice**, the most sensitive animal known to this type of brain injury. Not only do humans concentrate glutamate to a much greater degree, but it remains at an elevated level in the blood for much longer periods of time, exposing the unprotected portions of the brain to very toxic levels.

What makes all of this so disturbing in the case of children is that the damage done at the time of initial exposure produces no obvious outward effects. But when the animal (or person) reaches a later stage of development (adolescence or adulthood) the damage may present itself as an endocrine disorder or even possibly a learning disorder (autism, attention deficit disorder, dyslexia) or emotion control disorder (violent episodes, schizophrenia, paranoia). Hundreds of millions of infants and young children are at great risk and their parents are not even aware of it.

It was only through the diligent efforts of Dr. John Olney that the food industry was forced to halt the obvious use of excitotoxin food additives in baby foods. But, as we have seen, no one warned pregnant mothers that the MSG laced food they were eating could endanger the developing babies still in their womb. And more and more excitotoxin "taste enhancers" were being added to adult foods and even toddler foods all the time. Again, this was despite the rapid accumulation of research data demonstrating these previously known dangers and even new dangers associated with using excitotoxins in food.

But by this time MSG was not only being added to virtually every processed food, it was being promoted in cookbook recipes as well. In the sixties it was being sold in food stores in powdered form for this purpose. A whole generation had been, and continues to be, exposed to high doses of excitotoxins.

In 1969 James Schlatter, a bench biochemist working with a compound called aspartame as a possible cure for stomach ulcers, happened to lick his thumb while turning a page in his notebook. He was struck by the intense sweetness of the chemical that had inadvertently covered his thumb. From this serendipitous discovery was born a business that would reap 736 million dollars in sales for the NutraSweet® Company in 1988 alone. By 1989 G.D. Searle & Company, the manufacturer of Nutra-Sweet®, had reached a profitability that put it ninth on the Fortune 500 list.

Despite concerns over the safety of this new sweetener, including brain tumor induction in experimental animals, seizures, precipitation of head-aches, and an adverse effect on the developing brain, the FDA approved its use as an artificial sweetener. Sales began to grow immediately. The Nutra-Sweet® company spent over 60 million dollars on advertising alone during its first three years.

NutraSweet® hit the market at just the right time. Americans had become weight conscious and were looking for a sugar substitute, and it replaced the recently outlawed cyclamate. Soon, it surpassed saccharin in sales. In fact, NutraSweet® played a large role in making the soft drink business one of the fastest growing businesses in what had been a stagnant enterprise. Americans were guzzling diet colas under the mistaken belief that sugar consumption was the primary cause of obesity. But they were unaware of the serious health effects of excess aspartate consumption.

MSG had come under criticism periodically from various members of the medical profession, the research community, and consumer advocates. But by then the excitotoxin "taste enhancing" business had become a mul-tibillion dollar enterprise. The Ajinomoto company, the primary manufac-turer of MSG and hydrolyzed vegetable protein, in conjunction with a dozen American food manufacturers, decided to protect their interest by forming a powerful public relations firm known as the Glutamate Asso-ciation. The number one contributor to this "attack group" was the Ajinomoto Company of Japan.

The purpose of this group was not only to defend and promote the use of MSG and other " taste enhancers", but to attack anyone who dared to point out the adverse health effects of MSG. They did this by bringing their own scientists into any area where a serious question about safety had been raised. In most cases consumer advocates are knowledgeable people who lack the scientific background to withstand an assault by a scientist steeped in the jargon of the pure and applied chemist. These attacks could be cruel and overwhelming and only those with thick skin and determination could withstand the assault.

They went even further by hiring their own scientists to perform studies that would seem to confirm the safety of the products in question.

Sometimes these scientists were merely funded by the Searle company or the International Glutamate Technical Committee (an offshoot of Glutamate Association), and on other occasions the scientists worked full-time for the companies manufacturing and adding excitotoxins to the food. The bias of these studies is quite evident in many instances, as pointed out by neuroscientist and excitotoxin researcher, Dr. John Olney, as well as other scientists.

The attacks launched by the Glutamate Association on its detractors are often intimidating and ruthless. After all, billions of dollars are at stake. One would, from this behavior, naturally assume that the free enterprise system is unable to discipline itself and therefore we must turn to government for our protection. But it has been shown some time ago that government agencies often become the handmaidens for the companies they are supposed to regulate. This has been shown to be the case with the FDA.

It appears that the Glutamate Association has a cozy working relationship with the FDA. In fact, any time someone challenges the safety of MSG or hydrolyzed vegetable protein, the Glutamate Association is invited to give its defending testimony. If the FDA really wants an unbiased view it should seek the advice of scientists who have no connection at all to the manufacture and industrial use of MSG. But they rarely do.

Another way the FDA works with the Glutamate Association is by yielding to their lobbying efforts to change the labeling laws so that the words "monosodium glutamate" is not required on food labels unless it contains 100% pure MSG. Also MSG need not even be mentioned by any name if one product containing pure MSG is only used as an ingredient in another food. For example, if broth is used to make a soup, and the broth contains pure MSG, MSG does not have to be listed as an ingredient. But if the broth is sold alone, it must appear on the label.

As Dr. Schwartz has shown, substances labeled as "spices", "natural flavoring" and "flavoring" may contain anywhere from 30% to 60% MSG. But you as a consumer are denied this vital information. Your only recourse is to avoid all foods with these hidden label names. And as you will quickly discover, most manufactured foods contain one or more of these excitotoxin "taste enhancers".

So what should the FDA do? First, it should guarantee the consumer nutritional information by requiring the manufacturer to list all additives containing MSG and hydrolyzed vegetable protein and do so under these names and not disguised names. Second, it should conduct open hearings on the safety of these additives with scientific testimony from those not connected to the food manufacturing industry or to the manufacturers of MSG, NutraSweet® or hydrolyzed vegetable protein, or their representatives.

Should the FDA ban all such substances as food additives? This is a controversial subject. Libertarians would say "No". Consumer advocates would say "Absolutely". Actually, all that would be necessary would be to have an open forum on the subject to let the consumers decide. The problem today is that so little of this information is known by the general public. I am a strong advocate of reform by persuasion. If the general public is aware of the dangers involved and still decides to take the risk, so be it.

The problem with coercion is that far too often the conventional wisdom is wrong, as we have seen in the case of FDA approval of MSG and NutraSweet®. The public has grown to trust the wisdom of the government despite the fact that it has often been dreadfully wrong. We witnessed this during the great swine flu epidemic, the pandemic that never occurred. But the government forced thousands of Americans to take a vaccination that was not only unnecessary but that killed and crippled far more people than the swine flu did.

In the early fifties the government approved the Sabin Vaccine for polio. Millions were forcibly vaccinated. Years later it was discovered that the original vaccine contained a known cancer causing virus. The number of cancers developing in those vaccinated by this batch of tainted vaccine is still disputed.

And it was the FDA that banned the artificial sweetener cyclamate as a carcinogenic compound only to discover a decade later that the studies upon which this decision was based were seriously flawed. The same thing happened with saccharin. So government control of our food and drug industry can be just as harmful as their ignoring the dangers of these food toxins.

In fact, a case can be made for the idea that it is the faith built up by the public in the wisdom of the FDA that has allowed them to cover up the danger of MSG and the other excitotoxins. One of the most frequent retorts I receive when I lecture on this subject is, "If these chemicals are so dangerous why hasn't the FDA outlawed them?" People have placed so much faith in these guardian federal agencies that they ignore obvious dangers, no matter how much evidence supports such arguments.

Americans must learn to think for themselves. A good example of how government health agencies can create disasters of their own is seen in the case of dioxin. In 1982 the Environmental Protection Agency announced that the town of Times Beach, Missouri was an ecological time bomb. Its roads had been doused with dioxin "the most toxic man-made substance known", the EPA cried.

As a result of this declaration, the government ordered the town evacuated at a cost of 40 million dollars. All 480 acres were fenced off. Decontamination of the land was to take another ten years and cost an additional

120 million dollars. But now everything has suddenly changed. The chemical that was declared "the most toxic man-made chemical known" was recently found to be essentially safe and to pose little threat to humans. Vernon Houk, the man who initially made the decision to evacuate the town now announced that "he and others had seriously overestimated the hazards of dioxins." So how did they come to this startling new decision? It followed 400 million dollars worth of new government research on dioxins.

The point is that allowing government agencies to rule society based on scientific pronouncement can be a double-edged sword. While at times it can definitely save lives, it can also destroy them and even instill a false sense of security, as in the case of MSG and NutraSweet®.

Finally, we have seen that there are things that you can do to protect yourself. First, and most important, is to avoid foods containing excitotoxin additives. This not only requires skills in reading food labels but it also requires **willpower**. Many just cannot force themselves to give up their favorite brand of chips or pasta sauce. Second, there are ways to neutralize some of the harmful effects of excitotoxins. The anti-oxidant vitamins and minerals, magnesium, the branched chained amino acids, and zinc have all been shown to offer varying degrees of protection.

One should not assume that health food stores are safe havens from these excitotoxins. In fact, I have found that many products, including supplements as well as foods, contain one or more of these toxic compounds. For example, at least one product claiming to improve memory and boost brain power, contains large doses of glutamate and glutamine.

Several of the food products found in health food stores contain both MSG and hydrolyzed vegetable protein. Soybean milk, which naturally contains a high content of glutamate, frequently has glutamate added in the form of hydrolyzed vegetable protein. Kombu, miso, and soy sauce all contain MSG. One natural food distributor recently sent out a flyer attempting to allay consumer fears of added MSG in their products. In this flyer they make the statement that hydrolyzed vegetable protein is a natural source of "bound glutamate" and therefore is not dangerous. As we have seen this is not true. Sports supplements and weight loss products frequently contain either NutraSweet® or one of the other excitotoxins. Therefore be especially cautious in buying products from health food stores.

The person suffering from one of the neurodegenerative disease or at high risk for developing one of these diseases must be especially careful about ingesting excitotoxins. One may reduce the severity of the disease or slow the rate of progression of the disease. Individuals at risk for developing one of these disorders could possibly avoid developing the disease altogether. At this stage, however, this is only hypothetical since no long term extensive studies have been conducted to test this hypothesis.

Scientists are working to develop compounds that will offer protection against the excitotoxins without interfering with the normal functioning of the excitatory transmitter system in the brain. As you will recall, glutamate plays a vital role in the normal operation of the hypothalamic endocrine system, the motor portions of the brain, and the memory systems. Therefore the perfect protective molecule must preserve these systems but prevent their overactivation.

The fields of molecular biology, pharmacology, and nutritional sciences are growing at a rapid pace and it is only a matter of time before the magic bullet is found. Most likely, one of the most fruitful avenues of research will be in finding a way to repair the metabolic defect within brain cells that prevents them from supplying sufficient energy to protect themselves from excitotoxin damage. Until then we must protect ourselves and our loved ones from the harmful effects of excitotoxins by avoiding all foods and beverages containing these toxins.

8
Update

Since I began this book, much new information has surfaced concerning not only the lethal effects of excitotoxins on the nervous system, but also a growing list of ways to reduce the degree of such damage. It is obvious, despite denials from the food industry and its myriad supporters, that the scientific world is convinced that glutamate and aspartate are very toxic compounds to the nervous system. In fact, excessive excitotoxin accumulation within the injured brain constitutes the leading theory of a final common pathway for a multitude of disorders affecting the central nervous system, from strokes and trauma to neurodegenerative diseases and seizures.

In fact, there is only one point of contention that remains to be settled: Do the excitotoxins pass through the blood-brain barrier? There is overwhelming evidence that both glutamate and aspartate can enter even the protected brain from the unprotected parts of the brain, via the circumventricular organs. In the developing baby, we know that not only does glutamate pass through the placental barrier into the baby's brain but that drastic changes occur within the chemistry of the baby's immature brain that effect not only the child's future behavioral development, but also its capacity to learn complex information.[1,2,3] *I warn all pregnant women to avoid all forms of glutamate and aspartate, especially aspartame.* We know that ingestion of aspartame dramatically increases

---

[1] Frieder B and Grimm VE, Prenatal monosodium glutamate (MSG) treatment given through the mother's diet causes behavioral defects in rat offspring. **International J. Neuroscience** 23:117-126, 1984

[2] Frieder B and Grimm VE, Prenatal monosodium glutamate causes long-lasting cholinergic and adrenergic changes in various brain regions. **Journal of Neurochemistry** 48: 1359-1365, 1987

[3] Kubo T, et al, Neonatal glutamate can destroy the hippocampal CA1 structure and impair discrimination learning in rats. **Brain Research** 616: 311-314, 1993

brain levels of phenylalanine and methanol. Further, methanol is converted within the tissues of the brain into formic acid and formaldehyde, both powerful neurotoxins. So in the case of aspartame we have two powerful neurotoxins plus a powerful excitotoxin, all rolled in one.

PART I
PHARMACEUTICAL AGENTS

Experimentally, numerous agents (APV, DAA, and DAP, for example) have been used to block glutamate toxicity. One of the most commonly used has been a compound designated MK-801. Interestingly, it not only reduces the toxicity of glutamate on NMDA receptors but it also blocks the neurotoxicity of L-cysteine. This compound has been tested in both animals and humans with some significant success. But, it has some unfortunate drawbacks. For one, it not only blocks toxicity but it also blocks normal memory formation. Remember, glutamate is a neurotransmitter in the brain that initiates long-term potentiation in the temporal lobes necessary for laying down new memories. MK-801 is a non-selective NMDA type glutamate blocker. That is, it blocks pathological accumulation as well as normal levels of glutamate in brain tissue.

Because of this problem, pharmaceutical researchers have been searching for new compounds that are more selective. The commonly used antitussive dextromethorphan is a moderately powerful NMDA type glutamate blocker. I have used it successfully in a case of acute spinal cord disease. In a recent study of dextromethorphan used in surgical patients, clinicians at the Stanford Stroke Center found that using doses as high as 4mg per kilogram body weight were not only safe but they were able to attain brain levels that were significantly protective of the brain.[4] In fact, brain levels were sixty-eight times higher than serum levels. Neurological side effects were seen when using these high concentrations but resolved completely when the drug was stopped. At lower doses these patients experienced dizziness, slurring of speech, and loss of balance. Fatigue and hallucinations occurred with the highest doses. Again all of these side effects subsided when the dextromethorphan was stopped. One of the most

---

[4] Steinberg GK, et al. Dose escalation safety and tolerance study of the N-methyl-D-aspartate antagonist dextromethorphan in neurosurgery patients. **Journal of Neurosurgery** 84: 860-866, 1996

common side effects was a sense of euphoria very similar to feeling "drunk." Interestingly, ethyl alcohol is known to block NMDA type glutamate receptors.[5] The ability of ethanol to block LTP memory circuits may explain the memory blackouts seen in alcohol abuse.

Some of the anti-Parkinson's drugs are also glutamate blockers, such as procylidine and ethopropazine. There is growing evidence that excitotoxicity plays a key role in Parkinson's disease and that a successful therapy may be found utilizing a selective blockade of the involved glutamate receptors.

In the early seventies a new anesthetic, Ketamine, was implemented for the purpose of light anesthesia. Unfortunately, the agent had serious drawbacks. Patients often had combative hallucinations. It is now known that Ketamine is a powerful NMDA type glutamate blocker. This disturbing side effect can be blocked using another drug called scopolamine. Ketamine may be useful in reducing the damaging effects of various types of brain trauma including strokes.

Another interesting compound, developed by the Wellcome Foundation LTD, designated 619C89, suppresses glutamate release from the injured brain and has far fewer psychomotor and behavioral side effects than earlier NMDA antagonists. In stroke experiments, this compound has been shown to successfully suppress glutamate accumulation within thirty minutes and continues to protect the brain for twenty-four hours.[6] Not only is 619C89 safer, but it is also more effective in reducing toxic levels of glutamate and aspartate in strokes than is MK-801 by almost a factor of two. This compound holds great promise in reducing brain damage in strokes, subarachnoid hemorrhages, and brain trauma.

But, while 619C89 appears to be very effective in preventing the toxic accumulation of excitotoxins when their source is from within the brain itself, it would have little effect on excitotoxins entering the brain from the blood stream. Several approaches to this problem are possible. We know

---

[5] Lovinger DM, et al. NMDA receptor-mediated synaptic excitation selectively inhibited by ethanol in hippocampal slice from adult rat. **Journal of Neuroscience** 10: 1372-1379, 1990

[6] Tsuchida E, et al. A use-dependent sodium channel antagonist, 619C89 in reduction of ischemic brain damage and glutamate release after acute subdural hematoma in the rat. **Journal of Neurosurgery** 85:104-111, 1996

that excitotoxins do their damage to brain cells by initiating a series of destructive reactions involving special fatty acids found within the cell membrane. The process begins with the release of arachidonic acid which in turn passes through a series of enzymatic steps leading to the creation of a series of compounds known as eicosanoids.

Not all eicosanoids are "bad." Some serve useful purposes such as improving blood flow, stimulating immune function and reducing inflammation. The so-called bad eicosanoids have opposite effects. They can suppress immune function, impair blood flow, and promote inflammation. When the "bad" eicosanoids are produced in excess in brain cells one can see cellular destruction, massive free radical formation, and withering of synaptic connections. We know that glutamate markedly increases the release of arachidonic acid and, likewise, arachidonic acid may enhance glutamate release from hippocampal nerve terminals.[7] This produces a vicious cycle of destructive reactions within the cell.

Fortunately, we have several drugs that can reduce the production of some "bad" eicosanoids. One of the most commonly used of these drugs is aspirin. Another group of compounds, called non-steroidal anti-inflammatory drugs, also block some of these reactions. These include most of the commonly used arthritis drugs such as ibuprofen. Glucocorticoids are some of the most powerful eicosanoid blocking drugs known. By blocking "bad" eicosanoid production, one bypasses the negative effects of interfering with normal glutamate function. Unfortunately, the available drugs do not selectively block all of the "bad" eicosanoids. One group of particularly bad eicosanoids, called leukotrienes, are not blocked.

In Chapter six I discussed several studies that indicated that persons who took nonsteroidal anti-inflammatory drugs had a lower incidence of Alzheimer's disease. It is my opinion that these drugs block "bad" eicosanoid production. Remember, during this process of eicosanoid production, massive free radicals are also formed. This adds significantly to the damage done by excitotoxins. Drugs that block "bad" eicosanoid production also block much of the free radical production as well.

One of the most effective ways to block the production of harmful eicosanoids is to prevent the initial release of arachidonic acid from the cell

---

[7] Piomelli, D. Eicosanoids in synaptic transmission. **Critical Reviews in Neurobiology** 8: 65-83, 1994

wall, which begins the cascade of destruction within the cell. The enzyme that releases arachidonic acid is called phospholipase A2. Two drugs that block this enzyme are quinacrine and 4-bromophenacyl bromide (BPB). Experimentally, quinacrine can reduce toxicity caused by arachidonic acid by 92% and BPB by 68%.

Protection can also be obtained by attacking steps further down the line in this destructive reaction. The lipooxygenase enzyme stimulates the production of a series of harmful substances called leukotrienes. Inhibitors of this enzyme, such as nordihyroguaiaretic acid (NDGA) and phenidone, can reduce glutamate damage by 97% and 62% respectively. In fact, giving NDGA even twelve hours after glutamate will completely block any further toxicity.

Recent research has uncovered a very interesting group of compounds called 21-aminosteroids. One of the earlier of this group designated U-74006F (tririlazal mesylate) is known to be a potent antioxidant and lipid peroxidation inhibitor, both of which appear to play a central role in neurodegenerative diseases. A newer generation 21-aminosteroid designated U-89678 appears to be even more potent in its protection of neurons.[8] In a recent clinical trial it was found that subarachnoid hemorrhage patients (usually caused by ruptured aneurysms) experienced a significantly lower death rate and improved recovery when given the drug.

A more recent study found that the newer compound could not only significantly block iron-induced lipid peroxidation injury to neurons but could actually reduce damage to the blood-brain barrier by as much as 60%. This would protect the brain from glutamate and aspartate in the blood stream.

In the first edition of *Excitotoxins*, I only mentioned a class of glutamate receptors called the metabotropic receptors in passing. But, recent research has shed much more light on this important class of glutamate receptors. We now know that there are at least three types of metabotropic receptors, called types I, II, and III. Overactivity of type I

---

[8] Smith SL, et al. Protective effect of tririlazad mesylate and metabolite U-89678 against blood-brain barrier damage after subarachnoid hemorrhage and lipid peroxidative neuronal injury. **Journal of Neurosurgery** 84: 229-233, 1996

appears to be associated with excitotoxic lesions to the brain.[9] There is growing evidence that this class of receptor plays a major role in Parkinson's disease. Blocking this receptor with drugs appears to be neuroprotective. But types II and III metabotrophic receptors have an opposite effect. Activation of these receptors seem to actually protect specific brain cells. That is, drugs which stimulate these receptors are neuroprotective.

While the field of neuroprotection is relatively new, it is growing increasingly sophisticated. Other avenues being explored are a group of phospholipids normally found in the brain called gangliosides.[10] Early experiments seem to indicate that they may prevent, to some degree, glutamate damage to the brain. Another group of naturally occurring substances being explored as neuroprotectants are called nerve growth factors.

NUTRITIONAL PROTECTION

The area of nutritional protection is a wide open field. Unfortunately, the pharmaceutical industry has little interest in this area since many of these useful compounds cannot be patented as they are found commonly in nature. In general, besides reducing the concentration of excitotoxins themselves, there are three major areas in which nutritional supplements may help in preventing damage by excitotoxins: 1) reducing the production of "bad"eicosanoids; 2) reducing free radical damage and 3) improving energy production.

Reducing " Bad" Eicosanoids: Enter the Zone

I took this subtitle from an important book written by Dr. Barry Sears called, *The Zone: A Dietary Road Map*.[11] When I read his book I realized that Dr. Sears had discovered an important piece of the puzzle that could explain a multitude of disorders involved in the connection between

---

[9] Nicoletti F, et al. Metabotrophic glutamate receptors: a new target for the therapy of neurodegenerative disorders? **Trends in Neurosciences** 19: 267-271, 1996

[10] Manev H, et al. Protection by gangliosides against glutamate excitotoxity. **Advances in Lipid Research** 25: 269-288, 1993

[11] Sears B. **The Zone. A Dietary Roadmap**. Regan Books, 1995

hypoglycemia, insulin, and "bad" eicosanoid production. He makes the important point that one of our major nutritional myths is that we need to consume a large amount of carbohydrates to remain healthy. In fact, he shows just the opposite. Not only is most of our obesity related to carbohydrate excess, but many of the diseases that plague our society, such as cancer, arthritis, and cardiovascular diseases, are also related to this unhealthy practice.

Not only should we reduce our carbohydrate intake but we should also carefully select the type of carbohydrates that we do eat. Only recently did anyone ask the question, "Are all carbohydrates equal in terms of absorption from the gut?" The answer turned out to be, "No!" Carbohydrates are absorbed at highly variable rates. Some are absorbed very rapidly, and others relatively slowly. So why would this matter? Because the rate of absorption of carbohydrates determines the amount of insulin secreted in response from the pancreas. Carbohydrates rapidly absorbed by the gut flood the blood stream with glucose (all carbohydrates are converted to glucose). To handle this sudden load of sugar the pancreas has to secrete a large amount of insulin. In sixty million Americans there is a significant overshoot of insulin that, in turn, drives the blood sugar to levels that impair brain function. We experience this overshoot by intense hunger, tremulousness, and anxiety.

But, what Dr. Sears has shown is that the excess insulin also stimulates the production of "bad" eicosanoids, which severely damage cells, including brain cells. We know that hypoglycemia causes the brain to internally secrete excess amounts of glutamate, especially aspartate.[12] Further, as we have seen, these excitotoxins also stimulate the production of "bad" eicosanoids. At least two major studies have shown that the majority of Alzheimer's patients have hyperinsulinemia and hypoglycemia. The question that remains unanswered is, "Will altering the diet early in life prevent such neurodegenerative diseases?" Dr. Sears makes the important point that food should be viewed as a very powerful drug.

Another approach to reducing the amounts of "bad" eicosanoids limiting its precursor substance, arachidonic acid, in the diet. This can be done by avoiding egg yolks, organ meats (liver and most deli meats) and red

[12] Sandberg B, et al. Metabolically derived aspartate-elevated extracellular levels in vivo in iodoacetate poisoning. **Journal of Neuroscience Research** 13: 489-495, 1985

meats. It is also critical that you maintain a low fat diet, especially saturated fats, since these can produce a state of insulin resistance. Insulin resistance means that the cell will not respond to insulin even in very high concentrations. This is believed to be the cause of adult onset diabetes (type II diabetes).

Omega 3-fatty acids

The majority of fats in the American diet consist of what are called omega 6 polyunsaturated fatty acids. This includes the essential fatty acids linoleic and linolenic acids, which are high in corn, cotton, soya, safflower, and sunflower oils. While the popular trend, initiated by the American Heart Association, promotes the use of polyunsaturated oils, there is growing evidence that these oils promote the generation of "bad" as well as "good" eicosanoids. In fact, there is significant evidence that these oils may actually promote arteriosclerosis, and therefore, coronary artery disease and strokes.

Omega 3-fatty acids are derived primarily from coldwater fish. When the diet consists of a high proportion of these oils the generation of arachidonic acid is significantly reduced, thereby reducing the generation of "bad" eicosanoids. Experimental animal and human studies have both demonstrated a significant reduction in blood coagulation and, hence, in the incidence of both strokes and heart attacks.

We know that cell membranes are critical in receptor function, ion exchange, enzyme function, and nutrient entry into the cell. With aging, the cell membranes lose some of their fluidity and as a result these critical functions are impaired. It has been shown that omega 3-fatty acids can improve cell membrane fluidity. It is also know that dietary omega 3-fatty acid can change the composition of the cell membranes in a short period of time so that the major component of the membrane lipids are then comprised of the two types of oils found in fish oils, mainly eicosapentaenoic acid (EPA) and docosahexaenoic acid (DHA). These particular oils inhibit the production of arachidonic acid within the cell membrane. It is the activation and release of arachidonic acid from the cell membrane that triggers the production of eicosanoids, resulting in the production of prostaglandins and leukotrienes. Many of these products are quite toxic to cells and can generate massive amounts of free radicals, leading to damage to the cell's membranes as well as its genetic structure. As we have seen, this process plays a critical role in glutamate toxicity.

The bottom line is that omega 3-fatty acids (fish oils) can block the production of "bad" type eicosanoids.

Other studies have shown that feeding omega 3-fatty acids to animals can significantly improve nerve conduction within the optic nerve.[13] While no one has measured it, one could safely assume that neural conduction within other parts of the nervous system would improve as well. It is important to buy only quality products free of pesticide residues and mercury. Some brands have high concentrations of omega 3-fatty acids and should be preferred. Another warning, always keep your capsules in the refrigerator. Omega 3-fatty acids are unsaturated and subject to rancid destruction. Because of this, I would recommend taking at least 400iu of alpha-tocopherol per day with your capsules.

Effects of aging on the brain: Free radicals
It is now known that as we age our cells, including neurons, lose a significant amount of their ability to generate energy. As you will recall, most cells generate the majority of their energy from electrons passing through a series of enzymatic reactions within the mitochondria, known as the electron transport chain. These electrons are derived from the breakdown of glucose in Kreb's cycle.

The various steps in energy generation by the electron transport chain have been designated complex I through V as listed in table 5-1. Anything which blocks one of these enzymatic steps severely interferes with the cells' ability to produce energy, primarily in the form of ATP. But to better understand how energy deficits occur we must go back one more step.

Even before energy production declines another process begins to develop as we age—the cells began to accumulate free radicals in larger amounts. We know that free radicals can damage cell membranes, intracellular components, and even the DNA itself. One reason for this gradual and increasing accumulation of free radicals is the reduction in the cell's protective mechanisms. For example, we know that all cells contain three antioxidant enzymes—glutathione, catalase and superoxide dismustase—as well as a multitude of scavenging vitamins and minerals (Vitamins C, E, D, K, beta carotene, selenium, magnesium, and zinc). In

---

[13] Connor WE and Neuringer M. Importance of dietary omega-3 fatty acids in retinal function and brain chemistry. **Nutritional Modulation of Neural Function**, Academic Press,1988, pp 191-200

fact, even co-enzyme Q_{10} acts as a powerful free radical scavenger and a regenerator of antioxidant vitamin C and E.

As we age, there is a progressive decline in reduced glutathione, as well as the other antioxidants, within the cellular environment.[14] In part, this is due to the increased production of several oxygen radicals, such as superoxide and the hydroxide radical, which in essence overwhelm the antioxidant enzymes. A combination of decreased availability of the antioxidant enzymes, depletion of the dietary antioxidants, and increased generation of free radicals puts all cells at considerable risk of serious injury or death.

In humans, we know that lipid peroxidation, a process of free radical injury to cell membrane lipids, results in the accumulation of "age" pigments within the brain called lipofuscin. Animals fed diets low in vitamin E develop a dramatic increase in these "age" pigments.[15] Vitamin E supplementation markedly reduces brain lipofuscin.

One of the early findings in Parkinson's disease, as you will recall, is a dramatic fall in the glutathione levels within the neurons of the primary area of the brain affected, the substantia nigra. This is accompanied by a buildup of peroxides and the dangerous hydroxide radical. Iron accumulation within these affected neurons acts as a powerful free radical generator as well. A recent study also indicated that there may be an accumulation of copper in addition to iron.[16] Copper, too, is a powerful generator of free radicals. Interestingly, iron is also known to be increased in the frontal lobes in cases of Alzheimer's disease.[17] And, as one would expect, there is an increase in lipid peroxidation in cases of Alzheimer's

---

[14] Ando S, et al. Increased levels of lipid peroxides in aged rat brain as revealed by direct assay of peroxide values. **Neuroscience Letters** 113: 199-204, 1990

[15] Williams LR. Oxidative stress, age-related neurodegeneration, and the potential for neurotrophic treatment. **Cerebrovascular and Brain Metabolism Reviews** 7: 55-73, 1995

[16] Pall HS, et al. Raised cerebrospinal-fluid copper concentration in Parkinson's disease. **Lancet** Aug1: 238-241, 1987

[17] Williams LR. Oxidative stress, age-related neurodegeneration, and potential for neurotrophic treatment. **Cerebrovascular and Brain Metabolism Reviews** 7:55-73, 1995

disease. Microscopically, free iron seems to concentrate in and around the neuritic plaques common to Alzheimer's disease patients. Others have reported a significant reduction in brain levels of vitamin E, A and carotenoids in autopsied cases of the disease.

The buildup of free radicals within the neurons with aging not only affects energy production (complex I is especially sensitive to damage by free radicals) but also produces severe damage to the mitochondrial DNA.[18] Cells, you see, possess two types of genetic material. One found in the nucleus (that most think of) and another within the mitochondria. The latter is responsible for reproduction of the mitochondria within the cell.

Damage to mitochondrial DNA affects only the involved mitochondria and not the genetics of the cell itself. But, when that mitochondria reproduces itself the defect is passed on to the new mitochondria as well. Today, we know that there is a growing list of diseases caused by mitochondrial malfunction. We know that many of these diseases do not present themselves until later childhood or even adulthood. The explanation for this delay may lie in the fact that until greater than 60% of the mitochondria are affected no disease occurs. That may take many years or even decades.

It is known that mitochondrial DNA mutates at a rate ten times that of chromosomal DNA.[19] Most likely this is because the former lacks histones and repair enzymes. In the first study of its kind, Dr. Allen C. Bowling and co-workers demonstrated an age dependent impairment of electron transport chain enzymes in the primate cortex.[20] They found that complex I and IV in the brain were especially vulnerable to age-related damage; these are the same two complexes damaged in Alzheimer's disease, Parkinson's disease, and the Huntington's disorder. A portion of these two

---

[18] Olanow CW. A radical hypothesis for neurodegeneration. **Trends in Neuroscience** 16: 439-444, 1993

[19] Miguel J. An integrated theory of aging as the result of mitochondrial-DNA mutations in differentiated cells. **Archives of Gerontology and Geriatrics** 12: 99-117, 1991

[20] Bowling AC, et al, Age-dependent impairment of mitochondrial function in primate brain. **Journal of Neurochemistry** 60: 1964-1967, 1993

complexes are encoded in the mitochondrial DNA. Complex II, III and V were preserved, not surprisingly, since they are encoded by the chromosomal DNA only. Complex I is known to be very sensitive to destruction by the hydroxyl radical and complex IV to peroxide.

It is also of interest to note that glutamate not only damages the microtubules within the dendrites, even in sublethal doses, but it also damages the DNA as well.[21] Dr. S.E. Shephard and co-workers, in a most important research study, found that aspartame (NutraSweet), when nitrosated in the stomach, shows a significant mutagenicity,[22] causing damage to the genetic structure of the cell. In fact, they found that the nitrosated aspartame was quite toxic to cells themselves.

PROTECTING OUR NEURONS FROM FREE RADICALS
Since the primary defect causing neurons to have difficulty generating energy is related to free radical generation, our primary concern should be in how to restore the cell's ability to combat these accumulating free radicals. There are, in fact, several things that we can do.

N-Acetyl L-Cysteine (NAC)
In the first edition of *Excitotoxins: The Taste That Kills*, the relation between L-cysteine and excitotoxic brain injury was covered. Since then, a multitude of people have called or written to ask if N-acetyl-L-cysteine is also an excitotoxin. So here it is: **N-Acetyl L-cysteine is not an excitotoxin and even in high doses does not seem to damage the brain.** L-cysteine produces its damage by converting to cysteine sulfinic acid and cysteic acid, both of which are excitotoxins. Remember, excitotoxins produce their damage only when outside the cell (in the extracellular space). N-acetyl L-cysteine enters the cell and is converted to glutathione, a powerful antioxidant enzyme.

A multitude of studies have shown that NAC can significantly elevate glutathione levels in the tissues, including brain tissues. Not only can glutathione neutralize one of the most powerful of the free radicals, the

---

[21] Didier M, et al. Chronic glutamate toxicity causes DNA damage. **Neurology** 44 (Abstract) A236, 1994

[22] Shephard SE, et al. Mutagenic activity of peptides and the artificial sweetener aspartame after nitrosation. **Food Chemical Toxicology** 31:323-329, 1993

hydroxyl radical, it can also regenerate the free radical scavenging power of vitamin C as well. When vitamin C and E are exposed to free radicals they are oxidized and may become free radicals themselves. They must be reduced before they can become effective free radical scavengers once again.

While N-acetyl L-cysteine appears to be safe, even in large doses (4 to 6 grams), more study is needed to assure its long term safety. There may be better and safer ways to increase intracellular glutathione.

Single antioxidant vitamins vs multiple vitamins

Another frequently asked question is, "Would it be better to take a single antioxidant vitamin in high doses or several types of antioxidants in lower doses, since they all seem to do the same thing?" The answer is that it is better to take several different types of antioxidants. There are many different types of free radicals—peroxides, hydroxide radical, superoxide, and singlet oxygen—for example. The antioxidants each specialize in removing specific types of free radicals. For example, vitamin E scavenges the superoxide radical, hydroxyl radical and acts as a chain-breaking agent in the propagation phase of lipid peroxidation. But, for most forms of vitamin E, it does so only in the lipid fractions of the cell, that is the fatty membranes. Water soluble vitamin E appears to concentrate in the cytosol of the cell as well. Coenzyme Q_{10}, on the other hand, blocks both the initiation as well as the propagation of lipid peroxidation.

Vitamin C and beta carotene block free radicals within the watery parts of the cells (cytosol) and in the space outside the cell (extracellular space) but not in the lipid membranes. Also important to consider is the fact that vitamin C and coenzyme Q_{10} can recycle vitamin E, thereby restoring its antioxidant function.[23] Glutathione recycles vitamin C.

It is for these reasons that the antioxidant vitamins and minerals should be taken in combination. Clinical studies, as well as experimental animal studies, confirm this observation.

Excitotoxins as free radical generators

It needs to be emphasized that all excitotoxins—glutamate, aspartate, and L-cysteine—stimulate large amounts of free radicals within exposed

---

[23] Sato K, et al. Synergism of tocopherol and ascorbate on the survival of cultured brain neurons. **Neuroreport** 4: 1179-1182, 1993

neurons. In fact, in a recent paper, Catherine Bergeron stated that the best theory for excitotoxity in ALS was that it initiated oxidative stress and the arachidonic cascade (by phospholipase A_2), thereby generating enormous and overwhelming concentrations of free radicals in the anterior horn cells of the spinal cord.[24] This, in time, results in the progressive death of these motor neurons and the onset of progressive weakness.

Similar scenarios are carried out in the other neurodegenerative diseases, such as Alzheimer's, Parkinson's and Huntington's diseases. In all cases, we know that excess excitotoxic stimulation results in the buildup of free radicals within the involved neurons, eventually overwhelming the cell's ability to neutralize these harmful particles.

Directly stimulating mitochondrial energy production
Once the problem of excess free radical generation is corrected, we are still left with damaged mitochondria that are unable to produce a sufficient amount of energy for normal functioning and survival. A growing list of mitochondrial diseases are being recognized. Treatment of these diseases, until recently, has been hopeless. What changed all of this was the realization that these are metabolic defects and that by manipulating the cell's metabolism one might correct some of these defects.

One of the early treatments involved using riboflavin and L-carnitine. The results were quite surprising and gratifying. Many patients improved and for the first time became functionally independent.

Coenzyme Q_{10} plus niacinamide
We know that certain mitochondrial toxins can mimic these disorders. Dr. Flint Beal and colleagues, using animals, found that if these animals were given a mitochondrial toxin they consistently developed lesions deep in their brains.[25] But, if the animals were pretreated with a combination of coenzyme Q_{10} and niacinamide the lesions could be prevented. Coenzyme Q_{10} alone could prevent these neurons from losing their ATP energy

---

[24] Bergeron C. Oxidative stress: its role in the pathogenesis of amyotrophic lateral sclerosis. **Journal of Neurological Science** 129: 81-84, 1995

[25] Beal MF, et al. Coenzyme Q_{10} and niacinamide are neuroprotective against mitochondrial toxins in vivo. **Neurology** (Supplement 2) A177, 1994

molecules but could not prevent cell death. But, by combining it with niacinamide there was a significant increase in brain cell ATP levels, thereby preventing excitotoxic damage.

It is my own personal feeling that riboflavin and thiamine would also boost ATP production to a even greater degree when added to Coenzyme Q_{10} and niacinamide. The dosage used in most studies was 100 mg of each and 120 mg of Coenzyme Q_{10}.

Acetyl L-carnitine

This compound is a derivative of L-carnitine, a natural biochemical component of all cells. It differs in that it enters the cell easier and provides an acetyl group for the production of the neurotransmitter acetylcholine. In fact, acetyl-L-carnitine has neurotransmitter properties much like acetylcholine.[26] This remarkable compound has several useful properties. It is an antioxidant, it increases mitochondrial energy production, it stabilizes cell membranes, increases cholinergic transmission in the brain (involved in memory), and chelates iron.[27]

Experimentally, it has been shown to reverse hippocampal and prefrontal loss of neurons associated with aging and it significantly reduces lipofuscin pigment (age pigment) accumulation.[28] In addition, acetyl-L-carnitine reduces the receptor loss associated with aging of the brain and significantly improves learning and memory in aged animals and humans. If all this is not enough, this remarkable compound has also been shown to defend brain cells against lipid peroxidation, and increase cellular glutathione and ubiquinol (Coenzyme Q_{10}) concentration.

In Chapter five I explained how a chemical accidentally manufactured during the production of illicit drugs, called MPTP, produced a sudden

---

[26] Onofry M, et al. Central Cholinergic effects of levo-acetyl carnitine. **Drug Exp Clinical Research** 9: 161-169, 1983

[27] Calvani M, et al . Clues to the mechanism of action of acetyl-L-carnitine in the central nervous system. **Dementia** 2: 1-6, 1991

[28] Angelucci L, et al. Acetyl-L-carnitine in the rat's hippocampal aging: morphological, endocrine and behavioral correlates. In: Gorio A, et al, Eds. **Neural Development and Regeneration. Cellular and Molecular Aspects.** Berlin: Springer-Verlag, 1988: 57-66

explosive onset of full-blown Parkinson's disease in hundreds of young people. It is now know that acetyl-L-carnitine can block certain aspects of MPTP toxicity and restore the reduced glutathione in the affected substantia nigral neurons.[29] In addition, this compound can increase the inhibitory neurotransmitter GABA, which protects neurons against excess stimulation. Glutamic acid moderately inhibits acetyl-L-carnitine uptake into the brain.[30] This is another reason to avoid MSG in your food.

Incredibly, I believe this remarkable, yet expensive compound may safely be used in doses of 3 to 4 grams a day.

L-Carnitine

I am often asked if L-carnitine can do the same things as acetyl-L-carnitine. Unfortunately, it cannot. But, it can do some pretty important things in terms of protecting the brain.[31]

For example, in the aging brains of rats it has been demonstrated to reduce the deteriorating histological changes as well as slow down behavioral deterioration. L-carnitine improves long-term memory, discriminatory learning, spatial learning and seems to extend longevity. Most importantly, L-carnitine significantly improves cellular energy production, including that in brain cells.

One thing L-carnitine cannot do that acetyl L-carnitine can do is increase cellular glutathione levels. Also, acetyl L-carnitine is much better absorbed by neurons than is L-carnitine. One important property of L-carnitine is that it has been shown to reduce glutamate toxicity in a dose dependent fashion.[32] That is, the higher the dose of L-carnitine, the better the protection. As for safety, L-carnitine has few side effects. In some individuals higher doses (two or more grams) can induce diarrhea.

---

[29] Ruggero G, et al. Systemic acetyl L-carnitine elevates nigral levels of glutathione and GABA. **Life Sciences** 43:289-292,1988

[30] Burlina AP, et al. Uptake of acetyl-L-carnitine in the brain. **Neurochemical Research** 14: 489-493, 1989

[31] Slivka A, et al. Carnitine treatment for stroke in rats. **Stroke** 21: 808-811, 1990

[32] Felipo V, et al. L-carnitine increases the affinity of glutamate for quisqualate receptors and prevents glutamate neurotoxicity. **Neurochemical Research** 19: 373-377, 1994

Taurine

Taurine is an amino acid found in high concentrations in the brain and appears to function as a neuromodulator in the nervous system. A neuromodulator is a substance that controls other neurotransmitters by preventing too great a response. In essence, its function is to protect the brain. We know that taurine plays a major role in stabilizing nervous system excitability. The highest concentrations are found in the pituitary and pineal glands, the retina, cerebellum, olfactory bulb, and the striatum. One experiment that makes the case for the importance of taurine in protecting the brain was conducted using cats.[33] Two sets of cats were fed an identical concentration of L-cystine, but one group was fed a taurine-free diet and the other was given a small amount of taurine.

All nine cats fed the taurine-free diet plus the 5% L-cystine developed lethargy, inability to stand, rigidity of the neck and lower limbs, epileptic seizures, and eventually died. The cats fed a diet containing a small amount of taurine plus the L-cystine showed only minimal symptoms or were symptom free. None died. The animals were followed for years.

By adding taurine to tissues exposed to the excitotoxins kainic acid and quinolinic acid, complete protection could be afforded.[34] Infant diets and tube feedings used for hospitalized patients, until recently, were without taurine. Because of the strong association between brain damage and excitotoxins, manufacturers are now adding taurine to infant feedings.

Conclusions

It is becoming increasing evident that many if not all of the neurodegenerative diseases of the central nervous system begin with an impaired energy production system. This leaves the neuron vulnerable to excitotoxin injury. By using nutritional products to increase mitochondrial energy production this final destructive step is avoided. Interestingly, L-carnitine and acetyl L-carnitine can by-pass the defect in complex I that I have seen in Parkinson's disease and Huntington's disease. Riboflavin,

---

[33] Strurman JA, et al . Cystine neurotoxicity is increased by taurine deficiency. **NeuroToxicology** 10:15-28,1989

[34] Sansberg PR, et al. Chronic taurine effects on various neurochemical indicies in control and kainic acid lesioned neostriatum. **Brain Research** 161:367-370, 1979

niacinamide, thiamine, and vitamin K also improve mitochondrial energy production in cases of poor energy generation by the cells. A new compound on the scene, Alpha-lipoic acid holds even more promise.

FURTHER IMPROVING BRAIN FUNCTION NUTRITIONALLY

Phosphatidylcholine (Lecithin)
The nervous system consist of a multitude of complex phosphorus containing lipids, such as sphingomyelin, gangliosides, and cerebrosides. Not only do they form the insulation for the nerve pathways (myelin sheath) but they also make up the majority of the cell membranes.

One of the popular products sold in health food stores to improve memory function is lecithin. While in biochemical terms lecithin is synonymous with phosphatidylcholine, in most preparations it is a combination of phosphatidylcholine, phosphatidylethanolamine, and phosphatidylserine. Pure phosphatidylcholine is thought to improve memory by increasing the availability of choline for the production of the neurotransmitter, acetylcholine. While acetylcholine has many functions in the brain as a neurotransmitter it does play a major role in various aspects of memory.

Several experiments have shown that even in normal individuals, phosphatidylcholine can improve memory.[35] Experiments using this product to treat Alzheimer's patients has met with some minor success. The results are better when lecithin is combined with choline.

There is also interest in using lecithin to repair injuries to the insulation of nerves (in cases of multiple sclerosis, trigeminal neuralgia, stroke, and head injury, for example.) I have used lecithin in cases of brain injuries and strokes and have seen a significant improvement in these patients' outcomes. Others have reported similar results.

Lecithin capsules should be kept in the refrigerator at all times to prevent spoilage. It also makes them more palatable.

---

[35] Drachman DA and Sahakian BJ. Effect of cholinergic agents on human learning and memory. In, Baseau, et al (eds) **Nutrition and the Brain**. Vol 5, Raven Press, pp351-366 , 1979.

Phosphatidylserine

While previously all the attention has been given to its biochemical cousin, phosphatidylcholine, this phospholipid is being shown to have superior neurological properties. When fed to aging animals, it has been shown to significantly improve their passive-active avoidance reaction, spatial memory and other learning and memory tasks.[36]

In a recent study involving men 50 years or older suffering from serious memory loss not caused by Alzheimer's disease, it was found that giving 300mg of phosphatidylserine a day for three months significantly improved their memory function as measured by an extensive battery of tests.[37] Improvement was seen within three weeks of taking the product especially regarding name and face recognition and recall, telephone number recall, and misplaced object recall. Another interesting effect was the fact that these memory impaired men showed significant improvement in their ability to remember the details of a story that was read.

The exact mechanism for this improvement is not known. But, it is known that phosphatidylserine is a natural glutamate blocker. It has also been shown to improve cell membrane stability and fluidity. As we age our cell membranes become stiffer, interfering with their normal operation in a multitude of functions such as electrolyte exchange gradients, receptor function, and impulse generation. Phosphatidylserine appears to restore a more youthful composition to these vital membranes. This intriguing compound has also shown promise in Alzheimer's patients. Most improved on several measures of cognitive functions and the result appeared to be most dramatic in those having earlier stages of the disease.

Phosphotidylserine appears to be safe. Its only drawback is that it is very expensive. I would warn the reader to avoid products made from animal brains.

Dihyro-ergot compounds (Hydergine)

Hydergine is a combination product derived from a rye fungus, *claviceps purpurea*. The altered and purified form, called Hydergine, is manufactured by the Sandoz Pharmaceutical company. It is composed of three ergot compounds: dihydroergocornine, dihydroergocristine mesylate,

---

[36] Crook TH, et al. Effects of phosphatidylserine in age-associated memory impairment. **Neurology** 41: 644-649, 1991

[37] *Ibid*

and dihydroergocryptine mesylate. This group of compounds has useful properties in counteracting the effects of aging on the brain. It is known to increase brain blood flow as well as oxygen delivery and acts as a free radical scavenger. Clinical studies have demonstrated improved alertness and higher levels of intellectual function in young, healthy individuals.[38]

One of the more interesting properties of Hydergine, is its effect on the cAMP second messenger system within brain cells.[39] These are chemical messengers that travel within the cell by delivering information between neurotransmitters, hormones, and neuromodulators and the components within the cell. Hydergine interacts with cAMP in a way so as to prevent its level from falling too low or going too high.

This is important in that it helps economize the brain's ATP levels, thereby preventing a sudden drain on brain energy reserves during times of stress. It is suspected that in the aged brain, stress precipitated release of catecholamine hormones (epinephrine and norepinephrine) may tax the neuron's energy generating machinery to the point that it can no longer compensate for the demand.[40] This can result in energy depletion and subject the neuron to excitotoxic injury or even eventual death. Hydergine inhibits catecholamine stimulation of the neuron's metabolism. Another, perhaps even more important response, is Hydergine's effect on membrane stability. As stated above, aging severely impairs the cell membrane's composition resulting in a multitude of problems. As with any medication, consult your physician for dosage.

DMAE (Deanol)

Dimethylaminoethanol (DMAE) or deanol, is a natural substance found in anchovies and sardines and, to a limited extent, in the brain itself. DMAE is known to increase the production of choline in the brain and, as a result,

---

[38] Meier-Ruge W, et al. Workshop on advances in experimental pharmacology of Hydergine. **Gerontology** 24(suppl 1) 1-153, 1978

[39] Markstein R, et al. Dehydrotoxine on cyclic-AMP generating systems in rat cerebral cortex slices. **Gerontology** 24: (suppl 1) 94-105, 1978

[40] Markstein R, et al. The effect of Dehydroergotoxine, phentolamine and pindolol on catecholamine stimulated adenyl-cyclase in rat cerebral cortex. **FEBS Letters** 55: 275-277, 1975

increases the brain's production of acetylcholine. Early reports found that DMAE produced a sense of mood elevation and improved memory and learning ability, even in the young.[41] In one large study involving behavioral problems in children, it was found that DMAE supplementation reduced hyperactivity, increased attention span, and reduced irritability in 76% of girls and 66% of boys.[42] It may offer a better alternative than Ritalin in cases of attention deficit disorder.

The beneficial effects of DMAE usually require two to three weeks of supplementation. In most studies, maximal benefit was attained at least by six months. There are several reports of DMAE reducing daytime fatigue and giving one a sense of having more energy. Not only is sleep often sounder, but many report that individuals may require less sleep than before supplementation.

As with the other compounds, DMAE appears to stabilize cell membranes. Side effects are usually limited to spasms of the neck and jaw.

STABILIZING THE BLOOD-BRAIN BARRIER
The above items constitute a short list of supplements that have shown particular value in reversing the effects of aging on the brain and may offer protection from excitotoxin damage. There is a growing list of compounds and drugs that may offer even greater results. Finally, I would like to mention one other area of protection that is purely theoretical but, is backed up by strong research evidence, and that is nutritional products that may strengthen the blood-brain barrier.

It was a gentleman by the name of Bill Sardi who focused my attention on the concept and presented me with some startling research. Bill wrote a very interesting book entitled, **Nutrition and the Eyes**. But it was the second part of a two-part article he wrote for the *Townsend Newsletter for*

---

[41] Osvaido R. 2-dimethylaminoethanol (deanol): a brief review of its clinical efficacy and postulated mechanism of action. **Current Therapeutic Research** 16: 138-1242, 1974

[42] Oettinger L. the use of Deanol in the treatment of disorders of behavior in children. **Journal of Pediatrics** 3: 671-675, 1958

Doctors that attracted my attention.[43] Then, much to my surprise, Bill wrote to me and we discussed some of these ideas. So how is this connected to the brain?

Embryologically, the eyes develop as special extensions of the brain. And like the brain, the eyes have their own blood barrier system, much like the blood-brain barrier.

What Bill showed was that a special group of nutritional compounds tend to protect the eyes from damage by disease and from the changes of aging. These compounds are commonly known as flavonoids or bioflavonoids. A multitude of reports demonstrate that several of the flavones, quercetin, rutin and the flavanone, hesperidin, can significantly protect this retinal barrier and improve the strength of the capillaries in the eye. One would assume, since they have the same composition, that the blood-brain barrier would likewise be strengthened by flavone-flavanone supplementation. In general, these compounds are relatively cheap and non-toxic. It would be worthwhile to supplement those in danger of barrier disruption, such as hypertensives, diabetics and those with multiple sclerosis.

Two of the flavanone substances are of particular interest, quercetin and hesperidin. Both have been shown to be significant inhibitors of the eicosanoid generating enzyme delta lipoxygenase.[44] Quercetin was found to be a potent and prolonged inhibitor of proinflammatory arachidonic acid metabolism. Hesperidin, at higher concentrations, was found to inhibit the enzyme, phospholipase A_2, responsible for the release of arachidonic acid. This could not only be important in protecting the integrity of the blood-brain barrier, but in protecting the cells of the brain from excitotoxic damage, since it uses the same pathways.

---

[43] Sardi B. Diabetic retinopathy: Insulin and laser vs diet and nutritional supplements. Part II The real way to save sight. **Townsend Newsletter for Doctors**. May 1996, pp 66-75

[44] Welton AF, et al. Effect of flavanoids on arachidonic acid metabolism. **Plant Flavonoids in Biology and Medicine: Biochemical, Pharmacological, and Structure-activity Relationships**. pp231-242, 1986

Alpha-lipoic acid: Is it a miracle nutrient?

Alpha-lipoic acid, also called thiotic acid, is a natural component of tissues throughout the body. It has a multitude of functions, many of which play an important role in protecting the body against free radicals, heavy metal toxicity, and a number of age-related destructive changes in cells and tissues.[45] It appears to be the reduced form of alpha-lipoic acid, called dihydrolipoic acid or DHLA, that plays such a vital role in neutralizing free radicals.

Scientists consider the ideal "universal antioxidant" to have some of the following properties:

1. It should have a specific activity against free radicals;
2. It should chelate or bind oxygen reactive metals;
3. It should interact with other antioxidants;
4. It should have maximal absorption from the gut and be easily available to all tissues (bioavailable);
5. It should be able to enter both the membrane (lipid domain) and the cytosol (aqueous domain).

Reduced alpha-lipoic acid, DHLA, appears to meet virtually all of these criteria, making it a "universal antioxidant." As we have learned, one of the most potent free radicals known is the hydroxyl radical. DHLA not only scavenges this dangerous radical but also removes hypochlorous acid, singlet oxygen, and the superoxide radical. Another way DHLA reduces free radical formation is by its ability to chelate free iron and copper, both of which are very powerful free radical generators. It can scavenge the peroxyl radical and has been shown to protect DNA from single strand breaks caused by singlet oxygen.

One of the more interesting and vitally important characteristics of DHLA is that it appears to be able to regenerate other antioxidants. As mentioned before, when vitamin C and E are used to neutralize free radicals they themselves become oxidized. To be used as antioxidants, they must be returned to a reduced form. DHLA is a powerful regenerator of reduced ascorbate and tocopherol. It is this continuous process of recycling of vitamin C and E to their reduced form by DHLA that prevents the cell membrane from undergoing destructive lipid peroxidation. Alpha-lipoic acid has been shown to prevent the symptoms of both vitamin C and E

---

[45] Packer L, et al. Alpha-lipoic acid as a biological antioxidant **Free Radical Biology and Medicine** 19: 227-250, 1995

deficiency. Alpha-lipoic acid is also known to increase the levels of ubiquinol (coenzyme Q_{10}) during times of oxygen stress (free radical buildup). In addition, alpha-lipoic acid increases intracellular glutathione, another powerful antioxidant. As for bioavailability, following dietary supplementation, both alpha-lipoic acid and DHLA increase in all tissues.

Besides its function as a free radical scavenger and regenerator of other antioxidants, alpha-lipoic acid has also been shown to enhance glucose transport into cells as well, even without insulin. Normally glucose cannot enter a cell, except in the brain, unless insulin is present. What makes this especially important is that this could play a vital role in treating both forms of diabetes, type I or juvenile onset, and type II, adult onset.

Clinical Studies with Alpha-Lipoic acid and DHLA

The clinical studies using these two compounds have been very encouraging. In one study of people having type II diabetes, alpha-lipoic acid was shown to enhance glucose utilization by 50%. Another area of interest is in dealing with the complication of diabetes, particularly polyneuropathy and cataracts. Diabetic polyneuropathy is a disorder of the nerves in the arms and especially in the legs, causing severe burning pains and numbness, and sometimes affecting bladder and bowel function. The pains are quite incapacitating. Studies on patients having this disorder have shown that the majority have shown significant improvement of their symptoms on alpha lipoic acid supplementation.

Cataracts are known to be related to free radical damage to the lens of the eye. Experimental studies, using chemicals that induce cataracts in rats, demonstrated that alpha-lipoic acid prevented cataract formation.[46] Examination of the lenses of the supplemented animals also demonstrated significant elevations in glutathione, ascorbate, and vitamin E.

It is known that when the blood supply to the brain is temporally cut off and then restored minutes later the brain is flooded with free radicals, often leading to death of the animals. This would mimic the clinical situation seen with persons suffering from a sudden and prolonged cardiac arrest or from a massive stroke. Normally, the mortality from such

---

[46] Maitra I, et al. Alpha-lipoic acid prevents buthionine sulfoximine-induced cataract formation in new born rats. **Free Radical Biology and Medicine** 18: 823-829, 1995

experiments is as high as 80%. But when animals are pretreated with alpha-lipoic acid the mortality falls to 20%. This remarkable lowering of death rates in animals receiving alpha-lipoic acid is in part due to improved glutathione concentrations in the brain and the resulting reduction in lipid peroxidation.

Another effect of alpha-lipoic acid is its effect on the aging brain. In one study of memory loss seen in aging mice, alpha-lipoic acid supplementation improved performance to such an extent that twenty-four hours later the aged animals were performing better than the young animals.[47] Yet, when given to the younger animals it did not improve their memory.

It is tempting to think that the improved mental function in the aged brain may be secondary to the improved passage of glucose into the brain past dysfunctional glucose transporters.

Recently, Greenamyre and co-workers found that by treating animals with alpha-lipoic acid or DHLA for seven days they could significantly reduce (by 50%), either directly of indirectly, excitotoxic lesions caused by injecting a powerful excitotoxin or metabolic inhibitor deep into the brain.[48] The mechanism could be by alpha-lipoic acid's ability to either improve brain energy metabolism, or by its antioxidant effect, or both.

Alpha-lipoic acid, but not DHLA, was discovered to give profound protection against radiation injury to the blood forming tissues (hematopoetic tissue) in mice.[49] Survival in heavily irradiated mice increased from 35% to 90% when they were treated with alpha-lipoic acid. And in one of the largest human experiments in radiation exposure, the Chernobyl disaster, it was found that thousands of children, as well as

---

[47] Hartmann SSH, et al. The potent free radical scavenger alpha-lipoic acid improves memory in aged mice: putative relationship to NMDA receptor deficits. **Pharmacology, Biochemistry and Behavior** 46: 799-805, 1993

[48] Greenamyre JT, et al. The endogenous cofactors, thiotic acid and dihydrolipoic acid, are neuroprotective against NMDA and malonic acid lesions of striatum. **Neuroscience Letters**. 171: 17020, 1994

[49] Ramakrishnan N, et al. Radioprotection of hematopoetic tissues in mice by lipoic acid. **Radiation Research** 130: 360-365, 1992

adults, were living in zones of constant low-level radiation.[50] These children were found to have high levels of peroxidation products in their blood. But, the children treated with alpha-lipoic acid were found to have levels as low as that of unexposed, normal children. The addition of vitamin E to the alpha-lipoic acid lowered the levels of peroxidation products even further, while vitamin E alone had no effect.

Finally, alpha-lipoic acid, as a metal chelator, has been shown to offer complete protection against mercury poisoning in mice when given in a high dose. Similar protection was also seen in cases of arsenite poisoning in animals. But, the dose had to be in a high ratio to the poison. Cadmium poisoning is known to induce cellular membrane damage, lipid peroxidation, and depletion of cellular glutathione. In rats, alpha-lipoic acid was found to completely prevent cadmium-induced lipid peroxidation in the heart, brain, and testes.

As you can see alpha-lipoic acid is truly a remarkable compound. It may hold great promise, when used in combination with some of the other supplements, in preventing or even reversing the neurodegenerative diseases. More research is needed to answer this important question. Alpha-lipoic acid works best if it is taken on a daily basis, since in several experiments protection was afforded only if it had been taken well before the damaging event. Most likely, this is because it must be converted to its active reduced form, dihydrolipoic acid in order to give full protection.

The side effects associated with alpha-lipoic acid are usually few and minor. The Germans have been using it in larger doses for many years. Allergic skin reactions are possible and when given in very large intravenous doses it may lower the blood sugar to hypoglycemic levels.

PART II
WHAT DID THE FASEB REPORT REALLY SAY?

In July of 1995, the Life Sciences Research Office of the Federation of American Societies for Experimental Biology (FASEB) prepared what was to be a definitive report on the question of safety of monosodium glutamate for the Food and Drug Administration. The report is divided into two

---

[50] Korkina LG, et al. Antioxidant therapy in children affected by irradiation from the Chernobyl nuclear accident. **Biochemical Society Transactions** 21: 314S, 1993

major parts, an executive summary prepared by the FDA followed by the indepth analysis of the medical and research literature on MSG. The news media never got past the executive summary, which I am sure is what the FDA was counting on. And, as predicted, the evening news announced that the report from the experts on the panel concluded that when less than three grams was consumed, MSG appeared to be safe. In the June 1996 issue of *Nutrition Today* there is a statement by the Institute of Food Technologist which uses the very same selective reading done by the major media, giving the reader the impression that the FASEB report gives MSG a clean bill of health.[51]

In fact, that is not what the report said at all. The executive summary was couched in very clever terms. For example, on page vi they make the statement that, "no evidence exists to support the role of ingested glutamate in the etiology or exacerbation of these or any other long-term or chronic illness." At first look this seems to say that studies have been conducted to see if there is a causal link between MSG ingestion and worsening of these disorders, and that no link was found. But in truth, as the body of the report makes plain, no such studies have ever been done. No one has examined this vital question. But there is plenty of clinical, as well as research, evidence to support the very real danger of MSG ingestion in neurodegenerative diseases.

I have received calls from several patients suffering from ALS who have told me that their doctors, who staff some of the largest ALS clinics and research centers in the country, confidentially tell them to avoid MSG and aspartame. The reason they are reluctant to go public with this is because they fear ridicule by colleagues and the industry. This is reminiscent of doctors' responses to claims of the beneficial effects of vitamins less than a decade ago.

The defenders of MSG safety have always relied on the weak argument that glutamate is excluded from the brain by the blood-brain barrier. But the text of the FASEB report says the opposite. In fact, they cite a recent study done by Bogdanov and Wurtman (1994) in which they measured deep brain (striate) levels of glutamate following a dose of MSG. These researchers found that following the dose of MSG, striate levels of glutamate rose sharply and significantly (Page 29 of the report).

---

[51] Monosodium Glutamate. A Statement of the Institute of Food Technologist. **Nutrition Today** 31: 107, 1996

In this book I give three other references that confirm that brain levels of glutamate rise following elevations in blood glutamate. In fact, one researcher found that with chronic ingestion of glutamate, brain levels of glutamate were consistently elevated. This, of course, would more closely imitate the case in humans since they consume foods high in glutamate over many years, even a lifetime.

Then the report confirms something that I discuss in my book, that several areas of the brain possess no blood-brain barrier. The report concludes, "The net result is that certain areas of the brain may be vulnerable to acute, large magnitude fluctuations in plasma glutamate concentrations because of flooding from adjacent circumventricular organs." (Page 29) The report ignored the multitude of clinical conditions in which the blood-brain barrier can be damaged, such as during hypertension, diabetes, stroke, Alzheimer's disease, and head injury.

On page 43 of the report the expert panel notes that the nucleus solitarius (in the brain stem) is one area of the brain that might allow glutamate from the blood to affect the rest of the brain, since this nucleus regulates the blood vessels to the rest of the brain. Also, this nucleus is not protected by the blood-brain barrier. Again, no one has examined this important question.

On page 42 they further state, *"...in the absence of studies or corroborating evidence* linking symptoms or signs of adverse effects...it is not possible to link either acute or chronic consumption of MSG to glutamate mediated neurodegenerative diseases *at this time."* (Italics added) Note the two disclaimers: "In the absence of studies" and "at this time." This leaves the expert panel a way out should future studies discover such a link. They further protect themselves by stating on the same page, "Levels of ingested MSG might be sufficient to raise the concentration of blood glutamate and related compounds enough to change the levels of these amino acids in the brain, particularly in the circumventricular areas not protected by the blood-brain barrier."

. On pages 42 to 43 they go even further when they discuss the lack of protection for the pineal gland. "The elevated levels of glutamate and related compounds would then have adverse neuroexcitatory effects, be neurotoxic, and/or initiate a chain of metabolic events that would result in either neurotoxicity or the release of substances that would cause the neurological manifestations reportedly associated with MSG exposure." And on page 100 of the report they state, "In contrast, glutamate concentrations in the extracellular fluid in brain regions not protected by the blood-brain barrier will closely mirror changes in circulating glutamate concentrations."

This is an incredible admission. Are they saying that these areas of the brain not protected by the barrier are unimportant? Is the hypothalamus unimportant? What about the hippocampus? In addition, there is ample evidence that with chronic exposure to MSG in the diet glutamate will seep from the unprotected parts of the brain into the normally protected areas. Sort of a back door approach.

But the hedging goes even further. On page 46 they say that, "It is conceivable that the consumption of MSG in genetically or otherwise predisposed individuals can exacerbate a preexisting neurological condition." So what are some of these conditions that put people at risk when they ingest MSG? They would include Alzheimer's disease, ALS, Huntington's disease, Parkinson's disease, and olivopontocerebellar degeneration. Does this sound like the expert panel was saying that MSG added to food is safe?

What about brain lesions caused by MSG? The expert panel concluded on page 57 that after reviewing 43 different studies the weight of the evidence is "convincing" that MSG causes destructive lesions in the hypothalamus and a reduction in endocrine organ weights in all species studied. What we are talking about here are major alterations in the endocrine system that could result in a multitude of endocrine disorders such as infertility, menstrual difficulties, polycystic ovaries, and other reproductive problems. The hypothalamus also controls appetite, sleep-wake cycles, immunity, and a host of other vital functions.

On page 103 they conclude, "Theoretically, if blood levels seen in animals as a result of MSG challenge were achieved in humans, similar lesions and/or neuroendocrine effects could be expected to occur." Studies, even by defenders of MSG safety, have shown that, in fact, humans develop blood levels of glutamate much higher than that seen in animals, when given MSG in comparable doses. In fact, humans develop blood levels higher than any known species. So, in essence, what they are saying is that hypothalamic lesions in humans would be expected following MSG ingestion.

Regarding seizures, on page 65 they note that, "Motor disturbances and changes in seizure threshold have been noted in numerous studies." It is interesting to note that all of the newer anti-seizure medications are glutamate blocking drugs.

On page 66 the expert panel notes that there is convincing evidence that glutamate given to newborn rodents can cause behavioral and neurologic effects. This is discussed extensively in chapter four.

On pages 64 and 65 they state that there are numerous studies confirming the link between changes in brain chemistry and MSG exposure. This is particularly worrisome in children, since the reported neurochemical changes involve transmitters responsible for learning and memory and behavioral control.

The panel found that some infant feeding formulas contained very high levels of free glutamate. This was especially true of formulas made from casein hydrolysates. Today we are seeing MSG and or aspartame being added to a multitude of child related food products and medications such as vitamins, cold preparations, vaccines, and foods. There is sufficient evidence to condemn such a irresponsible practice.

MORE EVIDENCE

One extremely interesting part of the FASEB study was the clear demonstration by the expert panel of what can only be described as deception by the defenders of MSG safety. Of even more interest, is the fact that these startling revelations, also discussed in this book, are never mentioned in the FDA's executive summery.

The most obvious false claim by MSG defenders is that the blood-brain barrier excludes dietary glutamate from the brain. The body of the report points out in numerous citations that the blood-brain barrier can be breached at several sites in the normal brain. (See pages 28, 29,43-43, 96, 100 and 104 in the FASEB report.)

I would especially recommend that the reader study the section on pages 54 and 55 in which the expert panel reviews some of the deceptive tactics used by the defenders of MSG safety. For example, on page 54 is a discussion of the Reynolds, *et al* deception that can only be described as scientific fraud.

Another method used by the MSG defenders, which was pointed out by the FASEB review, is discussed on page 57. In several papers reviewed by the FASEB panel, the researchers claimed that their studies did not show brain lesions following MSG exposure in test animals, thus giving the impression that Dr. John Olney's work was invalid. But, the animals were anesthetized with a drug called Ketamine, which is known to be a powerful glutamate blocker. In fact, I use Ketamine to block glutamate toxicity in some of my neurosurgical patients. It was a well known fact that Ketamine had this property long before these MSG defenders designed their experiments. One can only conclude that the experiments were designed to have negative results so that the industry could site them as supporting the safety of MSG.

Summary

In conclusion, the actual body of the report is very good and supports much of what is in this book. But the FASEB expert panel did not go far enough. For example, the discussion on effects on the developing brain were severely deficient, especially in light of their finding of very high levels of free glutamate in some infant feeding formulas. I go into much more detail in Chapter four of this book.

I am also puzzled by the lack of data on actual amounts of glutamate added to processed foods. While several questionable studies on total consumption are cited, it seems to me to be a simple matter to obtain from each industry the actual amounts of glutamate and related excitotoxins that are being added to the foods at the time of processing. This would give us a much more accurate picture of free glutamate in the diet. I was also disappointed in their lack of discussion of the additive effects of excitotoxins in the diet. We know that even subtoxic doses of excitotoxins when added together can produce an ultimate toxic dose to the brain. This is especially important in evaluating not only differing forms of MSG in food, but the fact that large amounts of aspartame are also being consumed as well, which adds significantly to the danger.

I would have liked to see the expert panel come out with a much stronger condemnation of MSG as a food additive, especially in light of their conclusion that even oral doses of MSG have been shown to cause necrotizing brain damage in the hypothalamus and further that microscopically one sees "massive cytoplasmic breaks," "dissolution of cell contents," and "massive cell membrane breaks." Certainly our children deserve better.

Since I began the research in writing this book, an incredible amount of new material has surfaced concerning the harmful nature of free excitotoxins within the nervous system. Today, virtually all of the neurodegenerative diseases are now considered to be intimately related to the excitotoxic process. Seizures, headaches, strokes, brain injury, subarachnoid hemorrhage, and developmental brain disorders are all intimately related to excitotoxins. Yet we continue to add tons of free glutamate, aspartate, and cysteine to our food and drink. That is not a rational thing to do.

It is my opinion, after reviewing an enormous amount of medical and research literature, that monosodium glutamate, aspartame, and other excitotoxin dietary additives poise an enormous hazard to our health and to the development and normal functioning of the brain. To continue to add enormous amounts of excitotoxins to our food is unconscionable and will lead to suffering and ruined lives for generations to come. The civilized world, especially the United States, has become the largest experimental laboratory in history. The question that begs for an answer is, "Are we creating a nightmare world?"

Finally, even though I have discussed a multitude of nutrients and drugs that can provide some protection against excitotoxin damage, I am in no way encouraging you to use these supplements to justify a continued use of excitotoxic food additives. This is especially true for those at high risk for excitotoxic damage and for developing one of the neurodegenerative diseases.

Appendix I

HIDDEN SOURCES OF MSG

As discussed previously, the glutamate manufacturers and the processed food industries are always on a quest to disguise MSG added to food. Below is a partial list of the most common names for disguised MSG. Remember also that the powerful excitotoxins aspartate and L-cysteine are frequently added to foods and according to FDA rules require no labeling at all.

Additives that always contain MSG:[492]
Monosodium Glutamate
Hydrolyzed Vegetable Protein
Hydrolyzed Protein
Hydrolyzed Plant Protein
Plant Protein Extract
Sodium Caseinate
Calcium Caseinate
Yeast Extract
Textured Protein
Autolyzed Yeast
Hydrolyzed Oat Flour

Additives that frequently contain MSG:
Malt extract
Malt Flavoring
Bouillon
Broth
Stock
Flavoring
Natural Flavoring
Natural Beef or Chicken Flavoring
Seasoning

255

Spices
Additives that may contain MSG or excitotoxins:
Carrageenan
Enzymes
Soy Protein Concentrate
Soy Protein Isolate
Whey Protein Concentrate

Protease enzymes of various sources can release excitotoxin amino acids from food proteins.[493]

Glossary

Acetylcholine: A neurotransmitter used by the nervous system. It is synthesized from a substance found commonly in foods, called choline. It is thought to play a role in memory.

Amino acid: A group of compounds that make up the building blocks of proteins. Humans use approximately twenty-two different types of amino acids.

Antioxidant: (Free radical scavengers.) These are compounds that render free radicals harmless. They may be minerals, vitamins, or enzymes. Common examples include vitamin E, vitamin C, and beta-carotene.

Anterior horn cells: Special neurons found within the grey matter of the spinal cord that stimulate motor movement in the body.

Aspartate: An acidic amino acid used by the brain as a neurotransmitter. At higher doses it can injure or kill neurons and is then considered an excitotoxin.

ATP: Abbreviation for adenosine triphosphate, a high-energy compound that all cells in the body use for energy. It is generated by the metabolism of food.

Blood-brain barrier: This is a mechanical system that the brain uses to keep certain harmful compounds from entering the brain. The barrier is thought to exist in the walls of the capillaries within the brain.

Calcium channels: These are special microscopic pores found within the walls of cell membranes. They function to regulate the entry of calcium into the cell's interior.

Designer drugs: These are drugs that are especially designed by a chemist for the purpose of producing brain stimulation. For example, the drug "ecstasy" is a designer drug.

Electron transport system: This is the final common pathway in the production of energy in the cell during metabolism.

Excitatory amino acids: These are special amino acids (mostly acidic types) that when applied to neurons will cause them to become very excited. These include cysteine, aspartate and glutamate.

Excitotoxins: These are a group of excitatory amino acids that can cause sensitive neurons to die. Some of these compounds are found in nature and some are created artificially, such as kainate.

Fatty acid: These are building blocks of fats, just as amino acids are building blocks from proteins. When combined in various configurations they form specific types of fats.

Free radicals: These are highly reactive substances that can damage important parts of the cell such as the chromosomes and mitochondria. Scientifically they consist of atoms or compounds having an unpaired valence electron in their outer orbital. Examples include hydroxyl ions and superoxide.

Glia cells: These are special cells found throughout the nervous system. They do not conduct signals but rather act to supply energy and other supportive functions for the neurons. They include several specialized types of cells, such as the astrocyte, the oligodendroglia and the microglia.

Glucose transporter: This is a special mechanism within the cells lining the capillaries that make up the blood-brain barrier that is used to transport glucose into the brain. It does not require energy for its operation. The brain's energy supply is totally dependent on this mechanism.

Glutamate: This is an excitatory amino acid used by the brain as a neurotransmitter. When it is allowed to accumulate in concentrations higher than needed for this purpose it can become a powerful poison to special neurons in the nervous system. At these concentrations it is considered an excitotoxin.

Glutamine: This is a form of amino acid commonly found in foods. It is converted in the glia cells of the brain into glutamate. There are special enzymes within the glia cells that allow glutamine to be converted to glutamate when it is needed by the neurons for neurotransmission. When glutamate accumulates in a concentration higher than is normally safe for the brain, some is reconverted to glutamine and stored in the glia cells.

Grey matter: When the brain is sliced into sections one notices areas that have a gray appearance, such as the cortex and the nuclei deep within the brain. This gray appearance comes from the large number of neurons located in these areas.

Hippocampus: An area of the brain located in the temporal lobe. On cross section it has the appearance of a rolled up scroll. It appears to play a vital role in recent memory function.

Hypoxia: This means that an insufficient amount of oxygen is being supplied to the organs for whatever cause, such as failure of the lungs, severe anemia or impaired blood supply to the brain. When the supply of oxygen is completely cut off it is referred to as anoxia.

Kreb's cycle: This is a cyclic series of metabolic reactions that occurs in all cells of the body. Its function is to break down glucose and other substances into energy. It is also the source of other chemicals used in the cell. It is also referred to as the citric acid cycle.

L-BMAA: Chemical abbreviations for L-B-N-methylamino-L-alanine. This substance is normally found in the seed of the sago plant (Cycas circinalis) and has been shown to destroy glutamate type neurons. It has been linked to a special disorder found in natives who consume the sage seed flour in high concentrations. This disorder shows characteristics of Parkinson's disease, ALS, and Alzheimer's disease.

L-BOAA: A chemical abbreviation for L-B-N-oxalyamino-L-alanine, which is found in high concentrations in the chick pea. Persons eating a diet high in chick peas are known to develop a disorder in which portions of the spinal cord are destroyed.

LTP: Long termed potentiation. This is the mechanism that is thought to play a vital role in the development of memories. It involves circular pathways in the hippocampus that continue to fire for days or even weeks. Glutamate plays a significant role in initiation of LTP.

Mitochondria: This is a small microscopic bubble within all cells that is the center of energy metabolism. It contains critical enzymes which guide these reactions along so as to produce enormous amounts of energy for the cell in the form of high energy phosphate compounds such as ATP and phosphocreatinine.

MSG: Monosodium Glutamate. This is the sodium salt of glutamate. It has the same excitotoxic properties as pure glutamate. Other salts of glutamate, such as monopotassium glutamate, are also toxic to the system.

MPTP: The chemical abbreviation for 1-methyl-4-phenyl-1,2,3,6-tetra-hydropyridine. This powerful toxin can produce Parkinson's disease in man and other primates. It was accidentally manufactured by drug addicts as a designer drug.

Neurotransmitter: Also referred to as a transmitter. These are a group of chemicals that allow neurons to communicate to each other. The are secreted into the small cleft between the ends of the nerve fiber called the synapse.

Neuron: This is a nerve cell found within the central nervous system (the brain or the spinal cord).

Neuritic plaque: These are microscopic bodies found outside of the neuron. They consist of degenerating nerve endings surrounding a central core made of a protein substance called amyloid. These plaques are seen in aging brains and are especially numerous in cases of Alzheimer's disease.

Neurofibrillary tangles: These are abnormal neurons that are filled with a fibrous substance made of paired helical filaments. These filaments contain several characteristic proteins such as tau, phosphorylated neurofibrillary protein, MAP-2, and other peptides. They are characteristic of Alzheimer's disease. These tangles are seen to be numerous in the temporal lobes and parietal lobes of the brain.

Nuclei: These are clumps of gray matter found below the cortex of the brain. Examples of nuclei include the thalamus, putamen, and the substantia nigra.

Prostaglandins: These are a group of compounds found throughout the body. When acted on by enzymes in the cells they are converted into powerful chemicals that have various functions such as increasing blood flow, stimulating inflammation, immune suppression, and many other physiologic functions.

Receptors: These are special areas on the surface of neuron membranes that act as receptacles for chemical messengers. For example, glutamate receptors react only with glutamate or aspartate-type compounds. The receptor is like the lock and glutamate is like the specific key that opens that lock.

Striatum: These are a group of nuclei found deep within the brain that play a vital role in certain types of movements. They include the putamen, the caudate and the globus pallidus.

Substantia nigra: This is a group of small nuclei found within the brain stem. It is one of the major areas damaged in cases of Parkinson's disease.

White matter: This refers to the white substance of the brain found below the cortex. It gets its white appearance from the fatty sheath surrounding the nerve fibers coursing through it.

Notes

1. Hayashim, T. "Effects of Sodium Glutamate on the Nervous System." *Keio J. Med.* **3** (1954): 183-192.

2. Van Harreveld, A. and Mendelson, M. "Glutamate-Induced Contractions in Crustacean Muscle." *J. Cell Comp. Phys.* **54** (1959): 85-94.

3. Reynolds, W. A., *et al.* "Hypothalamic Morphology Following Ingestion of Aspartame or MSG in Neonatal Rodent and Primate: A Preliminary Report." *J. Toxicology Environmental Health* **2** (1976): 471-480.

4. Coyle, J.T., et al. "Excitatory Amino Neurotoxins: Selectivity, Specificity, and Mechanism of Action." *Neurosci. Res. Program Bulletin* **19**(1981): 4.

5. Bradford, H.F., Bennet, G.W., and Thomas, A.J. "Depolarizing Stimuli and the Release of Physiologically Active Amino Acids from Suspension of Mammalian Synaptosomes." *J. Neurochem.* **21**(1973): 495-505.

6. For a more in-depth understanding of receptors I would recommend the book *Basic Neurochemistry*, edited by G. Siegel, et al., New York:Raven Press, 1989. Also, Stanislav Reinis' and Jerome M. Goldman's book, *The Chemistry of Behavior: A Molecular Approach to Neural Plasticity.* New York:Plenum Press, 1982. See also the study by Siesjo, B.K., Bengtsson, F., et al. "Calcium, Excitotoxins, and Neuronal Death in the Brain." *Ann. NY Acad. Sci.* **568**(1989): 234-251.

7. Monaghan, D.T., Bridges, R.J., and Cotman, C.W. "The Excitatory Amino Acid Receptors: Their Classes, Pharmacology, and Distinct Properties in the Function of the Central Nervous System." *Ann. Rev. Pharm. & Toxic.* **29** (1989): 365-402. Actually, there are many subclasses of glutamate receptors. In fact, there is more than one type of NMDA receptor and this helps explain why different diseases are produced by exposure to a single-compound glutamate.

8. Watkins, J.C. and Evans, R.H. "Excitatory Amino Acid Transmitters." *Ann. Rev. Pharm. Toxic.* **21**(1981): 165-204.

9. Coyle, Joseph T., et al. "Excitatory Amino Acid Neurotoxins: Selectivity, Specificity, and Mechanism of Action." *Neurosci. Res. Prog. Bull.* **19**(1981): 347-349. For an excellent review of ion channels and their regulation see Lewis, D.L., Lechleiter, J.D., et al. "Intracellular Regulation of Ion Channels in Cell Membranes." *Mayo Clinic Proceedings* **65**(1990): 1127-1143.

10. Choi, D.W., "Glutamate Neurotoxicity, Calcium and Zinc." *Ann. NY Acad. Sci.* **568**(1989): 219-224.

11. Kleckner, N.W. and Dingledine, R. "Requirement for Glycine in Activation of NMDA Receptors Expressed in Xenopus Oocytes." *Sci.* **241**(1988): 835-837. In this study, it was shown that glycine appears to induce a conformational change in the receptor complex that is essential for opening of the channel or binding of glutamate to its receptor. Glycine is absolutely necessary for the action, including toxicity, of glutamate and aspartate.

12. Neiuwenhuys, R. *Chemoarchitecture of the Brain.* New York:Springer-Verlag, 1985.

13. Schwartz, G.R. *In Bad Taste: The MSG Syndrome.* Santa Fe:Health Press, 1988. This is the only book that discusses this most important syndrome. Dr. Schwartz has obtained the history of the development of MSG through the translation of original Japanese sources. I have summarized only a part of this most interesting history.

14. Weil-Malherbe, H. "Significance of Glutamic Acid for the Metabolism of Nervous Tissue." *Phys. Rev.* **30**(1950): 549-568. At this time, glutamate was not considered a neurotransmitter, but rather a metabolite. Even today other workers are experimenting with glutamic acid as a method of restoring memory and alterness in those suffering from Alzheimer's disease. Many health food stores sell concoctions containing glutamic acid and herbs, advertised as "mental alerters" and "brain boosters." I would caution the reader to avoid such concoctions.

15. Lucas, D.R. and Newhouse, J.P. "The Toxic Effect of Sodium L-Glutamate on the Inner Layers of the Retina." *Arch. Opthalmology* **58**(1957): 193-201.

16. Olney, J.W. "Brain Lesions, Obesity, and Other Disturbances in Mice Treated with Monosodium Glutamate." *Sci.* **165**(1969): 719-271. Humans also lack a blood-brain barrier in the hypothalamus, even as adults. It is for this reason that Dr. Olney and other neuroscientists are so concerned about the widespread and heavy use of excitotoxins, such as MSG, hydrolyzed vegetable protein, and cysteine, as food additives. In his experiments Dr. Olney found that high-dose exposure to MSG caused hypoplasia of the adenohypophysis of the pituitary and of the gonads, in conjunction with low hypothalamic, pituitary, and plasma levels of LH, growth hormone, and prolactin. When doses below toxic levels for hypothalamic cells were used, he found a rapid elevation of LH and a depression of the pulsatile output of growth hormone. In essence, these excitotoxins can cause severe pathophysiological changes in the central endocrine control system. Many of these dysfunctional changes can occur with subtoxic doses of MSG. One can speculate that chronic exposure to these neurotoxins could cause significant alterations in the function of the hypothalamus, including its non-endocrine portions.

17. Olney, J.W. "Toxic Effects of Glutamate and Related Amino Acids on the Developing Central Nervous System." In *Heritable Disorders of Amino Acid Metabolism*, edited by W.N. Nylan. New York:John Wiley, 1974.

18. Ibid.

19. Toth, L., Karascu, S., et al. "Neurotoxicity of Monosodium L-Glutamate in Pregnant and Fetal Rats." Act. *Neuropath.* (Berl) **75**(1987): 16-22. In this study, they found that a single dose of MSG when given to pregnant rats could cause acute necrosis of the area postrema in the fetuses. While the neuronal swelling was less pronounced in the embryos, the degeneration of the neurons was much more rapid than in adults. The area postrema has been shown to contain numerous glutamatergic neurons.

20. Olney, J.W. "Glutamate, A Neurotoxic Transmitter." *J. Child Neuro.* **4**(1989): 218-226.

21. Ibid.

22. Olney, J.W. "Excitotoxic Food Additives: Functional Teratological Aspects." *Prog.*

Brain Res. **18**(1988): 283-294. Dr. Olney found that human children are often exposed to acute MSG intakes in the range of 100 to 150 mg/kg just by eating prepared (manufactured) foods. In humans, this amount causes a twenty-fold elevation in their plasma glutamate levels. In comparison, mice develop only a four-fold increase in glutamate levels after a comparable dose. Remember, most of the initial research that has shown glutamate to be destructive of the brain was done using mice. Critics ignore this important fact.

23. Ibid.

24. Choi, D.W. "Glutamate Neurotoxicity: A three-stage process." In *Neurotoxicity of Excitatory Amino Acids*. FIDA Research Foundation Symposium Series, Vol. 4, edited by A. Guidotti, 235-242. New York:Raven Press, 1990.

25. Coyle, J.T., et al. "Excitatory Amino Acid Neurotoxins: Selectivity, Specificity, and Mechanisms of Action." *Neurosci. Res. Prog. Bull.* **19**(1981): 4.

26. The interested reader will find a more complete discussion of this process in the following references: Choi, D.W. "Glutamate Neurotoxicity: A Three-Stage Process." In *Neurotoxicity of Excitatory Amino Acids*, edited by A. Guidotti, (1990): 235-242.

27. Nairn, A.C., et al. "Protein Kinases in the Brain." *Ann. Rev. Biochem.* **54**(1985): 931-976.

28. The products created by these two reactions produce a series of substances called eicosanoids or prostaglandins. Some of these substances affect blood coagulation, blood vessel diameter, inflammatory responses, immune reactions, and a host of other physiological reactions. These important by-products play a vital role in a host of diseases. Aspirin and all of the other anti-inflammatory drugs (called non-steroidal anti-inflammatory drugs) act by inhibiting certain of these prostaglandins. It is interesting to note that the fish oil, omega-3-fatty acids, also have a profound effect on these prostaglandins. They do so by replacing arachnodonic acid, which initiates the reaction. In doing so, they produce a false transmitter that inactivates the destructive cellular reactions. Several of the anti-inflammatory drugs have been shown to greatly reduce this intracellular destructive process.

29. Demopoulos, H.G., Flamm, E.S., and Seligman, M.L. "Membrane Perturbations in Central Nervous System Injury: Theoretical Basis for Free Radical Damage and a Review of the Experimental Data." In *Neural Trauma*, edited by A.J. Popp, et al. New York: Raven Press, 1979. Other good reviews included: Imlay, J.A., and Linn, S. "DNA Damage and Oxygen Radical Toxicity." *Sci.* **240**(1988): 1302-1309; and Schmidley, J.W. "Free Radicals in Central Nervous System Ischemia." *Stroke* **21**(1990): 1986-1990.

30. Stadtman, E.R. "Protein Oxidation and Aging." *Sci.* **257**(1992): 1220-1224.

31. Ibid.

32. Schanne, F.A., Kane, A.B., et al. "Calcium Dependence of Toxic Cell Death: A Final Common Pathway." *Sci.* **206**(1979): 700-702.

33. Ibid.

34. Baethmann, A., Maier-Hauff, K., et al. "Release of Glutamate and of Free Fatty Acids in Vasogenic Brain Edema." J. *Neurosurgery* **70**(1989): 578-591. This is an excellent paper which demonstrates that not only does glutamate accumulate with brain injury but so does arachidonic acid. In fact, in this study, glutamate accumulated in the area of injury in concentrations 1000 to 1500 times normal. This was not transported from the plasma, but rather was secondary to local release of glutamate from the astrocytes. Arachidonic acid concentrations were higher than that seen in the plasma.

Remember, the release of arachidonic acid is triggered by glutamate. This study demonstrates that acute elevations of glutamate in the brain can result from trauma. Nutritionists are now recommending that glutamate and glutamine be added to tube feedings to promote better gut function in the traumatized and severely ill patient. This study should caution against this, especially in the neurosurgical patient, many of whom have impaired blood-brain barrier mechanisms.

35. Demopoulos, H.B., Flamm, E.S., and Seligmann, M.L. "Membrane Perturbations in Central Nervous System Injury: Theoretical Basis for Free Radical Damage and a Review of Experimental Data." In *Neural Trauma*, edited by Popp AJ, et al. New York:Raven Press, 1979.

36. Ibid.

37. Choi, D.E. "Glutamate Neurotoxicity and Diseases of the Nervous System." *Neuron* 1(1988): 623-634. This is an excellent review article which covers all aspects of glutamate toxicity.

38. McDonald, J.W. and Johnston, M.V. "Physiological Roles of Excitatory Amino Acids During Central Nervous System Development." *Brain Res.* 15(1990): 41-70.

39. Maragos, W.F., Greenamyre, J.T., et al. "Glutamate Dysfunction in Alzheimer's Disease: An Hypothesis." *TINS* 10(1987): 65-68.

40. Spencer, P.S., Nunn, P.B., et al. "Guam Amyotrophic Lateral Sclerosis-Parkinsonism-Dementia Linked to a Plant Toxin Excitant Neurotoxin." *Sci.* 237(1987): 517-522.

41. Plaitakis, A. "Glutamate Dysfunction and Selective Motor Neuron Degeneration in Amyotrophic Lateral Sclerosis: An Hypothesis." *Ann. Neurol.* 28(1990): 3-8.

42. Weiss, J.H. and Choi, D.W. "Differential Vulnerability to Excitatory Amino Acid-Induced Toxicity and Selective Neuronal Loss in Neurodegenerative Diseases." *Canadian J. Neurol. Sci.* 18(1991):394-397.

43. Greenamyre, J.T. and Young, A.B. "Excitatory Amino Acids and Alzheimer's Disease." *Neurobiology of Aging* 10(1989): 593-602.

44. Henneberry, R.D., Novelli, A., Cox, J.A., and Lysko, P.G. "Neurotoxicity at the N-Methyl-D-Aspartate Receptor in Energy-Compromised Neurons. An Hypothesis for Cell Death in Aging and Disease." *Ann. NY Acad. Sci.* 568(1989): 225-233.

45. Mayer, M.L., Westbrook, G.L., and Guthrie, P.B. "Voltage-Dependent Block by Magnesium of NMDA Responses in Spinal Cord Neurons." *Nature* 309(1984):261-263. Also see: Choi, D.W. "Glutamate Neurotoxicity and Disease of the Nervous System." *Neuron* 1(1988): 623-634; and Olney, J.W., Price, M.T., et al. "The Role of Specific Ions in Glutamate Neurotoxicity." *Neurosci. Let.* 65(1986): 65-71.

46. Siesjo, B.K., Bengtsson, F., et al. "Calcium, Excitotoxins, and Neuronal Death in the Brain." *Ann. NY Acad. Sci.* 568(1989): 234-251. The mitochondria also sequesters calcium ions and acts as a storage site. Both systems require energy for their operation.

47. Retz, J.C. and Coyle, J.T. "Kainic Acid Lesion of Mouse Striatum: Effects on Energy Metabolites." *Life Sci.* 27(1980): 2495-2500. They found that when kainate was injected directly into the rat striatum there was a significant drop in the concentration of phosphocreatine and ATP. Alteration in brain energy levels occurred as early as 30 minutes and were pronounced at 120 minutes. Lactate levels in the striatum were nearly doubled and glucose levels fell nearly fifty percent. [14C]-2-deoxyglucose autoradiography data shows that there is a marked increase in glucose utilization in the striatum, the overlying cortex, and the limbic structures within two hours of kainate

injection into the striatum. (Nicklas, W.J. "Glutamate Metabolism and its Compartmentation." In "Excitatory Amino Acid Neurotoxins: Selectivity, Specificity, and Mechanisms of Action." edited by J.T. Coyle, et al. *Neurosci. Res. Prog. Bull.* **19**(1981): 372-376.

48. Kuhn, T.S. "The Structure of Scientific Revolutions." In *International Encyclopedia of Unified Science*, Vol. 2(2). Chicago, IL:University of Chicago Press, 1970.

49. Rosenberg, P.A. and Aizenman, E. "Hundred-Fold Increase in Neuronal Vulnerability to Glutamate Toxicity in Astrocyte-Poor Cultures of Rat Cerebral Cortex." *Neurosci. Let.* **103**(1989): 162-168.

50. Stegink, et al. "Comparative Metabolism of Glutamate in the Mouse, Monkey and Man." In *Glutamic Acid: Advances in Biochemistry and Physiology,* edited by L.J. Filer, Jr., et al. New York:Raven Press, 1979.

51. Broad, W., Wade, N. *Betrayers of the Truth: Fraud and Deceit in the Halls of Science.* New York:Touchstone Books, 1982.

52. Ray, D.L. and Guzzo, L. *Trashing the Planet.* Wash., DC:Regnery Gateway, 1990.

53. Taken from a letter to the *Saturday Evening Post,* October 1990, written by John D. Buchholz, Research Association for the Glutamate Association, Atlanta, Georgia.

54. Olney, J.W. Prepared statement for the public meeting (April 1993) pertaining to adverse reactions to monosodium glutamate.

55. Shatz, C.J. "The Developing Brain." *Sci. Am.* September 1992: 61-67.

56. Ibid.

57. Mattson, M.P. "Neurotransmitters in the Regulation of Neuronal Cytoarchitecture." *Brain Res. Rev.* **13**(1988): 179-212.

58. Mattson, M.P., et al. "Outgrowth-Regulating Actions of Glutamate in Isolated Hippocampal Pyramidal Neurons." *J. Neurosci.* **8**(1988): 2087-2100.59

59. Ibid.

60. Mattson, M.P., Dou, P., and Kater, S.B. "Pruning of Hippocampal Pyramidal Neuron-Dendrite Architecture in Vitro by Glutamate and a Protective Effect of GABA Plus Diazepam." *Soc. Neurosci. Abstracts* **13**(1987): 367.

61. Cotman, C.W. "Specificity of Synaptic Growth in Brain: Remodeling Induced by Kainic Acid Lesions." *Progress in Brain Research* **51**(1979): 203-215.

62. Cline, H.T. "Activity-Dependent Plasticity in the Visual Systems of Frogs and Fish." *Trends in Neurosci.* **14**(1991): 104-111.

63. Pujol, J., et al. "When Does Human Brain Development End? Evidence of Corpus Callosum Growth up to Adulthood." *Ann. Neurol.* **34**(1993): 71-75.

64. Reinis, S. and Goldman, J.M. *The Development of the Brain: Biological and Functional Perspectives*, 211-212. Springfield, IL:Thomas Books, 1980.

65. Malenka, R.C. and Nicoll, R.A. "NMDA-Receptor Dependent Synaptic Plasticity: Multiple Forms and Mechanisms." *Trends in Neurosci.* **16**(1993): 521-526.

66. Eccles demonstrates this in his book, Eccles, J.C. *Understanding the Brain.* New York:McGraw Hill, 1973.

67. Beatte, M.S. and Bresnahan, J.C. "Neuronal Plasticity: Implications for Spinal Trauma." In *Head Injury: Basic and Clinical Aspects*, edited by R.G. Grossman and P.L Gildenberg, 57-68. New York: Raven Press, 1982.

68. Richardson, P.M. "Neurotrophic Factors in Regeneration." *Curr. Op. in Neurobio.* **1**(1991): 401-406.

69. Choi, D.W. "Glutamate Toxicity, Calcium and Zinc." *Ann. NY Acad. Sci.* **568**(1989): 219-224.

70. Lemire, R.J., et al. *Normal and Abnormal Development of the Human Nervous System.* Hagerstown, MD:Harper & Row, 1975. This is an excellent book which systematically covers the development of the brain and spinal cord, giving the reader an appreciation of the intricacies of neuronal development.

71. Garthwaite, J. "Glutamate, Nitric Oxide and Cell-Cell Signalling in the Nervous System." *Trends in Neurosci.* **14**(1991): 60-67. While this article chiefly concerns itself with the role of nitric oxide as a transmitter substance and a possible second messenger, it also mentions the importance of "activity-dependent" organization of afferent fibers in relationship to their target neurons during nervous system development. These, the author points out, involve appropriately timed signals from postsynaptic neurons to presynaptic elements. Nitric oxide may be a candidate for such a role in development of three-dimensional structures and the conformational creation of ion channels. There is a close association between glutamatergic neurons and nitric oxide. It appears that at least some glutamate type neurons stimulate cGMP within the neurons. It is known that in the embryonic rat cerebellum, NMDA receptors mediate "most, if not all of the cGMP responses to maximally effective concentrations of exogenous glutamate."

72. Olney, J.W. "Excitotoxic Food Additives: Functional Teratological Aspects." *Progress in Brain Research* **73**(1988): 283-294.

73. McDonald, J.W. and Johnson, M.V. "Physiological and Pathophysiological Roles of Excitatory Amino Acids During Central Nervous System Development." *Brain Res. Rev.* **15**(1990): 41-70.

74. Brody, J.R., et al. "Effect of Micro-Injections of L-Glutamate into the Hypothalamus on Attack and Flight Behavior in Cats." *Nature* **224**(1969): 1330.

75. Klingberg, H., Brankack, J., and Klingberg, F. "Long-Term Effects on Behavior After Postnatal Treatment with Monosodium L-Glutamate. *Biomed. Biochem. ACTA* **46**(1987): 705-711.

76. Olney, J.W., et al. "Glutamate-Induced Brain Damage in Infant Primates." *J. Neuropath. & Exp. Neur.* **31**(1972): 464-487.

77. It should be noted that brain concussion is associated with the accumulation of glutamate within the brain, especially in the area of the hippocampus. The source of this glutamate is the brain itself, called endogenous glutamate. It is thought that the high levels of glutamate produce the damage that eventually leads to the "punch drunk" syndrome.

78. Price, B.H., Daffner, K.R., et al. "The Compartmental Learning Disabilities of Early Frontal Lobe Damage." *Brain* **113**(1990): 1383-1393.

79. Kerr, G.R., Waisman, H.A. "Transplacental Ratios of Serum-Free Amino Acids During Pregnancy in the Rhesus Monkey." In *Amino Acid Metabolism and Genetic Variation*, edited by W.L. Nathal, 429-437. New York:McGraw Hill, 1967.

80. Stegnik, L.D., et al. "Placental Transfer of Glutamate and its Metabolites in the Primate." *Am. J. Obstet. Gynecol.* **122**(1975): 70-78.

81. Kerr, G.R. and Waisman, H.A. "Transplacental Ratios of Serum-Free Amino Acids During Pregnancy in the Rhesus Monkey" In *Amino Acid Metabolism and Genetic Variation*, edited by W.L. Nathal, 429-437. New York:McGraw Hill, 1967.

82. Olney, J.W. "Toxic Effects of Glutamate and Related Amino Acids on the Developing Central Nervous System." In *Heritable Disorders of Amino Acid Metabolism*, edited

by W.N. Nylan, 501-511. New York:John Wiley & Sons, 1974.

83. Pritchard J.A., MacDonald P.C., and Gant, N.F. *Williams Obstetrics*, 17th Ed., 443-444, Connecticut:Appleton-Century, 1989.

84. Wakai, S. and Hirokawa, N. *Cell Tissue Research* Vol. 195, 195-203, 1978. Also: Risau, W. and Wolburg, H. Letter to the Editor. *Trends in Neurosci.* 14(1991): 15.

85. Olney, J.W. "Excitotoxic Food Additives: Functional Teratological Aspects." In *Progress in Brain Res.* Vol. 73, New York:Elsevier Science Publications, 1988.

86. Reinis, S. and Goldman, J.M. "The Development of the Brain" *Biological and Functional Perspectives*, 211-213. Springfield, IL:Thomas Books, 1980.

87. Olney, J.W. "Glutamate, A Neurotoxic Transmitter." *J. Child Neurology* 4(1989): 218-225.

88 Pearce, I., et al. *FEBS Letters* 223(1987): 143.

89. Cotman, C.W., et al. "The Role of the NMDA Receptor in Central Nervous System Plasticity and Pathology." *J. NIH Res.* 1(1989): 65-74.

90. Stewart, P.A. and Hayakawa, E.M. *Dev. Brain Res.* 32(1987): 271-281.

91. For a representative sampling of the studies, see: Gay, V.L., and Plant, T.M. "N-Methyl-di-aspartate (NMDA) Elicits Hypothalamic GnRH Release in Prepuberal Male Rhesus Monkeys (Macaca mulatta)." *Endocrinology* 120(1987): 2289-2296; Gay, V.L., Plant, T.M. "Sustained Intermittent Release in Prepuberal Male Rhesus Monkeys." *Endocrinology* 48(1988): 147-152; and Nemeroff, C.B. "Effects of Neurotoxic Excitatory Amino Acids on Neuroendocrine Regulation." In *Excitotoxins*, edited by K. Fuxe, et al., 295-305. London:MacMillan Press, 1983.

92. Olney, J.W. "Excitotoxic Food Additives: Functional Teratological Aspects." *In Progress in Brain Research* Vol. 73, edited by C.J. Boer, et al., 283-294, 1988.

93. Olney, J.W., Cicero, T.J., et al. "Acute Glutamate-Induced Elevations in Serum Testosterone and Luteinizing Hormone." *Brain Res.* 112(1076): 420-424.

94. Plaitakis, A. "Glutamate Dysfunction and Selective Motor Neuron Degeneration in Amyotrophic Lateral Sclerosis: An Hypotheses." *Ann. Neur.* 28(1990): 3-8.

95. Olney, J.W., et al. *Brain Research* 112: 420-424.

96. Grayson, D.R., Szekely, A.M., and Cosa, E. "Glutamate-Induced Gene Expression in Primary Cerebellar Neurons." In *Neurotoxicity of Excitatory Amino Acids*, edited by A. Guidotti New York:Raven Press Ltd., 1990. This gene activation occurs via a second messenger system, inositol triphosphate and diacylglycerol, which have been activated by phospholipase C. Modification of a preexisting transcription factor induces an early response in certain genes.

97. McDonald, J.W. and Johnston, M.V. "Physiological and Pathophysiological Roles of Excitatory Amino Acids During Central Nervous System Development." *Brain Res. Rev.* 15(1990): 41-70.

98. Klingberg, H., Brankack, J., et al. "Long-Term Effects on Behavior after Post-natal Treatment with Monosodium L-Glutamate." *Biomed. Biochem. ACTA* 26(1987): 705-711. In this study they found that in normal rats, early post-natal removal of the eyes caused hyperactivity. MSG treated rats never developed this syndrome but rather had decreased motor activity. The MSG animals behaved like animals with "lowered intelligence".

99. Toth, L., Karcsu, S., et al. "Neurotoxicity of Monosodium L-Glutamate in Pregnant and Fetal Rats." *ACTA Neuropath* (Berl) 75(1987): 16-22.

100. Olney, J.W., Sharpe, L.G., and Feigin, R.D. "Glutamate-Induced Brain Damage

in Infant Primates." *J. Neuropath. Exp. Neur.* **31** (1972): 464-488. Also of interest is an earlier paper by Dr. Olney in which he found that the excitatory amino acid cysteine could cause widespread damage to the fetal brain, especially in the amygdala, cerebral cortex, hippocampus, and several neuronal groups in the thalamus.

101. "Citizens Alliance for Consumer Protection of Korea." *United Nations Childrens Fund (UNICEF)* (1986): 1-9.

102. Olney, J.W. "Glutamate, A Neurotoxic Transmitter." *J. Child Neur.* **4** (1989): 218-226.

103. Thurston, J.H. and Warren, S.K. "Permeability of the Blood-Brain Barrier to Monosodium Glutamate and Effects on the Components of the Energy Reserve in Newborn Mouse Brains." *J. Neurochem.* **18** (1971): 2241-2244.

104. Inouye, M. "Selective Distribution of Radioactivity in the Neonatal Mouse Brain Following Subcutaneous Administration of 14 C-Labeled Monosodium Glutamate." *Cong. Anom.* **16**(1976): 79-84.

105. Toth, E. and Lajtha, A. "Elevation of Cerebral Levels of Nonessential Amino Acids In Vivo by Administration of Large Doses." *Neurochem. Res.* **6**(1981): 1309-1317.

106. McDonald, J.W. and Johnson, M.V. *Brain Research Reviews* **15** (1990): 41-70; also, Brewer, G.J. and Cotman, C.W. "NMDA Receptor Regulation of Neuronal Morphology in Cultured Hippocampal Neurons." *Neurosci. Let.* **99**(1989): 268-273; and Mattson, M.P., et al. "Outgrowth-Regulating Actions of Glutamate in Isolated Hippocampal Pyramidal Neurons." *J. Neurosci.* **8**(1988): 2087-2100.

107. Murphey, T.H., et al. "Immature Cortical Neurons are Uniquely Sensitive to Glutamate Toxicity by Inhibition of Cystine Uptake." *FASEB* **6**(1990): 1624-1633.

108. Ibid.

109. For a more detailed treatment of brain metabolism see: Siesjo, B.K. "Regional Metabolic Rates in the Brain." In *Brain Energy Metabolism*, edited by B.K. Seisjo, 131-150. New York:John Wiley & Sons, 1978.

110. Olney, J.W. "Glutamate, A Neurotoxic Transmitter." *J. Child Neur.* **4**(1989): 218-226. Also see: Rothman, S.M. and Olney, J.W. "Glutamate and the Pathophysiology of Hypoxic-Ischemic Brain Damage." *Ann. Neur.* **19**(1986): 105-111; and Kochhar, A., Zivin, J.A., et al. "Glutamate Antagonist Therapy Reduces Neurological Deficits Produced by Focal Central Nervous System Ischemia." *Arch. Neur.* **45**(1988): 148-153. Of particular interest is a study which demonstrated that glutamate and aspartate are increased to very high levels in the extracellular spaces of the brain following global ischemia. This appeared to be time related. After 10 minutes of complete global ischemia glutamate and aspartate levels increase 4 to 8 fold and by 30 minutes they increased 100 fold. Exogenous glutamate or aspartate could add to this already elevated pool of excitotoxins, especially under conditions of stroke or acute hypertension: conditions where the blood-brain barrier would be broken down.

111. Iversen, L.L., et al. "Neuroprotective Properties of the Glutamate Antagonist MK-801 in Animal Models of Focal and Global Ischemia." In *Pharmacology of Cerebral Ischemia* edited by J. Krieglstein, 165-171. Boca Raton:CRC Press, Inc., 1988.

112. Siesjo, B.K., et al. "Calcium Excitotoxins, and Neuronal Death in the Brain." *Ann. NY Acad. Sci.* **568**(1989): 234-251.

113. Chen, M.H., et al. "Ischemic Neuronal Damage after Acute Subdural Hematoma in the Rat: Effect of Pretreatment with a Glutamate Antagonist." *J. Neurosurgery* **74**(1991): 944-950.

114. Welch, K.M.A., et al. "The Concept of Migraine as a State of Central Neuronal

Hyperactivity." *Neurologic Clinics* **8**(1990): 4.

115. Olney, J.W. "Excitotoxins and Neurological Diseases." *Proceedings of the International College of Neuropathologist.* Kyoto, Japan, 1990.

116. Weiss, J.H. and Choi, D.W. "Differential Vulnerability to Excitatory Amino Acid-Induced Toxicity and Selective Neuronal Loss in Neurodegenerative Diseases." *Canadian J. Neurological Sci.* **18**(1991): 394-397.

117. Marks, V, and Rose FC. "Hypoglycemia in Children." In *Hypoglycemia*, 288-289. Oxford:Blackwell Scientific Publications, 1981.

118. Olney, J.W. "Excitotoxins and Neurological Diseases." *Proceedings of the International College of Neuropath.* Kyoto, Japan, 1990. Also see: Olney, J.W. "Excitotoxic Food Additives: Functional Teratological Aspects." In *Progress in Brain Research*, edited by, C.J. Boer, et al., Vol. 73, 283-294. New York:Elsevier Science Publications, 1988.

119. Olney, J.W. "Glutamate, A Neurotoxic Transmitter." *J. Child Neurology* **4**(1989): 218-226.

120. Olney, J.W. "Brain Lesions, Obesity, and Other Disturbances in Mice Treated with Monosodium Glutamate." *Sci.* **165**(1969): 719-721.

121. Olney, J.W. "Glutamate-Induced Neuronal Necrosis in the Infant Mouse Hypothalamus. An Electron Microscopic Study." *J. Neuropath. Exp. Neurol.* **30**(1971): 75-90.

122. Bakke, J.L., Lawrence, N., et al. "Late Effects of Administering Monosodium Glutamate to Neonatal Rats." *Neuroendocrinology* **26**(1978): 220-228. Also see: Olney, J.W. "Applications of Neurotoxins in Neurobiology." In *Neurosciences Research Bulletin*, edited by J.T. Coyle, et al., Vol. 19(4), 385-388, 1981. Critics often claim that only high doses of MSG cause such endocrine lesions, but a study done by Dr. Ralph Dawson demonstrates that even low doses of MSG can have profound effects on endocrine development, especially in terms of sex hormone release, and hence the onset of puberty in females. (Dawson, R. "Development and Sex-Specific Effects of Low Dose Neonatal Monosodium Glutamate Administration on Mesobasal Hypothalamic Chemistry." *Neuroendocrinology* **42**(1986): 158-166.) This study is particularly interesting in that it demonstrates that repeated doses at low levels can produce profound lesions in the hypothalamus. Other studies have found that MSG treatment produced gonadal atrophy, decreased hypothalamic estrogen binding, alterations in plasma levels of LH and LHRH release, delayed vaginal opening, and disturbances in sexual behavior.

123 Bodnar, R.J., et al. "Neonatal Monosodium Glutamate: Effect upon Analgesic Responsivity and Immunocytochemical ACTH/Beta-Lipotropin." *Neuroendocrinology* **30**(1980): 280-284; Nagasawa, et al. "Irreversible Inhibition of Pituitary Prolactin and Growth Hormone Secretion and Mammary Gland Development in Mice by Monosodium Glutamate Administration Neonatally." *ACTA Endocrinologica* **75**(1974): 249-259; Olney, J.W. and Price, M.T. "Excitotoxin Amino Acids as Neuroendocrine Probes." In *Kainic Acid as a Tool in Neurobiology* McGeer, E.G., Olney, J.W., and McGeer, P.L., 125-138. New York:Raven, 1978.

124. Ibid.

125. Shimicu, K., Mizutari, A., and Inoue, M. "Electron Microscopic Studies on the Hypothalamic Lesions in the Mouse Fetus Caused by Monosodium Glutamate." *Teratology* **8**(1973): 105.

126. Olney JW. "Excitotoxic food additives:functional teratological aspects." *Progress in Brain Research* **73**(1988): 283-294.

127. Urbanski, H.F., Ojeda S.R., "Activation of Luteinizing Hormone Releasing

Advances the Onset of Female Puberty." *Neuroendocrinology* **48**(1987): 273-276.

128. MacDonald, M., Wilkinson, M. "Peripubertal Treatment with N-Methyl-D-Aspartic Acid on Neonatally with Monosodium Glutamate Accelerates Sexual Maturation in Female Rats, an Effect Reversed by MK-801." *Neuroendocrinology* **52**(1990): 143-149.

129. Gay, V.L. and Plant, T.M. "N-methyl-D-L-aspartate Elicits Hypothalamic Gonadotropin Releasing Hormone Release in Prepubertal Male Rhesus Monkeys (Macaca Mulatta)" *Endocrinology* **120**(1987): 2289-2296.

130. Rose, P.A. and Weick, R.F. "Evidence for Reorganization of Neuroendocrine Centers Regulating Pulsatile LH Secretion in Rats Receiving Neonatal Monosodium L-Glutamate Treatment." *J Endocrinology* **113**(1987):261-269.

131. Bakke, J.L., et al. "Late Endocrine Effects of Administering Monosodium Glutamate to Neonatal Rats." *Neuroendocrinology* **26**(1978): 220-228.

132. Sun, Y.M., et al. "Sex Specific Impairment in Sexual and Ingestive Behaviors of Monosodium Glutamate Treated Rats." *Physiology and Behavior* **50**(1991): 873-880.

133. Pizzi, W.J., et al. "Monosodium Glutamate Administration to the Newborn Reduces Reproductive Ability in Female and Male Mice." *Science* **196**(1977): 452-454.

134. Nemeroff, C.B. "Monosodium Glutamate-Induced Neurotoxicity: Review of the Literature and a Call for Further Research." In *Nutrition and Behavior*, edited by S.A. Miller, 177-211. The Franklin Institute Press, 1981. See also: Olney, J.W. and Sharpe, L.G. "Brain Lesions in an Infant Monkey Treated with Monosodium Glutamate." *Science* **166**(1969): 386-388.

135. Daikoku, S., et al. "Ontogenesis of Immunoreactive Tyrosine Hydroxylase-Containing Neurons in Rat Hypothalamus." *Developmental Brain Research* **28**(1986): 85-98.

136. Dawson, R., Jr., Simpkins, J.W., and Wallace, D.R. "Age and Dose-Dependent Effects of Neonatal Monosodium Glutamate (MSG) Administration to Female Rats." *Neurotoxicology and Teratology* **2**(1989): 331-337.

137. Olney, J.W. and Price, M.T. "Excitotoxic Amino Acids as Neuroendocrine Probes." In *Kainic Acid as a Tool in Neurobiology*, edited by E.G. McGreer, J.W. Olney and P.L. McGreer, 125-138. New York:Raven Press, 1978.

138. Olney, J.W. "Application of neurotoxins in neurobiology." In JT Coyle, et al. (eds), *Neurosciences Research Bulletin* **14:4**(1981): 384.

139. Stegink, LD, et al. "Comparative Metabolism of Glutamate in Mouse and Man." In *Glutamic Acid: Advances in Biochemistry and Physiology* edited by LJ Filner, et al, 85-102. Raven Press:New York, 1979.

140. Olney, J.W. "Excitatory Neurotoxins as Food Additives: An Evaluation of Risk." *Neurotox.* **2**(1980): 163-192.

141. Ibid.

142. Ibid.

143. Stegnik, LD, et al. Data submission by G.D. Searle to Public Board of Inquiry on aspartame. 4:13, 1979; also Stegink, et al. "Toxicology of Protein Hydrolysate Solutions: Correlation of Glutamate Dose and Neuronal Necrosis to Plasma Amino Acid Levels in Young Mice." *Tox.* **2**(1974): 285-299.

144. Allen, DH, et al. "Monosodium L-Glutamate-Induced Asthma." *J. All. Clin.*

Immunol. **80**(1980): 530-537.

145. Stegink LD, et al. Glutamic Acid: *Advances in Biochemistry and Physiology.* New York:Raven Press, 1979.

146. National Research Council. National Academy of Sciences, subcommittee report on safety and suitability of MSG and other substances in baby foods. Washington DC, 1970.

147. Olney JW, *Neurotoxicology* **2** (1980): 163-192.

148. Nemeroff, CB. *Nutrition and Behavior,* 177-211. The Franklin Press, 1981.

149. Paull. W.K. "An Autoradiographic Analysis of Arcuate Neuron Sensitivity to Monosodium Glutamate." *Anat. Rec.* **181**(1975): 445.

150. Rietvelt W.J., et al. "The Effect of Monosodium Glutamate on the Endogenous Peroxidase Activity in the Hypothalamus Arcuate Nucleus in Rats." *Ob. Gyn.* **7**(1979): 573.

151. Bodnar, R.J., et al. "Neonatal Monosodium Glutamate: Effect Upon Analgesic Responsivity and Immunocytochemical ACTH/Beta-lipotropin." *Neuroendo.* **30**(1980): 280-284.

152. Thurston, J.H. and Warren, S.K. "Permeability of the Blood-Brain Barrier to Monosodium Glutamate and Effects on the Components of the Energy Reserve in Newborn Mouse Brain." *J. Neurochem.* **18**(1971): 2241-2244.

153. Van Den Pol, A.N., Wuarin, J.P. and Dudek, F.E. "Glutamate, the Dominate Excitatory Transmitter in Neuroendocrine Regulation." *Sci.* **250**(1990): 1276-1278. Immunoreactive axons were found in synaptic contact with dendrites and cell bodies throughout the hypothalamus. This included the magnocellular, parvocellular, paraventricular, supraoptic, and arcuate nuclei, all of which make up the final common pathway for the neuroendocrine system. Interestingly, there is low-level binding of glutamate receptors in the hypothalamus, demonstrated using autoradiographic techniques. Hypothalamic neurons show less dendritic branching, so that its neurons are more concentrated. This acts to magnify the effects of the glutamate neurons on the hypothalamic nuclei, so that fewer receptors are needed. The number of glutamate neurons far outnumber those using amine, peptides, or other neurotransmitters.

154. Olney, J.W. "Excitatory Neurotoxins as Food Additives: An Evaluation of the Risk." *Neurotox.* **2**(1980): 163-192.

155. Dawson, R., Simpkins, J.W., and Wallace, D.R. "Age and Dose-Dependent Effects of Neonatal Monosodium Glutamate (MSG) Administration to Female Rats." *Neurotox. Terato.* **11**(1989): 331-337. Observed that ontogenesis and the migration of dopaminergic neurons in the hypothalamus were altered by MSG in the neonatal rat. MSG has the ability to act as a growth factor that influences the differentiation of neurons and could possibly result in abnormal connections.

156. Aruffo, C., Freszt, R., et al. "Low Doses of L-Monosodium Glutamate Promote Neuronal Growth and Differentiation in Vitro." *Dev. Neurosci.* **9**(1987): 228-239.

157. Reynolds, W.A., et al. "Hypothalamic Morphology Following Ingestion of Aspartame or MSG in the Neonatal Rodent and Primate: A Preliminary Report." *J. Tox. Env. Hlth.* **2**(1976): 471-480.

158. Calne, D.B., Michael, D.M. and Zigmond, J. "Compensatory Mechanisms in Degenerative Neurologic Diseases: Insights from Parkinsonism". *Arch. Neurol.* **48**(1991): 361-363. Also see discussions in Coyle, J.T., et al. "Excitatory Amino Acid Neurotoxins: Selectivity, Specificity, and Mechanisms of Action." *Neurosci. Res. Bull.* **19**(1981): 4.

159. Whitehouse, P.J."Understanding the Etiology of Alzheimer's Disease: Current Approaches." *Neurol. Clin.* May 1986: 427-437. As our technology becomes more sophisticated so does our assurance that prions are not the cause of these degenerative diseases. Searches for other latent viruses have thus far been negative.

160. Nandy, K. "Brain-Reactive Antibodies in Aging and Senile Dementia." In *Alzheimer's Disease: Senile Dementia and Related Disorders*, vol. 7, edited by R. Katzman, et al, 503-512. New York:Raven Press, 1978.

161. Kurland, L.T. "Amyotrophic Lateral Sclerosis and Parkinson's Disease Complex on Guam Linked to an Environmental Neurotoxin." *Trnd. Neurosci.* 11(1988): 51-54.

162. Ibid.

163. Ibid. See also: Laquer, G.L. *Fed. Proc.* 23(1964): 1386-1388.

164. Spencer, P.S., Nunn, P.B. and Hugon, J. "Guam Amyotrophic Lateral Sclerosis-Parkinsonism-Dementia Linked to a Plant Excitant Neurotoxin." *Sci.* 237(1987): 517-522.

165. Kurland, L.T. "An Appraisal of the Neurotoxicity of Cycad and the Etiology of Amyotrophic Lateral Sclerosis on Guam." *Fed Proc* 31(1972): 1465-1538.

166. Garruto, R.M., Gajdusek, D.C. and Chen, K.M. "Amyotrophic Lateral Sclerosis among Chamorro Migrants from Guam." *Ann. Neurol.* 8(1980): 1540-1542.

167. Dastur, D.K. *Fed. Proc. Fed. Am. Soc. Exp. Biol.* 23(1964): 1368.

168. Spencer, P.S., Nunn, P.B. and Hugon, J., et al. "Guam Amyotrophic Lateral Sclerosis-Parkinsonism-Dementia Linked to a Plant Excitant Neurotoxin." *Sci.* 237(1987): 517-522.

169. Garruto, R.M. and Yase, Y. "Neurodegenerative Disorders of the Western Pacific: The Search for Mechanisms of Pathogenesis." *Trnd. Neurosci.* 9(1986): 368-374. This is an excellent review paper.

170. For a review of the connection between aluminum and Alzheimer's disease see: Murray, J.C., Tanner, C.M. and Sprague, S.M. "Aluminum Neurotoxicity: A Reevaluation." *Clin. Neuropharm.* 14(1991): 179-185.

171. Garruto, R.M. and Yase, Y. "Neurodegenerative Disorders of the Western Pacific: The Search for Mechanisms of Pathogenesis." *Trnd. Neurosci.* 9(1986): 368-374.

172. Glick, J.L. "Dementias: The Role of Magnesium Deficiency and an Hypothesis Concerning the Pathogenesis of Alzheimer's Disease." *Med. Hypoth.* 31(1991): 211-225. This is a most intriguing paper, which makes a good case for the importance of magnesium in protecting the brain, even though the author sees another etiology for Alzheimer's disease than excitotoxins. But the paper does demonstrate that low magnesium is a consistent finding in all of these neurodegenerative disorders. Remember, magnesium protects the neurons, at least when not depolarized, against excitotoxicity.

173. Henneberry, R.C. "Energy-Related Neurotoxicity at the NMDA Receptor: A Possible Role in Alzheimer's Disease and Related Disorders." *Prog. Clin. Bio. Res.* (1989): 143-156.

174. Carruto, R.M. and Yase, Y. "Neurodegenerative Disorders of the Western Pacific: The Search for Mechanisms of Pathogenesis." *Trnd. Neurosci.* 9(1986): 368-374.

175. Kumamoto, T., et al. "ACTA" *Histochem Cytochem* 8(1975): 294-303.

176. Henneberry, R.C., et al. *Prog. Clin. Bio. Res.* (1989): 143-156.

177. Henneberry, R.C. *Prog. Clin. Bio. Res.* (1989): 143-156.

178. Glick, J.L. *Med. Hypo.* 31(1991): 211-225.

179. Ballard, P.A., Tetrud, J.W. and Langston, J.W. "Permanent Human Parkinsonism due to 1-methyl-4-phrenyl-1,2,3,6-tetrahydropyridine (MPTP): Seven Cases." Neuro. 35(1984): 949-956. And Davis, G.C., Williams, et al "Chronic Parkinsonism Secondary to Intravenous Injection of Meperidine Analogues." *Psych. Res.* 1(1979): 249-254.

180. Burns, R.S., et al. "The Neurotoxicity of 1-methyl-45-phrenyl-1,2,3,6-tetrahydropyridine in the Monkey and Man." *Can. J. Neuro. Sci.* 11(1984): 166-168.

181. Markey, S.P. "MPTP: A New Tool to Understand Parkinson's Disease." *Discus. Neurosci.* vol iii, 4(1986).

182. It is now known that a large number of spontaneously occurring Parkinson's cases will eventually become demented. Interestingly, MPTP appeared to cause serious damage to the cognitive functions, even when motor symptoms were minor. It appears that the striatum plays a role in cognitive function in humans. Stern, Y., Tetrud, J.W., et al. "Cognitive Change Following MPTP Exposure." *Neurol.* 40(1990): 261-264.

183. For a complete discussion of MPTP, especially its biochemical role in striate destruction, see: Markey, S.P. *Discus. Neurosci.* vol iii, 4(1986).

184. Ibid.

185. Tetrud, J.W. and Langston, J.W. "The Effects of Deprenyl (Selegiline) on the Natural History of Parkinson's Disease." *Sci.* 245(1989): 519-522.

186. Ibid.

187. The Parkinson Study Group. "Effect of Deprenyl on the Progression of Disability in Early Parkinson's Disease." *NEJM* 321(1989): 1364-1371. This study also included a secondary study of alpha-tocopherol (Vitamin E), which showed promise in slowing the course of Parkinson's disease.

188. Murphey, T.H., Schnaar, R.L. and Coyle, J.T. "Immature Cortical Neurons are Uniquely Sensitive to Glutamate Toxicity by Inhibition of Cystine Uptake." *FASEB* 4(1990): 1624-1633. They also found that vitamin E was able to block the toxicity associated with low cystine.

189. Przedborski, S., et al. "Transgenic Mice with Increased Cu/Zn-Superoxide Dismutase Activity Are Resistant to N-Methyl-4-Phenyl-1,2,3,6-Tetrahydropyridine Induced Neurotoxicity." *J. Neurosci.* 12(1992): 1658-1667.

190. Turski, L., Stephens, D.N. "Excitatory Amino Acid Antagonist Protect Mice Against MPP+ Seizures." *Synapse* 10 (1992): 120-125.

191. Marttila, R.J., Lorentz, H. and Rinne, U.K. "Oxygen Toxicity Protecting Enzyme in Parkinson's Disease: Increase of Superoxide Dismutase-like Activity in the Substantia Nigra and Basal Nucleus." *J. Neurol. Sci.* 86(1988): 321-331.

192. Mayeux, R., Yaakov, S., et al. "An Estimate of the Prevalence of Dementia in Idiopathic Parkinson's Disease." *Arch. Neurol.* 45(1988): 260-262.

193. Sonsalla, P.K., Kicklas, W.J. and Heikkila, R.E. "Role for Exitatory Amino Acids in Methamphetamine-Induced Nigrostriatal Dopaminergic Toxicity." *Sci.* 243(1989): 398-400.

194. Ibid.

195. Ibid.

196. Nieuwenhuys, R. *Chemoarchitecture of the Brain*, 48-51. New York:Springer-Verlag, 1985.

197. Sonsalla, P.K., et al. *Sci.* 243: 398-400.

198. Olney, J.W., Zorumski, C.F. and Stewart, G.R. "Excitoxicity of L-Dopa and

6-OH-DOPA: Implications for Parkinson's and Huntington's Diseases." *Exp. Neuro.* **108**(1990): 269-272.

199. Ricaurte, G., et al. "Hallucinogenic Amphetamine Selectively Destroys Brain Serotonin Terminals." *Sci.* **229**(1985): 986-988.

200. Olney, J.W. and Scharpe, L.G. "Brain Lesions in an Infant Rhesus Monkey Treated with Monosodium Glutamate." *Sci.* **166**(1969): 386-388. This again shows how important it is to know the different sensitivity of species before interpreting results and extrapolating them to humans. Mice have a similar sensitivity to excitotoxins as humans and most of these studies have been done on rats and mice. It would be unethical to use humans for these studies even though the food industry utilizes the largest human study ever known to modern science—the public.

201. In fact, by removing this protective pump, neurons are made one hundred times more sensitive to the toxic effects of glutamate. Experimentally this is done by placing neurons in isolation in culture media, without astrocytes being present. The same thing can be accomplished simply by removing the energy from the system. This is, in effect, what happens during cases of severe hypoglycemia. Pathologically, the pattern of neuron loss in cases of fatal hypoglycemia is very close to that seen with exposure to MSG.

202. Evans, D.A., et al. "Prevalence of Probable Alzheimer's Disease in Persons Aged 85 and Older." *JAMA* **262**(1989): 2551-2556.

203. Lilienfeld, D.E., Chan, E., et al. "Two Decades of Increasing Mortality from Parkinson's Disease among the US Elderly." *Arch. Neurol.* **47**(1990): 731-734.

204. There are numerous studies demonstrating a breakdown of the blood-brain barrier under a multitude of pathological and even physiological conditions. See: Tornheim, PA, et al. "Acute Response to Experimental Blunt Head Trauma." *J. Neurosurg.* **60**(1984): 473-480; Robinson, J.S. and Moody, R.A. "Influence of Respiratory Stress and Hypertension upon the Blood-Brain Barrier." *J. Neurosurg.* **53**(1980): 666-673; Peterson, E.W., et al. "The Blood-Brain Barrier Following Experimental Subarachnoid Hemorrhage." *J. Neurosurg.* **58**(1983): 338-344; and Ushio, Y., et al. "Alterations of Blood-Brain Barrier by Tumor Invasion into the Meninges." *J. Neurosurg.* **55**(1981): 445-449.

205. Alafuzoff, I., et al. "Albumin and Immunoglobulin in Plasma and Cerebrospinal Fluid, and the Blood-Cerebrospinal Fluid Barrier Function in Patients with Dementia of Alzheimer-Type and Multi-Infarct Dementia." *J. Neuro. Sci.* **60**(1983): 465-472.

206. Wallin, A., et al. "Blood-Brain Barrier Function in Vascular Dementia." *ACTA. Neurol. Scand.* **81**(1990): 318-322.

207. Banks, W.A. and Kastin, A.J. "Peptides and the Senescent Blood-Brain Barrier." *Neurobiology of Aging* **9**(1988): 48-49.

208. Ibid. Also see, Pardridge, W.M. "Does the Brain's Gatekeeper Falter in Aging?" *Neurobiology of Aging* **9**(1988): 44-46.

209. This is also true of neurons that have been damaged sublethally from whatever cause. It appears that these cells have a defective DNA repair mechanism. In these studies lymphoid cells were used and not brain cells. See: Robbins, J.H., Otsuka, F., et al. "Parkinson's Disease and Alzheimer's Disease: Hypersensitivity to X-Rays in Cultured Cell Lines." *J. Neuro. Neurosurg. Psy.* **48**(1985): 916-923. Also see for a more generalized discussion: Robison, S.H. and Bradley, W.G. "DNA Damage and Chronic Neuronal Degenerations." *J. Neurol. Sci.* **64**(1984): 11-20.

210. Markey, S.P. "MPTP: A New Tool to Understand Parkinson's Disease." *Discus. Neurosci.* **111**(1986): 11-51.

211. Markus, H.S., et al. "Increased Prevalence of Undernutrition in Parkinson's

Disease and its Relationship to Clinical Disease Parameters." *J. Neural. Transmiss.* **5**(1973): 117-125.

212. Levi, S., et al. "Increased Energy Expenditure in Parkinson's Disease." *BMJ* **301**(1990): 1256-1257.

213. Costill, D.L. "Fats and Carbohydrates as Determinants of Atheletic Performance." In *Nutrition and Athletic Performance*, edited by W. Haskell, 21. Also, *Proceedings of the Conference on Nutritional Determinants in Athletic Performance*. San Francisco, Sept 24-25, 1981. Also Bergstrom, J., et al. "Diet-Muscle Glycogen and Physical Performance." *ACTA. Physiol. Scand.* **71**(1967): 140.

214. Schwartz, G.R. *The MSG Syndrome*, 2. Santa Fe:Health Press, 1988.

215. Reif-Lehrer, L. "A Questionnaire Study of the Prevalence of Chinese Resturant Syndrome." *Federal Proceedings* **36**(1977): 1617-1623.

216. Ghadimi, H., Kumars, S. and Abaci, F. "Studies on Monosodium Glutamate Ingestion. Biochemical Explorations of Chinese Resturant Syndrome." *Biochem. Med.* **5**(1971): 447-456.

217. See the following studies: Henneberry, R.C., et al. *Ann. N.Y. Acad. Sci.* **568**(1989): 225-233; Henneberry, et al. *Prog. Clin. Bio. Res.* (1989): 143-156; Takasaki, Y., *Tox. Let.* **4**(1979): 205-210.

218. "Medical Mailbox," edited by Cory SerVaas. *The Saturday Evening Post.* Oct 1990, 98-99.

219. McLaughlan, J.M., et al. "Blood and Brain Levels of Glutamic Acid in Young Rats Given Monosodium Glutamate." *Nutr. Rep. Int.* **1**(1970): 131-138.

220. Himwich, W.A., et al. "Ingested Sodium Glutamate and Plasma Levels of Glutamic Acid." *J. Appl. Physiol.* **7**(1954): 196-201.

221. Olney, J.W., et al. "Glutamate-Induced Brain Damage in Infant Primates." *J. Neuropathol. Exp. Neurol.* **31**(1972): 464.

222. Steginks, L.D., et al. "Effect of Sucrose Ingestion on Plasma Glutamate Concentrations in Humans Administered Monosodium L-Glutamate." *Amer. J. Clin. Nutr.* **43**(1986): 510-515.

223. Schapira, A.H.V., et al. "Mitochondrial Complex I Deficiency in Parkinson's Disease." *J. Neurochem.* **54** (1990): 823-827.

224. Schapira, A.H.V., et al. "Anatomic and Disease Specificity of NADH CoQ Reductase (Complex 1) Deficiency in Parkinson's Disease." *J. Neurochem.* **55**(1990): 2142-2145.

225. Novelli, J.A., et al. "Glutamate Becomes Neurotoxic via the N-methyl-D-aspartate Receptor when Intracellular Energy Levels are Reduced." *Brain Res.* **451**(1988): 205-212.

226. Ballinger, S.W., et al. "Mitochondrial DNA may Hold a Key to Human Degenerative Diseases." *J. NIH Res.* **4**(1992): 62-66.

227. Klockgether, T., Turskill, et al. "The AMPA Receptor Antagonist NBQX has Anti-Parkonsonian Effects in Monoamine Depleted Rats and MPTP-Treated Monkeys." *Ann. Neurol.* **30**(1991): 717-723.

228. Klockgether T., Turski, L. "NMDA Antagonist Potentiate Anti-Parkinsonian Actions of L-DOPA in Monoamine-depleted rats." *Ann. Neurol.* **28**(1990): 539-546.

229. Olney, J.W., et al. Anti-Parkinsonian Agents are Pencyclidine Agonist and N-methyl-aspartate Antagonist." *Euro. J. Pharm.* **142**(1987): 319.

230. Bormann, J. "Memantine is a Potent Blocker of N-methyl-D-aspartate

(NMDA) Receptor Channels." *Euro. J. Pharm.* **166**(1989): 591-592.

231. Dexter, D.T., et al. "Basal Lipid-Peroxidation in Substantia Nigra is Increased in Parkinson's Disease. *J. Neurochem.* **52**(1989): 381-389.

232. Domenico, E., et al. "Excitatory Amino Acid Release and Free Radical Formation may Cooperate in the Genesis of Ischemia-Induced Neuronal Damage." *J. Neurosci.* **10**(1990): 1035-1041.

233. Parkinson Study Group. "DATATOP: A Multicenter Controlled Clinical Trial in Early Parkinson's Disease." *Arch. Neuro.* **46**(1989): 1052-1060.

234. Shouldon, I., Fahn, S. and Langston, W. "Symposium on the Etiology, Pathogenesis, and Prevention of Parkinson's Disease." *Arch. Neuro.* **45**(1988): 807-811.

235. Dexter, D.T., et al. "Increased Iron Content in Post-Mortum Parkinsonian Brain." *Lancet* ii(1987), 219-220.

236. Jenner, P., et al. "Oxidative Stress as a Cause of Nigral Cell Death in Parkinson's Disease and Incidental Lewy Body Disease." *Ann. Neurol.* **32**(1992): 282-287.

237. Ibid.

238. Inouye, M. "Selective Distribution of Radioactivity in the Neonatal Mouse Brain Following Subcutaneous Administration of 14 C-labeled Monosodium Glutamate." *Congen. Anom.* **16**(1976): 79-84.

239. Olney, J.W. *Prog. Brain Res.* **73**(1988): 283-294. Also Olney, J.W. *J. Child. Neurol.* **4**(1989): 218-226.

240. Burkhards, C., et al. "Neuroleptic Medications Inhibit Complex I of the Electron Transport Chain." *Ann. Neurol.* **33**(1993): 512-517.

241. Caine, D.B. "Is Idiopathic Parkinsonism the Consequence of an Event or a Process?" *Neuro.* **44**(1994): 5-10.

242. Williams, D.B. and Windebank. "Motor Neuron Disease (Amyotrophic Lateral Sclerosis)" *Mayo. Clin. Proc.* **66**(1991): 55-82. This article offers an excellent review of ALS.

243. Veltema, A.N., Roos, R.A.C., et al. "Autosomal Dominant Adult Amyotrophic Lateral Sclerosis. A Six Generation Dutch Family." *J. Neurol. Sci.* **97**(1990): 93-115.

244. Kurland, L.T. *TINS* **11**(1988): 51-54.

245. Spencer, P.S., et al. *Sci.* **237**(1987): 517-522.

246. Plaitakis, A. and Caroscio, J.T. "Abnormal Glutamate Metabolism in Amyotrophic Lateral Sclerosis." *Ann. Neuro.* **22**(1987): 575-579.

247. Plaitakis, A. and Caroscio, J.T. "Abnormal Glutamate Metabolism in Amyotrophic Lateral Sclerosis." *Ann. Neuro.* **22**(1987): 575-579.

248. Plaitakis, A., Berl, S. and Yahr, M.D. "Neurological Disorders Associated with Deficiency of Glutamate Dehydrogenase." *Ann. Neuro.* **15**(1984): 144-153.

249. Liu, D., Thangnipon, W. and McAdoo, D.J. "Excitatory Amino Acids Rise to Toxic Levels upon Impact to the Rat Spinal Cord." *Brain Res.* **547**(1991): 344-348.

250. Patten, B.M., Harati, Y., et al. "Free Amino Acid Levels in Amyotrophic Lateral Sclerosis." *Ann Neuro* **3**(1978): 305-309.

251. Plaitakis, A., Constantakakis, E., Smith, J. "The Neuroexcitotoxic Amino Acids Glutamate and Aspartate are Altered in the Spinal Cord and Brain in Amyotrophic Lateral Sclerosis." *Ann Neurol* **24**(1988): 446-449.

252. Citizens Alliance for Consumer Protection of Korea. "A Study of the Use of MSG in Korea." *United Nations Childrens Fund (UNICEF)*(1986) 1-9.

253. "Glutamate Toxicity and Spinal Neuron Degeneration in Amyotrophic Lateral Sclerosis." An interview with Jeffery Rothstein, MD, PhD. *Neurosciences Forum* 3(1993): 7.

254. Plaitakis A., Berl S., Yahr M. "Neurological Disorders Associated with Deficiency of Glutamate Dehydrogenase." *Ann Neurol* 15(1984): 144-153.

255. Olney, J.W. *J. Child Neurol* 4(1989): 218-226.

256. Plaitakis A., et al. "Pilot Trial of Branched-Chain Amino Acids in Amyotrophic Lateral Sclerosis." *Lancet* 1(1988): 1015-1018.

257. Whether this is true or not is up for speculation. The incidence of the disease is approximately 4 to 8 per 100,000 population in the United States and 10% of this figure in Japan. There are areas that seem to cluster the disease, such as Lake Maracaibo, Venezuela. Since the disease is transmitted as an autosomal dominate hereditary disorder, intermarriage plays a vital role in such clustering of cases. *Merritt's Textbook of Neurology* edited by Lewis P. Rowland. Philadelphia:Lea & Febiger, 1989.

258. Young, A.B., Timothy J., et al. "NMDA Receptor Losses in the Putamen from Patients with Huntington's Disease." *Science* 241(1988): 981-983. Studies indicated that the striatal afferent pathways are largely spared, which means that the injury is not a non-specific one that destroys everything in the area. We also see decreases in striatal glutamate decarboxylase (GAD) as well as GABA and substance P. In this study it was found that [3H]-glutamate binding to NMDA receptors in tris-acetate in the presence of quisqualate was decreased by 93% in the putamen and [3H]-TCP binding was decreased by 67% in Huntington's disease. In Huntington's disease the medium sized spiny striatal neurons containing GABA and enkephalin, project to the lateral pallidum and are lost very early in the disease. Also lost early are cells containing the neuromodulators and transmitters, GABA and substance P that project to the substantia nigra pars reticulata. GABA and substance P containing neurons that project to the substantia nigra pars compacta and to medial pallidum are affected later in the disorder. Somatostatin and acetylcholine interneurons are relatively spared. Interestingly, animal studies confirm that when glutamate type excitotoxins are given (such as NMDA) they destroy the GABA and substance P containing neurons and spare the somatostatin and acetylcholine type neurons, just as is seen in the clinical disease.

259. Coyle, J.T. "Structure-Activity Relationships for Neurotoxicity." In *Excitatory Amino Acid Neurotoxins: Selectivity, Specificity, and Mechanism of Action*, edited by J.T. Coyle, et al. *Neurosci. Res. Pro. Bull.* 19(4)(1981):359; see Table 3, which lists the various excitotoxins in order of toxic potential.

260. Ibid, p 355.

261. Young, A.B., et al. *Science* 241(1988): 981-983.

262. Biziere, K. and Coyle, J.T. "Influence of Cortico-Striatal Afferents on Striatal Kainic Acid Neurotoxicity." *Neurosci Letters* 8(1978): 303-310. See also Coyle, J.T. *Neurosci Res Pro Bull* 19(4)(1981): 389-391.

263. Ibid, p 390.

264. Young, A.B., et al. *Science* 241(1988): 981-983.

265. It produces both the GABA losses and the selective neuronal sparing seen in Huntington's disease. Quniolinic acid is also known to act at the NMDA receptor. In some cases of Huntington's disease virtually all of the NMDA receptor neurons were lost. Ibid.

266. Retz, K.C. and Coyle, J.T. "Acute Effects of Kainic Acid on Energy States in the Striatum of the Mouse." *Soc Neurosci Abstr* 6(1980): 444.

267. Mazziotta, J.C. "PET Scanning: Principles and Applications." *Discussions in Neurosciences* **11(1)**(1985): 39-40.

268. Ibid.

269. In another study it was found that patients exposed to MPTP, who did not develop symptoms of Parkinson's disease, had low metabolism of within their striatum. (Stern, T., et al. *Neurol* **40**(1990): 261-264.) Again, this demonstrates that neurons can be damaged without evidence of pathological damage being seen on microscopic examination. This would throw into disrepute many of the studies claimed by the critics of MSG toxicity, who cite studies demonstrating no pathological damage with exposure. It is obvious that MSG and the other excitotoxins can produce sublethal, and pathologically indistinguishable, injury to neurons. As our means of measuring subtle damage becomes more sensitive, the harmful effect of excitotoxins will become more obvious.

270. Olney, J.W. and deGubareff "Glutamate Neurotoxicity and Huntington's Chorea." *Nature* **271**(1978): 557-559.

271. Lipton, S.A., and Rosenberg, P.A. "Excitatory Amino Acids as a Final Common Pathway for Neurologic Disorders." *N Engl J Med* **330**(1994): 613-622.

272. *Impact of Alzheimer's Disease on the Nation's Elderly.* Joint Hearing Subcommittee on Aging. Ninety-sixth Congress, Second session. July 15, 1980.

273. For an excellent review of the metabolic changes with aging I would suggest the chapter, "Aging in the Nervous System" by Carl W. Cotman and Christine Peterson, in, *Basic Neurochemistry. Molecular, Cellular, and Medical Aspects* edited by George J. Siegel, et al. New York:Raven Press.

274. Duara R., et al. "Human Brain Glucose Utilization and Cognitive Function in Relation to Age." *Annals Neurology* **16**(1984): 702-713.

275. Samorajski, T. "Neurochemical Changes in the Aging Human and Nonhuman Primate Brain." In, *Psychopharmacology of Aging* edited by C. Eisdorfer and W.E. Fann, pp.145-168. New York:SP Medical and Scientific Books, 1980.

276. Cotman, C.W. and Peterson, C. "Aging in the Nervous System." In, *Basic Neurochemistry* edited by G. J. Siegel, et al., 523-540. New York:Raven Press, 1989.

277. McGreer P.L., McGreer E.G., and Suzuki, S.E. "Aging and Extrapyramidal Function." *Arch Neurol* **34**(1977): 33-35.

278. Iqbal, K., et al. "Neurofibrous Proteins in Aging and Dementia" in *Aging of the Brain and Dementia* (Aging Vol. 13), edited by L. Amaducci, et al., pp 39-48. New York:Raven Press, 1980.

279. It has been consistently shown that the dendritic trees of elderly brains (average age 80) show more extensive branching than cases of demented elderly (average age 51). Computerized studies of dendritic trees in the hippocampus of aging individuals indicates that there are two populations of neurons: one that is undergoing a process of progressive loss of dendritic spines and another that demonstrates dendritic spine growth. During the process of normal aging the latter is predominate. See Bowen, D.M. "Biochemical Evidence for Nerve Cell Changes in Senile Dementia" In *Aging of the Brain and Dementia (Aging*, Vol. 13) edited by L. Amaducci, et al., 127-138. New York:Raven Press, 1980. Also see reviews: Donlin, M., Long. "Aging in the Nervous System." *Neurosurg.* **17**(1985):348-354. Smith, C.B. "Aging and Changes in Cerebral Metabolism." *TINS* **7**(1984): 203-208 and "Aging Research Matures." *TINS* **5**(1982): 217.

280. For an excellent discussion of the pathophysiology, biochemistry, and possible origin of these tangles see: Bignami, A. et al (eds), "Molecular Mechanisms of Pathogenesis of Central Nervous System Disorders." In *Discus. in Neurosci. FESN* **III**(1986).

281. Ibid., 42-46.

282. An excellent review of dendritic function, growth and maturation can be found in Lund, R.D. *Development of Plasticity of the Brain*, Chap. 11, 166-182. New York:Oxford University Press, 1978.

283. Hershey, L.A. "Dementia associated with stroke." *Stroke* 21(1990): 9-11.

284. Tanne, J.H. "At the Frontiers of Medical Science." *The NYU Physician* 42(1986): 19-21. See also "The Role of Folate and Vitamin B_{12} in Neurotransmitter Metabolism and Degenerative Neurological Changes Associates with Aging." *Life Sciences Research Office Federation of Amer. Soc. Exper. Biol.* May 19-20 (1988).

285. Karnaze, D.S. and Carmel, R. "Low Serum Cobalamin Levels in Primary Degenerative Dementia: Do Some Patients Harbor Atypical Cobalamin Deficiency States?" *Arch. Inter. Med.* 147(1987): 429-431; see also related article, Lindenbaum, et al. *New. Engl. J. Med.* 318(1988): 1720-1728.

286. Ikeda, T., et al. "Vitamin B_{12} Levels in Serum and Cerebrospinal Fluid of People with Alzheimer's Disease." *Acta. Psych. Scand.* 82(1990): 327-329.

287. Rother, J., et al. "Hypoglycemia Presenting as Basilar Artery Thrombosis." *Stroke* 23(1992): 112-113.

288. Maragos W.F., et al. "Glutamate Dysfunction in Alzheimer's Disease: an Hypothesis." *TINS* 10(1987): 65-68. See also Foster, A.C. "Physiology and Pathophysiology of Excitatory Amino Acid Neurotransmitter Systems in Relation to Alzheimer's Disease." In *Advances in Neurology*, edited by Richard J. Wurtman, et al. Vol. 51, 97-102. New York: Raven Press, 1990.

289. DeBoni, U. and Crapper-McLachlan, D.R. "Controlled Induction of Paired Helical Filaments of the Alzheimer-type in Cultured Human Neurons by Glutamate and Aspartate." *J. Neurol. Sci.* 68(1985):105-118.

290. Koh, J.Y., Yang, L.L. and Cotman, C.W. "B-amyloid Protein Increases the Vulnerability of Cultured Neurons to Excitotoxic Damage." *Brain Res.* 533(1990):315-320.

291. Mattson, M.P., et al. "B-amyloid Peptides Destabilize Calcium Homeostasis and Render Human Cortical Neurons Vulnerable to Excitotoxicity." *J. Neurosci.* 12(1992):376-389.

292. Wolozin, B. and Davies, P.D. "Alzheimer-Related Neuronal Protein A68: Specificity and Distribution." *Ann. Neurol.* 22(1987): 521-526.

293. Ibid.

294. Mattson, M.P. "Antigenic Changes to Those Seen in Neurofibrillary Tangles are Elicited by Glutamate and Ca +2 Influx in Cultured Hippocampal Neurons." *Neuron* 2(1990): 105-117. See also Sindou, P.S., et al. "A Dose-Dependent Increase of Tau Immunostaining is Produced by Glutamate Toxicity in Primary Neuronal Cultures." *Brain Res.* 572(1992): 242-246.

295. DeBoni, U. and Crapper-McLachlan, D.R. "Paired Helical Filaments of the Alzheimer Type in Cultured Neurons." *Nature* 271(1978): 566-568.

296. DeBoni, U., and McLachlan, D.R.C. "Controlled Induction of Paired Helical Filaments of Alzheimer's type in Cultured Human Neurons by Glutamate and Aspartate." *J. Neurol. Sci.* 68(1985): 105-118.

297. Mattson, M.P., et al. "B-amyloid Peptides Destabilize Calcium Homeostasis Render Human Cortical Neurons Vulnerable to Excitotoxicity." *J. Neuro. Sci.* 12(1992): 376-389. See also Koh, J.Y., et al. "B-amyloid Protein Increases the Vulnerability of Cultured Cortical Neurons to Excitotoxic Damage." *Brain Res.* 533(1990): 315-320.

298. Penfield, W. and Jasper, H. *Epilepsy and the Functional Anatomy of the Human*

Brain. Boston:Little, Brown & Co., 1954.

299. Ibid, p. 137.

300. Ibid, p. 513.

301. Maragos, W.F., et al. *TINS* **10**(1987): 65-68.

302. For the reader interested in a more complete discussion of long-term potentiation and memory I would suggest: Swanson, L.W., et al. "Hippocampal Long-term Potentiation: Mechanisms and Implications for Memory." *Neurosci. Res. Prog. Bull.*, Vol 20, No. 5, 1982.

303. Foster, A.C. "Advances in Neuro." *Alzheimer's Disease, Vol. 51.*, 197-202. New York:Raven Press, 1990.

304. Morris, R.G.M., et al. "Selective Impairment of Learning and Blockade of Long-term Potentiation by an N-methyl-D-aspartate Receptor Antagonist, AP5." *Nature* **319**(1986): 774-776.

305. Monaghan, D.T., Bridges R.J., Cotman, C.W. "The Excitatory Amino Acid Receptors: Their Classes, Pharmacology, and Distinct Properties in the Function of Central Nervous System." *Ann. Rev. Pharm.* **29**(1989): 365-402.

306. Weiss, J.H. and Choi, D.W. "Differential Vulnerability to Excitatory Amino Acid-induced Toxicity and Selective Neuronal Loss in Neurodegenerative Diseases." *Can. J. Neurol. Sci.* **18**(1991): 394-397.

307. Greenamyre, J.T., and Maragos, W.F. "Neurotransmitter Receptors in Alzheimer's Disease." *Cerebrovas. Brain Meta. Rev.* **5**(1993): 61-94.

308. For a more in depth examination as to how this technique works and early result of examination of various brain disorders, see Mazziotta, J.D. "Pet Scanning: Principles and Applications." *Discus. Neurosci.*, Vol 11, No. 1, Jan-March 1985.

309. Greenamyre, J.T., et al. J. Neurochem. 48(1987): 543-551. See also Greenamyre, J.T., and Yound, A.B. "Excitatory Amino Acids and Alzheimer's Disease." *Neurobio. Aging* **10**(1989): 593-602.

310. Ellison, D.W., et al. "A Postmortem Study of Amino Acid Neurotransmitters in Alzheimer's Disease." *Ann. Neuro.* **20**(1986): 616-621.

311. Agnoli, A., et al. "Effect of Cholinergic and Anticholinergic Drugs on Short-Term Memory in Alzheimer's Dementia: A Neuropsychological and Computerized Electroencephalographic Study." *Clin. Neuropharm.* **6**(1983): 311-323.

312. Irle, E. and Markowitsch, H.J., "Basal Forebrain-Lesioned Monkeys are Severely Impaired in Task of Association and Recognition Memory." *Ann. Neuro.* **22**(1987): 735-742.

313. Smith, C.M. and Swash, M. "Effects of Cholinergic Drugs on Memory in Alzheimer's Disease." In *Aging of the Brain and Dementia*, Aging, Vol. 13, 295-304, edited by L. Amaducci, et al. New York:Raven Press, 1980.

314. Arendash, G.W., et al. "Long-Term Neuropathological and Neurochemical Effects of Nucleus Basalis Lesions in the Rat." *Sci.* **238**(1987): 952-956.

315. Agnoli, A. et al. *Clin. Neuropharm.* **6**(1983): 311-323.

316. Greenamyre, J.T., Young, A.B. "Excitatory Amino Acids and Alzheimer's Disease." *Neurobio. Aging* **10**(1989): 593-603.

317. Ibid.

318. Foster, A.C. "Physiology and Pathophysiology of Excitatory Amino Acid Neurotransmitter Systems in Relation to Alzheimer's Disease." In *Advances in Neurology*, Vol 51: Alzheimer's Disease, 97-102. Edited by Richard J. Wurtman, et al. New York:Raven Press, 1990.

319. Greenamyre, J.T., et al. "Dementia of the Alzheimer's Type: Changes in Hippocampal L-[3H] Glutamate Binding." *J. Neurochem.* **48**(1987): 543-511.

320. Maragos, J., et al. "Glutamate Dysfunction in Alzheimer's Disease: An Hypothesis." *TINS* **10**(1987): 65-68.

321. Olney, J.W. "Glutamate, a neurotoxic transmitter." *J. Child. Neuro.* **4**(1989): 218-226.

322. Coyle J.T., et al. "Excitatory Amino Acids Neurotoxins: Selectivity, Specificity, and Mechanisms of Action." *Neurosci. Res. Prog. Bull.* **19**(1981).

323. Foster, A.C. "Physiology and Pathophysiology of Excitatory Amino Acid Neurotransmitter Systems in Relation to Alzheimer's Disease." *Advances in Neurology: Alzheimer's Disease* Vol 51, edited by Richard J. Wurtman, et al. New York:Raven Press, 1990.

324. Greenamyre, J.T. and Young, A.B. "Excitatory Amino Acids and Alzheimer's Disease." *Neurobio. Aging* **10**(1989): 593-602.

325. Greenamyre, J.T., et al. "Dementia of the Alzheimer's-Type: Changes in Hippocampal L-[3H] Glutamate Binding." *J. Neurochem.* **48** (1987): 543-551.

326. Arendash, G.E., et al. *Sci.* **238**(1987): 952-956.

327. Sofroniew, M.V., Pearson, R.C.A. *Brain Res.* **339**(1985): 186-190.

328. Akhlaq, A., et al. "Increased Activities of Lipolytic Enzymes in Alzheimer's Disease." *Adv. Neuro.* **51**(1990): 127-129.

329. Murphey, T., et al. "Arachidonic Acid Metabolism in Glutamate Neurotoxicity." *Ann. NY Acad. Sci.* **559**(1989): 474-477.

330. McGeer, P.L., et al. "Anti-Inflammatory Drugs and Alzheimer's Disease." *Lancet* **28**(1990): 335.

331. Breiter, J.C.S., et al. "Inverse Association of Anti-Inflammatory Treatments and Alzheimer's Disease: Initial Results of Co-Twin Control Study." *Neuro.* **44**(1994): 227-232.

332. Pellegrini-Giampietro, D.E., et al. "Excitatory Amino Acid Release and Free Radical Formation may Cooperate in the Genesis of Ischemia-Induced Neuronal Damage." *J. Neurosci.* **10**(1990): 1035-1041.

333. Mattson, M.P. *J. Neurosci.* **12**(1992): 376-389.

334. Greenamyre, J.T. and Young, A.B. "Excitatory Amino Acids and Alzheimer's Disease." *Neurobio. Aging* **10**(1989): 593-602.

335. DeBoni, U. and Crapper-McLachlan, D.R. "Controlled Induction of Paired Helical Filaments of the Alzheimer's-Type in Cultured Human Neurons by Glutamate and Aspartate." *J. Neuro. Sci.* **68**(1985): 105-118.

336. Spencer, P.S., et al. "Guam Amyotrophic Lateral Sclerosis-Parkinsonism-Demential Linked to a Plant Excitant Neurotoxin." *Sci.* **237**(1987): 517-522.

337. Spencer, P.S. "Etiology of Alzheimer's Disease: A Western Pacific View." Wurtman, R.J., et al (eds.), 79-82. *Advances in Neurology: Alzheimer's Disease: Vol. 51.* New York:Raven Press, 1990.

338. Cambell, L.W., Hao, S.Y., Landfield, P.W. "Aging-Related Increases in L-like Calcium Currents in Rats Hippocampal Slices." *Soc. Neurosci. Abs.* **15**(1989): 260.

339. For a fuller discussion of the brain's metabolism I would suggest: Clarke, D.D., et al. "Intermediary Metabolism." In, *Basic Neurochemistry*, edited by Siegal, et al, 541-564. New York:Raven Press, 1989. Also Siesjo. "Brain Energy Metabolism." New York: John Wiley & Sons, 1978.

340. Olney J.W., "Excitotoxins and Neurological disease." *Proceedings of the Interna-*

tional College of Neuropathologist. Kyoto, Japan, 1990; also see Wieloch, T. "Hypoglycemia-Induced Neuronal Damage Prevented by N-methyl-D-aspartate Antagonist."
Sci. **230**(1985): 681-683.

341. Benveniste, H., et al., "Elevation of the Extracellular Concentrations of Glutamate and Aspartate in Rat Hippocampus During Transient Cerebral Ischemia Moni-
tored by Intracerebral Microdialysis." *J. Neurochem.* **43**(1984): 1369-1374. See also
Riikonen R.S., Kero P.O., Simell, O.G., "Excitatory Amino Acids in Cerebrospinal
Fluid in Neonatal Asphyxia." *Ped. Neuro.* **8**(1992): 37-40.

342. Takasaki, Y. "Protective Effect of Mono and Disaccharides on Glutamate-
Induced Brain Damage in Mice." *Toxicology Letters* **4**(1979): 205-210. Stegink and
coworkers have also shown that sucrose can reduce the concentration of glutamate in
the blood stream following an oral dose of MSG. Stegink, L.D., et al. "Effect of Sucrose
Ingestion on Plasma Glutamate Concentrations in Humans Administered Monosodium L-Glutamate." *Amer J. Clin Nutr* **43**(1986): 510-515.

343. Henneberry, R.C. "The Role of Neuronal Energy in the Neurotoxicity of Excitatory Amino Acids." *Neurobiology of Aging* **10**(1989): 611-613 and also Rosenberg, P.A.
and Aizenman, E. "Hundred-Fold Increase in Neuronal Vulnerability to Glutamate
Toxicity in Astrocyte-Poor Cultures of Rat Cerebral Cortex." *Neuroscience Letters*
103(1989): 162-168.

344. Bazzano, G., D'Elia, A., Olson, R.E. "Monosodium glutamate: Feeding of
Large Amounts to Man and Gerbils." *Science* **169**(1970): 1208-1209.

345. Chadimi H., Kumar S., Abaci F. "Studies on Monosodium Glutamate Ingestion: Biochemical Exploration of Chinese Restaurant Syndrome." *Biochemical Medicine* **5**(1971): 447-456.

346. Reif-Lehrer, L. "A Questionnaire Study of the Prevalence of Chinese Restaurant
Syndrome." *Federal Proceedings* **36**(1977): 1617-1623.

347. Reif-Lehrer, L. and Stemmermann, M.G. "Monosodium Glutamate Intolerance
in Children." *N Engl J Med* **293**(1975): 1204-1205.

348. LaManna, J.C. and Harik, S.I. "Regional Comparisons of Brain Glucose Influx."
Brain Research **326**(1985): 299-305.

349. Ibid.

350. Henneberry, R.C. "The Role of Neuronal Energy in the Neurotoxicity of Excitatory Amino Acids." *Neurobio Aging* **10**(1989): 611-613.

351. Foster, N.L., et al. "Cortical Abnormalities in Alzheimer's Disease." *Ann Neuro*
16(1984): 649-654.

352. Ibid.

353. Ibid.

354. Duara, R., et al. "Human Brain Glucose Utilization and Cognitive Function in
Relation to Age." *Ann. Neuro.* **16**(1984): 702-713.

355. Bucht, G., et al. "Changes in Blood Glucose and Insulin Secretion in Patients
with Senile Dementia of Alzheimer's Type." *Acta. Medica. Scand.* **213**(1983): 387-392.

356. Fujisawa, Y., Sasaki, K., Akiyama, K. "Increased Insulin Levels after OGTT Load
in Peripheral Blood and Cerebrospinal Fluid of Patients with Dementia of Alzheimer's
Type." *Bio. Psych.* **30**(1991): 1219-1228.

357. Kalaria, R.N., et al. "The Glucose Transporter of the Human Brain and Blood-
Brain Barrier." *Ann. Neuro.* **24**(1988): 757-764.

358. Ibid.

359. Kalaria, R.N. and Harik, S.I. "Reduced Glucose Transporter at the Blood-Brain

Barrier and in the Cerebral Cortex in Alzheimer's Disease." *J. Neurochem.* **53**(1989): 1083-1088.

360. Harik, S.I. and LaManna, J.C., "Altered Glucose Metabolism in Microvessels from Patients with Alzheimer's Disease." *Ann. Neuro.* **26**(1991): 91-94.

361. Foster, N.L., et al. "Cortical Abnormalities in Alzheimer's Disease." *Ann. Neuro.* **16**(1984): 649-654.

362. Ibid.

363. Scheibel, A.B., Duong, T., Jacobs, R. "Alzheimer's Disease as a Capillary Dementia." *Ann. Med.* **21**(1989): 103-107.

364. Orlova, M.L. "Angioarchitectonics of the Cerebral Cortex and the Blood-Brain Barrier in Alzheimer's Disease." *Neurosci. Behav. Physio.* **19**(1989): 498-503.

365. Kalaria, R.N. "The Blood-Brain Barrier and Cerebral Microcirculation in Alzheimer's Disease." *Cerebrovas. Brain Meta. Rev.* **4**(1992): 226-260.

366. Kalaria R.N., et al. "Serum Amyloid P in Alzheimer's Disease: Implications for Dysfunction of the Blood-Brain Barrier." *Ann. NY Acad. Sci.* **640**(1991): 145-148.

367. Creasey, W.A. and Malawista, S.E. "Monosodium L-glutamate— Inhibition of Glucose Uptake in Brain as a Basis for Toxicity." *Biochem. Pharm.* **20**(1971): 2917-2920.

368. Toth, E., and Lajtha, A. "Elevation of Cerebral Levels of Nonessential Amino Acids In Vivo by Administration of Large Doses." *Neurochem. Res.* **6**(1981): 1309-1317.

369. Mann, V.M., et al. *Brain* **115**(1992): 333-342.

370. Parker, W.D., Filley, C.M., Parks, J.K. "Cytochrome Oxidase Deficiency in Alzheimer's Disease." *Neuro.* **40**(1990): 1302-1303.

371. Sheu K-F, R., et al. "An Immunological Study of the Pyruvate Dehydrogenase Deficit in Alzheimer's Disease Brain." *Ann. Neuro.* **17**(1985): 444-449.

372. Greenamyre, J.T., et al. "Dementia of the Alzheimer's Type: Changes in Hippocampal L-[3H] Glutamate Binding." *J. Neurochem.* **48**(1987): 543-551.

373. Sheu K-F, R., et al. *Ann. Neuro.* **17**(1985): 444-449.

374. Sims, N.R., et al. "Altered Glucose Metabolism in Fibroblast from Patients with Alzheimer's Disease." *NEJM* **313**(1985): 638-639.

375. Blass, J.P., Zemcov, A. "Alzheimer's Disease—a Metabolic Systems Degeneration?" *Neurochem. Path.* **2**(1984): 103-114.

376. Gibson, G.E., et al. "Reduced Activities of Thiamine-Dependent Enzymes in the Brains and Peripheral Tissues of Patients with Alzheimer's Disease." *Arch. Neuro.* **45**(1988): 836-840.

377. LaManna, J.C. and Harik, S.I. "Regional Comparisons of Brain Glucose Influx." *Brain Res.* **326**(1985): 299-305.

378. Gibson, G.E., et al. *Arch. Neuro.* **45**(1988): 836-840.

379. Blass, J.P., Baker, A.C., Ko L-W, "Alzheimer's Disease:Inborn Error of Metabolism of Late Onset?" *Advances in Neurology,* Vol. 51: Alzheimer's Disease, edited by Wurtman RJ, et al. New York:Raven Press, 1990.

380. Wisniewski, H., Terry, R.D. "Morphology of the Aging Brain, Human and Animal." *Prog. Brain Res.* **40**(1973): 167-186.

381. Henneberry, R.C., et al. "Energy-related Neurotoxicity at the NMDA Receptor: A Possible Role in Alzheimer's Disease and Related Disorders." In *Alzheimer's Disease and Related Disorders,* 143-156, Alan R. Liss, Inc., 1989.

382. Procter, A.W., et al. *J. Neurochem.* **50**(1988): 790-802.

383. Greenamyre, J.T. "Neuronal Bioenergetic Defects, Excitotoxicity and Alz-

heimer's Disease: Use it and Lose it." *Neurobio. Aging* 12(1991): 334-336.

384. Maragos, W.F., et al. "Glutamate Dysfunction in Alzheimer's Disease: An Hypothesis." *Trends Neurosci.* 10(1987): 65-68.

385. Choi, D.W. "Bench to Bedside: the Glutamate Connection." *Sci.* 258(1992): 241-246.

386. Weiss, J.H. and Choi, D.W. "Differential Vulnerability to Excitatory Amino Acid-induced Toxicity and Selective Neuronal Loss in Neurodegenerative Diseases." *Can. J. Neuro. Sci.* 18(1991): 394-397.

387. Toth, E. and Lajtha, A. *Neurochem. Res.* 6(1981): 1309-1317.

388. Pardridge, W.M. "Does the Brain's Gatekeeper Falter in Aging?" *Neurobio. Aging* 9(1988): 144-146.

389. Elovaara, et al. "Serum and Cerebrospinal Fluid Proteins and the Blood-Brain Barrier in Alzheimer's Disease and Multi-Infarct Dementia." *Euro. Neurol.* 26(1987): 229-234.

390. Scheibel, A.B. and Duong, T. "On the Possible Relationship of Cortical Microvascular Pathology to Blood-Brain Barrier Changes in Alzheimer's Disease." *Neurobiol. Aging* 9(1988): 41-42.

391. Bennow, K., et al. "Blood-Brain Barrier Disturbance in Patients with Alzheimer's Disease is Related to Vascular Factors." *Acta. Neuro. Scand.* 81(1990): 323-326.

392. Banks, W.A. and Kastin, A.J. "Peptides and the Senescent Blood-Brain Barrier." *Neurobiol. Aging* 9(1988): 48-49.

393. Inoue, T., et al. "Hyperosmotic Blood-Brain Barrier Disruption in Brains of Rats with Intracerebrally Transplanted RG-C6 Tumor." *J. Neurosurg.* 66(1987): 256-263.

394. Martinez-Vila, E., et al. "Placebo-Controlled Trial of Nimodipine in the Treatment of Acute Ischemic Cerebral Infarction." *Stroke* 21(1990): 1023-1028.

395. Barkay, L. "Changes in Barrier in Pathological States." In, *Brain Barrier Systems. Progress in Brain Research*, vol 29 edited by A. Lajtha and D.H. Ford, 315-341, 1968.

396. Smith, Q.R. "Transport of Calcium and Other Metals Across the Blood-Brain Barrier: Mechanisms and Implications for Neurodegenerative Disorders." *Advances in Neurology Vol 51.* edited by Richard J Wurtman, et al, 217-222. New York:Raven Press, 1990.

397. Mooradian, A.D. "The Effect of Aging on the Blood-Brain Barrier. A review." *Neurobio. Aging* 9(1988): 31-39.

398. Perl, T.M. et al. "An Outbreak of Toxic Encephalopathy Caused by Eating Mussels Contaminated with Domoic Acid." *NEJM* 322(1990): 1775-1780.

399. Quilliam, M.A., Wright, J.L.C. "The Amnesic Shellfish Poisoning Mystery. *Anal. Chem.* 61(1989): 1053a-1059a.

400. Teitelbaum, J.S., et al. "Neurologic Sequelae of Domoic Acid Intoxication due to the Ingestion of Contaminated Mussels." *NEJM* 322(1990): 1781-1787.

401. Ibid.

402. Ibid.

403. Ibid.

404. Ibid.

405. Stewart, G.R., et al. "Domoic Acid: A Dementia-Inducing Excitotoxic Food Poison with Kainic Acid Receptor Specificity." *Exper. Neuro.* 110(1990): 127-138.

406. Quillam, M.A., Wright, J.L.C. *Anal. Chem.* 61(1989): 1053a-1059a.

407. Perl, T.M., et al. *NEJM* **322**(1990): 1775-1780.

408. Teitelbaum, J.S., et al. *NEJM* **322**(1990): 1781-1787.

409. Perl, T.M., et al. *NEJM* **322**(1990): 1775-1780.

410. Novelli, A., et al. "Domoic Acid-Containing Toxic Mussels Produce Neurotoxicity in Neuronal Cultures through a Synergism between Excitatory Amino Acids." *Brain Res.* **577**(1992): 41-48.

411. Stewart, G.R., et al. *Exp. Neurol.* **110**(1990): 127-138.

412. Teitelbaum, J.S., et al. *NEJM* **322**(1990):1781-1787.

413. Novelli, A., et al. *Brain Res.* **577**(1992): 41-48.

414. Perl, T.M., et al. *NEJM* **322**(1990): 1775-1780.

415. Dickens, B.F., et al. "Magnesium Deficiency in Vitro Enhances Free Radical-Induced Intracellular Oxidation and Cytotoxicity in Endothelial Cells." *Fed. Euro. Biochem. Soc.* **311**(1992): 187-191.

416. Ibid.

417. Freedman, A.M., et al. "Erythrocytes from Magnesium-Deficient Hamsters Display an Enhanced Susceptibility to Oxidative Stress." *Am. J. Physiol.* **31**(1992): c1371-c1375.

418. Chutkow, J.G., Grabow, J.D. "Clinical and Chemical Correlations in Magnesium-Deprivation Encephalopathy of Young Rats." *Am. J. Physiol.* **2223**(1972): 1407-1414. See also Chutkow, J.G. "Clinical Chemical Correlations in the Encephalopathy of Magnesium Deficiency: Effect of Reversal on Magnesium Deficiency." *Mayo. Clin. Proc.* **49**(1974): 244-247.

419. Dorup, I., et al. "Oral Magnesium Supplementation Restores the Concentration of Magnesium, Potassium and Sodium-Potassium Pumps in Skeletal Muscle of Patients Receiving Diuretic Treatment." *J. Inter. Med.* **223**(1993): 117-123.

420. Langley, W.F. and Mann, D. "Central Nervous System Magnesium Deficiency." *Arch. Intern. Med.* **151**(1991): 593-596.

421. Langley, W.F. and Mann, D. *Arch. Intern. Med.* **151**(1991): 593-596.

422. Kubota, J. "How Soils and Climate Affect Grass Tetany." *Crops and Soils* **33**(1981): 15-17.

423. Allsop, T.F., Pauli, J.V. "Responses to Lowering of Magnesium and Calcium in the Cerebrospinal Fluid of Unanesthetized Sheep." *Aust. J. Biol.* **28**(1975): 475-481.

424. Kubota, J. *Crop Soils* **33**(1981): 15-17.

425. Durlach J. "Magnesium Depletion and Pathogenesis of Alzheimer's Disease." *Magnesium Research* **3**(1990): 217-218.

426. Korf, J., et al. "Cation Shifts and Excitotoxins in Alzheimer's Disease and Experimental Brain Damage." *Prog. Brain Res.* **70**(1986): 213-226.

427. Perl, D.P., Broady, A.R. "Detection of Aluminum by Sem-x-ray Spectrometry within Neurofibrillary Tangle-Bearing Neurons of Alzheimer's Disease." *Neurotox.* **1**(1980): 133-137.

428. Perl, D.P., Broady, A.R. "Alzheimer's Disease: X-Ray Spectrometric Evidence of Aluminum Accumulation in Neurofibrillary Bearing Neurons." *Sci.* **208**(1980): 297-299.

429. Siegal, N. "Aluminum Interactions with Biomolecules: The Molecular Basis for Aluminum Toxicity." *Am. J. Kidney. Dis.* **6**(1985): 353-357.

430. Ebel, H., Gunther, T. "Magnesium Metabolism: A Review." *J. Clin. Chem. Biochem.* **18**(1980): 257-270.

431. Cohen, P.G. "Hypomagnesemic Encephalopathy." *Magnesium* **4**(1985): 203.

432. Ibid.

433. Landfield, P.W. "Preventive Approaches to Normal Brain Aging and Alzheimer's Disease." In *Treatment Development Strategies for Alzheimer's Disease.* Edited by T. Crook, et al., 221-243.

434. Korf, J., et al. "Cation Shifts and Excitotoxins in Alzheimer and Huntington Disease and Experimental Brain Damage." *Prog. Brain Res.* **70**(1986): 213-226.

435. Glick, J.L. *Medical Hypotheses* **31**(1990): 211-225.

436. Lum, G. "Hypomagnesemia in Acute and Chronic Patient Populations" *Am. J. Clin. Pathol.* **97**(1992): 827-830.

437. Deloncle, R. and Guillard, O. "Mechanism of Alzheimer's Disease: Arguments for a Neurotransmitter-Aluminum Complex Implication.: *Neurochem. Res.* **15**(1990): 1239-1245.

438. Olney J.W., et al. "Cysteine-Induced Brain Damage in Infant and Fetal Rodents." *Brain Res.* **45**(1972): 309-313.

439. Ibid.

440. Olney, J.W., et al. "L-Cysteine, a Bicarbonate-Sensitive Endogenous Excitotoxin." *Sci.* **248**(1990): 596-598.

441. Ibid.

442. Weiss, J.J. and Choi, D.W. "Beta-N-methylamine-L-alanine Neurotoxicity: Requirement for Bicarbonate as a Cofactor." *Sci.* **241**(1988): 973-975.

443. Heafield, M.T., et al. "Plasma Cysteine and Sulphate Levels in Patients with Motor Neurone, Parkinson's and Alzheimer's Disease." *Neurosci. Let.* **110**(1990): 216-220.

444. Olney, J.W., et al. "Brain Damage in Mice from Voluntary Ingestion of Glutamate and Aspartate." *Tox.* **2**(1980): 125-129.

445. I would refer the reader to several articles reporting partial success in various diseases associated with electron transport defects. Bresolin, N., et al. "Ubidecarenone in their Treatment of Mitochondrial Myopathies: A Multicenter Double-blind Trial." *J. Neurol. Sci.* **100**(1990):70-78; Wijburg, F.A., et al. "Familial NADH: Q1 oxidorectase (complex I) Deficiency: Variable Expression and Possible Treatment." *J. Inherited Metabol. Dis.* **12**(1989): 349-351; Bernsen, P.L.J.A., et al. "Successful Treatment of Pure Myopathy, Associated with Complex I Deficiency with Riboflavin and Carnitine." *Arch. Neurol.* **48**(1991): 334-338.

446. Glick, J.L. "Dementias: The Role of Magnesium Deficiency and an Hypothesis Concerning the Pathogenesis of Alzheimer's Disease." *Med. Hypo.* **31**(1990): 211-225.

447. Nadler, J.V., "Evidence that Kainate Produces Epileptogenic Lesions": Coyle, J.T., et al (eds). *Neurosci. Res. Prog. Bull.* **19** (1981): 369-372.

448. Black, T.P. and Klawans, "Convulsive Disorders: Mechanisms of Epilepsy and Anticonvulsant Action." *Clin. Neurophar.* **13**(1990): 121-128. Also see Stasheff, S.F., et al, "NMDA Antagonist Differentiate Epileptogenesis from Seizure Expression in an in vitro Model." *Science* **245**(1989): 648-651.

449. Wurtman, R.J., "Aspartame: Possible Effects on Seizure Susceptibility." *Lancet* Nov 9 (1984): 1060.

450. Walton, R.G., "Seizure and Mania After High Intake of Aspartame." *Psychosomatics* **27**(1986): 218-220.

451. Hayashi, T. "Effects of Sodium Glutamate on the Nervous System." *Keio. J. Med.* **3**(1954): 183-192.

452. Camfield, P.R., et al. "Aspartame Exacerbates EEG Spike-Wave Discharge in Children with Generalized Absence Epilepsy." *Neurol.* **42**(1992): 1000-1003.

453. Pinto, J. and Maher, T.J. "Administration of Aspartame Potentiates Pentylenetetrazol- and Flurothyl-Induced Seizures in Mice." *Neuropharm.* **27**(1988): 51-59.

454. Guiso, G., et al. "Effect of Aspartame on Seizures in Various Models of Experimental Epilepsy. *Toxicol. Appl. Pharmacol.* **96**(1988): 485-493.

455. Dailey, J.W., et al. "Aspartame Fails to Facilitate Pentylenetetrazol-Induced Convulsions in CD-1 Mice." *Toxicol. Appl. Pharmacol.* **98**(1989): 475-486.

456. Coulombe, R.A. and Sharma, R.P. "Neurobiochemical Alterations Induced by the Artificial Sweetener Aspartame (Nutrasweet®)." *Toxicol Appl Pharmacol* **83** (1986): 79-85.

457. Schneiderman, J.H. and MacConald, J.F."Excitatory Amino Acid Blockers Differentially Affect Bursting of in vitro Hippocampal Neurons in Two Pharmacological Models of Epilepsy." *Neurosci.* **31**(1989): 593-603.

458. Johns, D.R. "Migraine Provoked by Aspartame." *NEJM* Aug 14, 1986.

459. Schiffman, et al. "Aspartame and Headache (Letters)." *NEJM* **318**(1988): 1201-1202.

460. Ibid, 1200-1202, 1988.

461. Chen, M., et al. "Ischemic Neuronal Damage after Acute Subdural Hematoma in the Rat: Effects of Pretreatment with a Glutamate Antagonist." *J. Neurosurg.* **74**(1991): 944-950. In this study they found that pretreatment of the animal with a glutamate blocker significantly reduced the size of the ischemic zone beneath the subdural hemorrhage. Also the paper by Faden, et al. "The Role of Excitatory Amino Acids and NMDA Receptors in Traumatic Brain Injury." *Sci.* **244**(1989): 798-800.

462. Nilsson, P. et al. "Changes in Cortical Extracellular Levels of Energy-Related Metabolites and Amino Acids Following Concussive Brain Injury in Rats." *J. Cerebral Blood Flow and Metabolism* **10** (1990): 631-637.

463. Olney, J.W. "Glutamate, a Neurotoxic Transmitter." *J. Child. Neurol.* **4**(1989): 218-226.

464. Ibid.

465. Baker, A.J., et al. "Excitatory Amino Acids in Cerebrospinal Fluid Following Traumatic Brain Injury in Humans." *J. Neurosurg.* **79**(1993): 369-372.

466. Kuroda, Y., et al. "Transient Glucose Hypermetabolism After Acute Subdural Hematoma in the Rat." *J. Neurosurg.* **76**(1992): 471-477.

467. Cummings, J.L., et al. "Amnesia with Hippocampal Lesions After Cardiopulmonary Arrest." *Neurol* **34**(1984): 679-681.

468. Shimada, N., et al. "Differences in Ischemia-Induced Accumulation of Amino Acids in the Cat Cortex." *Stroke,* **21**(1990): 1445-1451.

469. Katayama, Y., et al. "Massive Increases in Extracellular Potassium and the Indiscriminate Release of Glutamate Following Concussive Brain Injury." *J. Neurosurg.* **73**(1990): 889-900.

470. Krebs, et al. "Distribution of Glutamine and Glutamic Acid in Animal Tissues." *Biochem. J.* **44**(1949): 889-900.

471. Simon, R.P., et al. "Blockade of N-methyl-D-aspartate Receptors May Protect Against Ischemic Damage in the Brain." *Science* **226**(1984): 850-852.

472. Hadley, M.N., et al. "The Efficiency of Intravenous Nimodipine in the Treatment of Focal Cerebral Ischemia in a Primate Model." *Neurosurg.* **25**(1989): 63-70.

473. Germano, et al. "The Therapeutic Value of Nimodipine in Experimental Focal Cerebral Ischemia." *J. Neurosurg.* **67**(1987): 81-87.

474. Yang, G., et al. "Reduction of Vasgenic Edema and Infarction by MK-801 in Rats After Temporary Focal Cerebral Ischemia." *Neurosurg.* **34**(1994): 339-345.

475. Rothman, S.M. and Olney J.W. "Glutamate and the Pathophysiology of Hypoxic-Ischemic Brain Damage." *Ann. Neurol.* **19**(1986): 105-111.

476. Altura, B.M. and Altura, B.T. "Pharmacologic Inhibition of Cerebral Vasospasm in Ischemia, Hallucinogen Ingestion, and Hypomagnesemia: Barbiturates, Calcium Antagonist, and Magnesium." *Amer. J. Emerg. Med.* **2**(1983): 180-190.

477. Marier, J.R. "Magnesium Content of the Food Supply in the Modern World." *Magnesium* **5**(1986): 1-8.

478. Wieloch T. "Hypoglycemia-induced Neuronal Damage Prevented by an N-methyl-D-aspartate Antagonist." *Sci.* **230**(1985): 681-683.

479. Pulsinelli, W.A. and Cooper, A.J.L. "Metabolic Encephalopathies and Coma." In *Basic Neurochemistry*, edited by G. Siegel, et al. 777-778. New York:Raven Press, 1989.

480. Lipton, S.A., et al. "Synergistic Effects of HIV Coat Protein and NMDA Receptor-Mediated Neurotoxicity." *Neuron.* **7**(1991): 111-118.

481. Heyes, M.P. et al. "Quinolinic Acid in Cerebrospinal Fluid and Serum in HIV-1 Infection: Relationship to Clinical and Neurological Status." *Ann. Neurol.* **29**(1991): 202-209.

482. Kubera, M., et al. "Effect of Monosodium Glutamate on Cell-Mediated Immunity." *Pol. J. Pharmacol. Pharm.* **43**(1991): 39-44; also see Belluardo, N., et al. "Effects of Early Destruction of the Mouse Arcuate Nucleus by Monosodium Glutamate on Age-Dependent Natural Killer Activity." *Brain Res.* **534**(1990): 225-233.

483. Besedovsky, H. and Sorkin, E. "Network of Immune-Neuroendocrine Interactions." *Clin. Exp. Immunol.* **27**(1977): 1-12.

484. Study E-33, 34, Cross Reference E-87, Master File 134 for Aspartame, FDA Hearing Clerk's Office.

485. The data for this section comes largely from in-depth and carefully conducted analysis done by Dr. John W. Olney as a prepared statement before the Aspartame Board of Inquiry of the FDA; Part III.

486. National Cancer Institute SEER Program Data.

487. Ibid.

488. Roberts, H.J. *Aspartame (NutraSweet®) Is it Safe?* Philadelphia: The Charles Press, 1990.

489. Jellinger, K.A., et al. "Primary Central Nervous System Lymphomas: An Update." *J. Cancer Res. Clin. Onc.* **119**(1992): 7-27.

490. Desmeules, M., et al. "Increasing Incidence of Primary Malignant Brain Tumors: Influence of Diagnostic Methods." *J. Nat. Cancer Inst.* **84**(1992): 442-445.

491. Shaw, P.T. "Excitatory Amino Acid Receptors, Excitotoxicity, and the Human Nervous System." *Curr. Op. Neuro. Neurosurg.* **6**(1993): 414-422.

492. This partial list was obtained from Jack and Adrienne Samuels, compiled from their extensive research into the field of excitotoxin food additives.

493. For more information about the hidden sources of MSG I would suggest reading *In Bad Taste: The MSG Syndrome* by George R. Schwartz, M.D. (Health Press, 1988) and contacting the NOMSG Consumer Group, P.O. Box 367, Santa Fe, NM, 87504.

Index

References to figures are cited in **boldface**.

A

O

Obesity, 80, 82, 88, 217
Olivopontocerebellar atrophy (OPCA), 91, 123-24
Olney, John W.
on excitotoxins, 38, 230n16
research by, xix, 35, 36, 54-55, 56-57, 66-67, 74, 79, 106, 131, 183, 184, 211-12, 216, 218
testimony of, 36-37, 55-56
Omega-3-fatty acids, 188, 202, 203
Oxytocin, 87

P

Paired helical filaments, 142, 143, 154
Parathyroid glands, 98, 179
Pardridge, William M., 169
Parietal lobes, 5, 18, 136
Parkinson, James, 103
Parkinson's disease, 39, 91, 92, 94, 95, 97, 137, 215
dementia and, 103, 104, 117
described, 12, 103-4, 106-12, 114, 115-16
excitotoxins and, xxi, 104-5, 106, 118
metabolic rate and, 110, 165
MSG and, 106, 116-18
sudden, 100, 101
Pauling, Linus, 195
Paull, W. K., 86
Penfield, Wilder, 6-7, 144
Pentylenetetrazol, 196
Phagocytic cells, **81**
Phencyclidine, 57
Phenylalanine, 26, 68, 88, 196, 197
Phenylketonuria, 88
Phosphates, 189, 208
Phosphocreatine, 23, 72, 130
Phosphocreatinine, 50, 104
Phospholipase C, 44, 235n96
Pituitary gland, 13-14, **13**, 197
MSG and, 79, 82
Placental barrier, 68, 70
penetration of, 75-76
Plaitakis, Andreas, 120, 121
Plant toxins, 92-96
Plasticity, 61, 62, 63-64, 66-68, 73, 135
Pregnant women
excitotoxins and, 73-79

MSG and, 37, 61, 68, 88-90, 216
Primary lymphoma, 214
Prions, 92, 148, 240n159
Prolactin, 79, 80
Prostaglandins, 152, 188, 228
Prostaglandin synthesis, **45**
Proteins, 25, 134, 143-44
structure and shape of, 24
Puberty, 13, 80

Q

Quinolinic acid, 127, 130, 210, 245n265
Quisqualate receptors, 29, 49, 50, 87, 144, 183, 189
destruction of, 147, 151

R

Ray, Dixy Lee, 54
Recreational drugs, 99-100, 190, 225
Reinis, Stanislav, 61
Reproduction, 63, 80-81
abnormalities of, 82-83
Reproductive hormones, 36, 80
Reynolds, W. A., 56-57
Rheumatoid arthritis, 152
Rietvelt, W. J., 86
Roberts, H. J., 214
Rose, Clifford, 78
Rothstein, Jeffery, 122
Rush, Benjamin, 139

S

Sabin Vaccine, 219
Samuels, Adrienne, 200, 201
Samuels, Jack L., 200
Scheibel, Arnold B., 162, 169
Schiffman, Susan S., 198-99, 200
Schizophrenia, 18, 66, 71, 197, 216
Schlatter, James, 216-17
Schwartz, George, 34, 230n13 MSG and, 55, 111, 218
Scopp, Alfred, 201
Second messengers, 44, **44**
Seizures, 66, 78, 158, 176, 190
excitotoxins and, 191-203
Selenium, 47, 188
Serine, 26, 183

INDEX FOR CHAPTER 8

About the Author

Russell L. Blaylock, M.D. is a board-certified neurosurgeon who completed his medical training at the Louisiana State University School of Medicine in New Orleans, Louisiana. Afterwards he spent five years of neurosurgical training at the Medical University of South Carolina in Charleston. There he worked with the eminent neurosurgeon, teacher and researcher Dr. Ludwig G. Kempe. Together they published over a dozen scientific papers.

Dr. Blaylock, a clinical assistant professor at the University of Mississippi Medical Center, has written and illustrated three chapters in medical textbooks and a patient booklet on multiple sclerosis. For the past sixteen years he has had a busy private neurosurgical practice. During the course of his practice he has treated many cases of neurodegenerative diseases.

In March of 1989 his father succumbed to the ravages of Parkinson's disease. This began him on his journey to help others avoid this terrible experience, resulting in the writing of this book.

Russell L. Blaylock, M.D., is a member of the Congress of Neurological Surgeons, the American Association of Neurological Surgeons, Southern Neurosurgical Society, The American Nutritionist Association, the American Society for Parenteral and Enteral Nutrition, and the Society of Neurosurgical Anesthesia and Critical Care.

Dr. Blaylock enjoys art and drew all of the illustrations in this book. He lives in Madison, Mississippi with his wife, Diane, and their two children, Ron and Damien.